Respiratory Infections

LUNG BIOLOGY IN HEALTH AND DISEASE

Executive Editor

Claude Lenfant

Former Director, National Heart, Lung, and Blood Institute
National Institutes of Health
Bethesda, Maryland

The opinions expressed in these volumes do not necessarily represent the views of the National Institutes of Health.

Respiratory Infections

Edited by
Sanjay Sethi
University at Buffalo, State University of New York
Buffalo, New York, USA

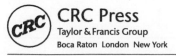

CRC Press
Taylor & Francis Group
Boca Raton London New York

CRC Press is an imprint of the
Taylor & Francis Group, an **informa** business

CRC Press
Taylor & Francis Group
6000 Broken Sound Parkway NW, Suite 300
Boca Raton, FL 33487-2742

First issued in paperback 2017

ISBN-13: 978-1-4200-8034-6 (hbk)
ISBN-13: 978-1-138-11489-0 (pbk)

Library of Congress Cataloging-in-Publication Data

Respiratory infections / edited by Sanjay Sethi.
    p. ; cm. — (Lung biology in health and disease ; 232)
    Includes bibliographical references and index.
    ISBN-13: 978-1-4200-8034-6 (hb : alk. paper)
    ISBN-10: 1-4200-8034-2 (hb : alk. paper) 1. Respiratory infections. I. Sethi,

Sanjay. II. Series: Lung biology in health and disease ; v. 232.
    [DNLM: 1. Respiratory Tract Infections. W1 LU62 v.232 2009 /WF 140 R434435 2009]

    RC740.R462 2009
    616.2—dc22

                                                                        2009039532

Visit the Taylor & Francis Web site at
http://www.taylorandfrancis.com

and the CRC Press Web site at
http://www.crcpress.com

Introduction

This new volume, *Respiratory Infections*, in the series of monographs, Lung Biology in Health and Disease, is edited by Sanjay Sethi and authored by a cadre of international experts with worldwide reputation. The volume brings to the forefront of medicine and clinical practice an area of critical importance, that is, the close link between pulmonary infection and chronic respiratory disease, but a link that may not be fully appreciated by the practicing community.

Public health officials in most parts of the world are now well aware that chronic diseases are the major cause of disability and death. According to the World Health Organization, in 2005 there were 68 million deaths worldwide; 35 million or 60% of these deaths were due to chronic diseases. This is indeed a dramatic shift in the causes of death considering that in the 1950s, two-thirds of the worldwide deaths were due to infectious diseases. While of all the chronic diseases, cardiovascular diseases hold the first position, other categories of chronic disease have seen major increases in their worldwide prevalence in the last three or four decades. One of these categories is respiratory diseases. As reported by the WHO program Global Alliance against Chronic Respiratory Diseases (1), hundreds of millions of patients suffer from asthma, chronic obstructive pulmonary diseases, idiopathic pulmonary fibrosis, and scores of other chronic respiratory diseases. It is noteworthy that according to WHO, "chronic diseases have not simply displaced acute infectious diseases in developed countries. Rather these countries now experience a prolonged and protracted double burden of disease" (2).

In his preface to this volume, Dr Sethi comments that "respiratory infections remain a very major cause of morbidity and mortality on a global basis," and that the patients are primarily seen by primary care physicians. It is therefore critical that these physicians are well informed about respiratory diseases, including respiratory disease infections. During the last three to four decades, the increase in prevalence of chronic respiratory disease has been accompanied by a huge and successful research effort to uncover the pathogenesis of these conditions and to develop appropriate treatments for the nonmicrobial pathogenic alterations of lung function.

However, the question appears to be whether the respiratory tract infection that parallels, sometimes precedes, or follows the lung damage of non-infectious origin receives the attention and care that is warranted. The response appears to be "probably not," simply because it may not be recognized that pulmonary infections "are an overlap area of medicine, falling in the purview of both infectious disease and pulmonary medicine." This volume is a remedy, not to say a solution to the problem, because it provides a vehicle for a better, more comprehensive approach to caring for patients who suffer from a pulmonary disease with a pulmonary infection that may be the cause, the consequence, or simply the exacerbation of the pulmonary disease.

I am grateful to Dr Sethi and the contributors to this volume for the opportunity to present it to the readership of the series of monographs Lung Biology in Health and Disease.

Claude Lenfant, MD
Vancouver, Washington, U.S.A.

References

1. Bousquet J, Dahl R, Khaltaev N. Global alliance against chronic respiratory diseases. Eur Respir J 2007; 29:233–234.
2. Yach D, Hawkes C, Gould CL, et al. The global burden of chronic diseases: overcoming impediments to prevention and control. JAMA 2004; 291:2616–2622.

Preface

Respiratory tract infections continue to be major cause of morbidity and mortality on a global basis, despite tremendous advances in medicine. Affected patients are usually first seen by primary care practitioners; however, infectious disease and pulmonary specialists are also often consulted. A thorough knowledge of respiratory infections is therefore essential for the broad spectrum of health care practitioners. Such knowledge should include information on not only microbial pathogens and antimicrobials but also on clinical presentation, pathophysiology, treatment guidelines, and the approach to complicated clinical situations. It is quite amazing that in spite of the importance and complexity of respiratory infections, few sources are currently available for comprehensive, up-to-date information on their management.

Respiratory tract infections are an overlap area of medicine, falling in the preview of both infectious disease and pulmonary medicine. This likely underlies the current fragmentation of published information regarding respiratory tract infections. Infectious disease textbooks and monographs tend to focus narrowly on the pathogens and antibiotic management, while pulmonary textbooks and monographs tend to concentrate on nonantimicrobial treatment and compromised lung function. These textbooks and monographs also fail to provide the relevant knowledge base for a practicing physician to distinguish between the various respiratory tract infection syndromes. The clinical presentation of the various respiratory tract infections overlap, and a practicing physician often expends (or should expend) considerable time and effort to distinguish between the various syndromes to make an accurate diagnosis. Only then can appropriate management be provided.

This book is an attempt to build bridges between these different perspectives on respiratory tract infections to provide comprehensive but clinically relevant knowledge to health care practitioners from different backgrounds. A syndrome-based approach is adopted wherever possible in this book to assist the practicing physician to readily distinguish clearly between the various syndromes. For each clinical syndrome, the specific chapters provide, in a consistent format, discussions about the definition, clinical presentation, etiopathogenesis and the diagnostic, treatment, and prevention approaches. Complications and difficult management scenarios are all too common in respiratory tract infections. For each syndrome, a discussion of such case scenarios is presented. For example, for acute exacerbations of chronic obstructive pulmonary disease, management of patients who experience recurrent exacerbations is discussed.

The initial chapters of this book address some important general issues, including normal lung defense mechanisms for respiratory pathogens, microbial pathogenetic mechanisms, and special considerations for antimicrobial use in respiratory infections. Subsequent chapters address the respiratory infection syndromes in a uniform manner to provide a comparative contextual framework for the reader. The last few chapters address the future, with a look at emerging infections, diagnostic modalities, and therapies.

It is my belief that this book will be useful not only for pulmonologists but also for infectious disease, critical care physicians, trainees, and allied health care practitioners. Though clinically oriented, it should provide researchers in the field to use this book as a state-of-the art summary of data relevant to their research.

Sanjay Sethi

Contributors

Rosemary Boyton National Heart and Lung Institute, Imperial College London, London, U.K.

Alexandra Chroneou Lahey Clinic Medical Center, Burlington, Massachusetts, U.S.A.

Brendan J. Clark University of Colorado Health Sciences Center, Denver, Colorado, U.S.A.

Donald E. Craven Lahey Clinic Medical Center, Burlington, and Tufts University School of Medicine, Boston, Massachusetts, U.S.A.

Charles L. Daley National Jewish Health and University of Colorado Health Sciences Center, Denver, Colorado, U.S.A.

Himanshu Desai University at Buffalo, State University of New York, Buffalo, New York, U.S.A.

Didier Dreyfuss Institut National de la Santé et de la Recherche Médicale, INSERM U722, Paris; UFR de Médecine Paris Diderot – Paris 7, and Assistance Publique–Hôpitaux de Paris, Hôpital Louis Mourier, Service de Réanimation Médicale, Colombes, France

Ali A. El Solh State University of New York at Buffalo School of Medicine and Biomedical Sciences, and School of Public Health and Health Professions, Buffalo, New York, U.S.A.

Elbio Mariano Esperatti Universitat de Barcelona, CIBER de Enfermedades Respiratorias (CIBERES) and Insitut d'Investigacions Biomèdiques August Pi i Sunyer (IDIBAPS), Barcelona, Spain

Thomas M. File, Jr. Northeastern Ohio Universities College of Medicine, Rootstown; and Summa Health System, Akron, Ohio, U.S.A.

Pieter S. Hiemstra   Leiden University Medical Center, Leiden, The Netherlands

Rana Kaplan   Memorial Sloan-Kettering Cancer Center and Weill Medical College of Cornell University, New York, New York, U.S.A.

Paul King   Monash Medical Centre/Monash University, Clayton, Melbourne, Victoria, Australia

Thomas J. Kufel   Veterans Affairs Western New York Healthcare System and University at Buffalo, State University of New York, Buffalo, New York, U.S.A.

Alan J. Lesse   Veterans Affairs Western New York Healthcare System and University at Buffalo, State University of New York, Buffalo, New York, U.S.A.

Chi-Chiu Leung   Tuberculosis and Chest Service, Department of Health, Hong Kong, China

Tom Lim   University of Calgary, Calgary, Alberta, Canada

John H. MacGregor   University of Calgary, Calgary, Alberta, Canada

Christopher H. Mody   University of Calgary, Calgary, Alberta, Canada

David R. Murdoch   University of Otago and Canterbury Health Laboratories, Christchurch, New Zealand

Timothy F. Murphy   University at Buffalo, State University of New York and Veterans Affairs Western New York Healthcare System, Buffalo, New York, U.S.A.

Michael S. Niederman   Winthrop University Hospital, Mineola, and Stony Brook University, Stony Brook, New York, U.S.A.

Jean-Damien Ricard   Institut National de la Santé et de la Recherche Médicale, INSERM U722, Paris; UFR de Médecine Paris Diderot – Paris 7, and Assistance Publique–Hôpitaux de Paris, Hôpital Louis Mourier, Service de Réanimation Médicale, Colombes, France

Damien Roux   Institut National de la Santé et de la Recherche Médicale, INSERM U722, Paris; UFR de Médecine Paris Diderot – Paris 7, France

Ruxana T. Sadikot   Department of Veterans Affairs, Jesse Brown VA Hospital, and University of Illinois at Chicago, Chicago, Illinois, U.S.A.

Clare Sander   National Heart and Lung Institute, Imperial College London, London, U.K.

Sanjay Sethi   Veterans Affairs Western New York Healthcare System and University at Buffalo, State University of New York, Buffalo, New York, U.S.A.

Antoni Torres Marti   Universitat de Barcelona, CIBER de Enfermedades Respiratorias (CIBERES) and Insitut d'Investigacions Biomèdiques August Pi i Sunyer (IDIBAPS), Barcelona, Spain

Dorothy A. White   Memorial Sloan-Kettering Cancer Center and Weill Medical College of Cornell University, New York, New York, U.S.A.

Wing-Wai Yew   Grantham Hospital, Hong Kong, China

Nikolaos Zias   Lahey Clinic Medical Center, Burlington, Massachusetts, U.S.A.

Contents

1

The Scope of Respiratory Tract Infections

MICHAEL S. NIEDERMAN
Winthrop University Hospital, Mineola, and Stony Brook University, Stony Brook, New York, U.S.A.

I. Introduction

Advances in modern medicine notwithstanding, respiratory tract infections remain a major source of morbidity, mortality, and medical costs in our society. In fact, as a consequence of the current capacity of modern medicine to apply novel life-sustaining therapies, a number of new patient populations have emerged with specific impairments in their ability to fight infection, and these individuals have an enhanced risk for one specific infection: pneumonia. Patients at risk for pneumonia include not only previously healthy individuals but also those with increased threat, such as the elderly—especially those with complex chronic illness—and those with novel forms of immunosuppressive illness as the result of organ transplantation or an HIV infection.

The problem of respiratory infection has not been eliminated by the development of new therapies, which have generally lagged behind the evolution in hosts and the changing nature of the etiologic pathogens. In the past 30 years, we have seen the emergence of antibiotic resistance among such common organisms as *Streptococcus pneumoniae* (multidrug resistance), *Staphylococcus aureus* (methicillin resistance), *Hemophilus influenzae* (β-lactamase production), enteric gram-negatives (extended spectrum β-lactamases and others), and *Mycobacterium tuberculosis* (extensively drug-resistant strains). In addition, new organisms causing respiratory infection have been identified, including *Legionella pneumophila*, hantavirus, severe acute respiratory syndrome coronavirus, *Chlamydophila pneumoniae*, and *Moraxella catarrhalis*. Efforts to improve diagnosis have not improved disease management, and prevention efforts, most notably vaccine development, have had only limited success.

II. Definitions of the Different Types of Respiratory Infections

The respiratory tract can be anatomically divided into an upper and lower system, with the vocal cords serving as the dividing line (Table 1). Infections of the upper respiratory tract include the common cold, sinusitis, otitis media, pharyngitis, tonsillitis, and epiglottitis. Influenza is a viral infection that can involve the epithelial cells of both the upper and lower respiratory tracts, and some patients have predominantly upper respiratory infection symptoms, while others have more marked lower airway signs and symptoms. This chapter focuses primarily on lower respiratory tract infections.

Infections of the lower respiratory tract can involve the airways, lung parenchyma, or pleural space. When infection involves the large airways, it is termed bronchitis, and symptoms include cough, sputum production, and often bronchospasm with wheezing.

Table 1 Classifications of Respiratory Tract Infection

Anatomic
  Upper respiratory tract
    Common cold
    Sinusitis
    Otitis media
    Pharyngitis
    Tonsillitis
    Epiglottitis
  Lower respiratory tract
    Bronchitis
    Bronchiectasis
    Bronchiolitis
    Pneumonia
      Lobar
      Bronchopneumonia
    Lung abscess
    Pleural space/empyema
Place of Origin
  Community acquired
  Nosocomial
  Health care associated

If the infection involves smaller, more peripheral airways, it is termed bronchiolitis, which primarily occurs in children, but recently a subacute illness in adults, possibly initiated by an infectious agent, has been recognized and is termed "bronchiolitis obliterans with organizing pneumonia." In addition, a chronic form of this illness has been described in Japan and is termed "diffuse panbronchiolitis" (1).

The airways can be infected acutely or chronically, and the latter infections include bronchiectasis and chronic bronchitis. Bronchiectasis is often a consequence of preceding respiratory infection or congenital defects in airway clearance of mucus and bacteria, as can occur with cystic fibrosis and immotile cilia syndrome. Symptoms result from chronic infection complicated by multiple episodes of superimposed acute infection in proximity to the diseased airways. Bronchiectasis is characterized pathologically by abnormal and permanent dilation of subsegmental airways, which are inflamed and usually filled with secretions (1). It is these areas of stagnant secretions that frequently become infected. Similarly, chronic bronchitis, a disease usually caused by cigarette smoking, is often complicated by bouts of acute infectious bronchitis that complicate chronic symptoms of daily cough and sputum production.

Pneumonia is an infection of the gas-exchanging units of the lung, most commonly caused by bacteria, but occasionally by viruses, fungi, parasites, and other infectious agents. In the immunocompetent individual, it is characterized by a brisk filling of the alveolar space with inflammatory cells and fluid. If the alveolar infection involves an entire anatomic lobe of the lung, it is termed "lobar pneumonia," and multilobar illness can be present in some instances and may lead to more severe clinical manifestations. When the alveolar process occurs in a distribution that is patchy and adjacent to bronchi, without filling an entire lobe, it is termed a "bronchopneumonia."

From a clinical perspective, pneumonias have been classified as being "typical" or "atypical," depending on their mode of clinical presentation. Although the typical pneumonia syndrome is characterized by sudden onset of fever, chills, pleuritic chest pain, and productive cough, this type of presentation can be expected only if the patient has an intact immune response system and if the infection is due to a bacterial pathogen such as *S. pneumoniae, H. influenzae, Klebsiella pneumoniae, S. aureus,* aerobic gram-negative bacilli, or anaerobes. If a patient is infected by one of these organisms but has an impaired immune response, the classic pneumonia symptoms may be absent, as can be the case with the elderly and debilitated patient. The atypical pneumonia syndrome, characterized by preceding upper respiratory symptoms, fever without chills, non-productive cough, headache, myalgias, and mild leukocytosis, is often the result of infection with viruses, *Mycoplasma pneumoniae, C. pneumoniae, Legionella* spp. and other unusual infectious agents (such as psittacosis and Q fever). In clinical practice it is often very difficult to use this type of classification to predict the microbial etiology of pneumonia. In fact, clinical features may be at best only 40% accurate in distinguishing *M. pneumoniae,* pneumococcus, and other pathogens (2).

When a parenchymal lung infection leads to the breakdown of lung tissue, it may lead to tissue necrosis and cavity formation, and this type of infection is termed a lung abscess. These infections usually result when a patient aspirates a highly virulent pathogen into the lung in the absence of effective clearance mechanisms, and the eti-ologic agents include anerobes, *S. aureus, K. pneumoniae, Escherichia coli, Pseudo-monas aeruginosa.* Empyema is an infection of the pleural space characterized by grossly purulent material and usually caused by extension of parenchymal infection outside the lung and is caused by anaerobes, gram-negative bacilli, *S. aureus,* and occasionally tuberculosis.

Another classification system that is applied to pneumonia relates to the place of origin of the infection. When the infection occurs in patients living in the community, it is termed community acquired pneumonia (CAP), while it is called nosocomial pneu-monia if it arises in patients who are already in the hospital (3,4). When nosocomial pneumonia develops in a patient who has been on mechanical ventilation for at least 48 hours, this is termed ventilator-associated pneumonia (VAP). However, the distinc-tion between these different types of infection is becoming increasingly blurred because of the complexity of patients who reside out of the hospital. When pneumonia develops in patients who come from a nursing home, in those receiving chronic hemodialysis and in those admitted to the hospital in the past three months, this is termed "health care–associated pneumonia" (HCAP). Because of their contact with the health care environment, these patients may already be colonized with multidrug resistant (MDR) organisms when they arrive at the hospital (4,5). Patients who develop pneumonia while receiving immunosuppressive therapy or who have an abnormal immune system are referred to as compromised hosts, and the infectious possibilities will vary with the nature of the immune defect. Thus, although the bacteriology of each type of pneumonia is unique, the relationship between bacteriology and the place of origin of infection is a reflection of several factors, including the comorbid illnesses present in the patient, their host-defense status, and their environmental exposure to specific pathogens.

In recent years, particularly with the application of immunosuppressive therapy for a variety of illnesses, with the emergence of the acquired immunodeficiency syn-drome (AIDS), and with an increasing number of institutionalized elderly individuals, tuberculosis and fungal and parasitic lung infections have emerged once again as important and common infections. Mycobacterial illnesses frequently complicate AIDS or occur in nursing homes, and fungal infections may emerge from a dormant state in patients living in endemic areas when a disease such as AIDS develops. From 1985 to 1992, the incidence of tuberculosis increased in the United States, but this trend has since reversed, with the case rate falling below 10 per 100,000. In fact, from 1993 to 2003, the incidence of tuberculosis fell by 44% (6,7). Certain populations are at increased risk for tuberculosis, particularly blacks, Hispanics, and immigrant populations. In 2003, the white, non-Hispanic population accounted for 19% of reported cases of tuberculosis (6,7). An additional concern today is the emergence of multidrug-resistant and extensively drug-resistant tuberculosis, a phenomenon that is particularly common in certain locations, such as large cities in the Northeastern United States and in many less developed countries around the world.

III. Epidemiology
A. Community-Acquired Pneumonia

In 2004, pneumonia, along with influenza, was the eighth leading cause of death in the United States, the sixth leading cause of death in those over age 65, and the leading cause of death from infectious diseases (6). Patients with CAP are primarily managed out of the hospital, but those admitted to the hospital consume the greatest proportion of economic resources. In a study using insurance and Medicare (Currently the Center for Medicare Services, CMS) data from 1994, the investigators found that over 5.6 million people were diagnosed with CAP in the United States, but the majority, 4.6 million, was treated out of the hospital (8). Data from 2005 showed that there were 1.3 million hospitalizations for pneumonia in the United States, more in females than in males and approximately 60% in those over the age of 65 (6). The cost of care for patients with CAP in the United States has been estimated to be over $40 billion in 2005, including both direct and indirect costs (6). The elderly account for a disproportionate amount of this cost, largely because they often require inpatient treatment, reflecting a high frequency of comorbid illness. Although those over age 65 account for only about one-third of all cases of CAP, they are responsible for 60% of those hospitalized with CAP and for more than half of all costs for this illness (8).

CAP has a seasonal variability, with a rise in frequency during the winter months, paralleling the times of influenza and viral infection, illnesses that can interfere with host defense and predispose to secondary bacterial pneumonia. Certain pathogens, such as *Legionella* spp. are more common in late summer and early fall, reflecting the waterborne sources of this organism. The reported mortality of CAP varies with the population being evaluated, ranging from less than 5% among outpatients to 12% among all hospitalized CAP patients, but rising to over 30% among those admitted to the ICU (9). The elderly have both an increased incidence of pneumonia and an increased mortality, compared with younger populations. In a large community-based study, the overall incidence of CAP was 266.8 cases per 100,000, but those aged 18 to 44 had an incidence of 92 cases per 100,000 population, compared with a rate of 1014 cases per 100,000 in those over age 65 (10). The mortality of CAP was 8.8% overall, but was only 4.5% in those aged 18 to 44, compared with 12.5% in those over age 65. The high frequency and enhanced mortality of pneumonia in older patients are well known, but controversy still continues about whether this is a consequence of aging itself, or the result of the comorbid illnesses that become increasingly common in the aging population. Recently, it has become apparent that elderly patients with CAP have long-term mortality consequences following acute pneumonia. In a study of over 150,000 Medicare patients admitted to the hospital for CAP, the in-hospital mortality rate was 11%, while at one year, these patients had over a 40% mortality rate, a rate that was higher than a matched population of Medicare patients admitted with other diagnoses (11).

B. Nosocomial Pneumonia

Nosocomial pneumonia is the leading cause of death from hospital-acquired infections, particularly in those managed in the intensive care unit. The frequency of VAP increases with the duration of mechanical ventilation, although the risk is greatest early in the course of ventilation. In a prospective study of 1014 mechanically ventilated patients, Cook and colleagues found that 177 patients developed VAP defined by strict clinical or microbiologic criteria (12). The mean time of onset was nine days, with the median time of onset being seven days after ICU admission. However, when the daily hazard rate of infection was calculated, it was estimated to be 3.3% at day 5, 2.3% at day 10, and 1.3% at day 15, documenting a dramatic decline in pneumonia risk over time. Since the risk of pneumonia was so high early after intubation, pneumonias beginning within the first five days (early onset infection) accounted for 50% of all VAP episodes, and the natural history and pathogens associated with this infection differ from VAP of late onset (4). Endotracheal intubation is present in at least 85% of patients who develop pneumonia in the ICU, and the intubation process itself contributes to the risk of infection. When patients with acute respiratory failure are managed with noninvasive ventilation, nosocomial pneumonia is less common (13).

Although 50% to 66% of all tracheostomized patients will develop nosocomial pneumonia, the daily risk (after tracheostomy) is lower than for patients with short-term endotracheal intubation. The explanation for this may be the self-selection process of generally healthier patients who are able survive long enough to undergo tracheostomy. Kollef et al. examined 521 patients requiring mechanical ventilation and compared the 51 who received tracheostomy with the 470 who did not (14). Those requiring tracheostomy had a higher incidence of nosocomial pneumonia prior to tracheostomy, but those who had a tracheostomy had a significantly lower hospital mortality rate (13.7%) than those not requiring it (26.4%). This suggests that tracheostomized individuals are a population better able to recover, and perhaps resist the development and impact of pneumonia, than patients who are too ill to live long enough to undergo tracheostomy.

The mortality rate of VAP can exceed 50%, but many of these patients are chronically and acutely ill and not all are dying as a direct result of pneumonia, but rather from their underlying illness. However, at least a third to a half of all the deaths in patients with VAP are the result of the pneumonia itself, and this "attributable mortality" is greater in medical than in surgical patients, in those infected with certain high-risk pathogens (*P. aeruginosa*, *Acinetobacter* spp. and *S. aureus*), and in those who receive initial inappropriate antibiotic therapy (15). In fact, in one study, when patients were given appropriate therapy for VAP, the attributable mortality rate was only about 20% compared with an attributable mortality of 60% in those who received initial inadequate therapy (15). Many retrospective studies have shown that the appropriateness of initial therapy is a major determinant of mortality in patients with VAP, but this goal may be harder to achieve as patients in ICUs are infected with increasingly more drug-resistant pathogens, and as a result, it is harder to choose an effective empiric therapy (16). This has been a particular problem for infections with *P. aeruginosa, Acinetobacter* spp, and *S. aureus* (17). In addition to its mortality impact, HAP increases the length of hospitalization on average by seven to nine days per patient, and the risk of prolonged hospitalization may be even longer with pathogens such as methicillin-resistant *S. aureus* (MRSA) (18). The impact of VAP on hospital stay has also been documented in tracheostomized patients, with Georges et al. showing an increased duration of ventilation in patients who developed VAP either early or late after tracheostomy (19).

C. Acute Infective Exacerbations of Chronic Bronchitis
Bronchitis—infection of the large bronchi—can be caused by either viruses or bacteria. In children, more than 40% of episodes of acute bronchitis are viral and the remainder is bacterial. Viral bronchitis in children may lead to transient or even persistent airway hyperreactivity and thereby may be a risk factor for subsequent adult asthma. Chronic bronchitis is an adult disease characterized by a persistent inflammatory state of the large airways, generally caused by cigarette smoking, and found in 12.5 million Americans (20,21). Bronchiolitis is an acute infection, usually viral, of the small airways that occurs in children usually between the ages of one month and one year, with an attack rate in this age group of six to seven cases per 100 children per year (1).

Patients with chronic bronchitis have chronic recurrent cough with sputum production for at least three months, during two consecutive years, and this disease is usually a consequence of cigarette smoking. Patients with chronic bronchitis usually have underlying chronic obstructive lung disease, of which the bronchitis can be a component, and they have two to four acute exacerbations per year, characterized by increased dyspnea, increased sputum production, and increased sputum purulence. At least half of all exacerbations are bacterial in origin, and others may be viral or allergic, or may be due to chemical tracheobronchitis. When exacerbations are due to bacterial infection, the common pathogens are *H. influenzae, M. catarrhalis,* and the pneumococcus, all of which are commonly antibiotic resistant, thus adding complexity to the choice of therapy. Controversy has persisted for years about the need to use antibiotics during acute exacerbations and about whether it matters which antibiotic is used (22). New data, using serologic and bacteriologic typing methods, have suggested that at least some exacerbations result from a change in bacterial surface epitopes, which allow organisms like *H. influenzae* to elude host defenses and lead to infection. In order for the infection to resolve, the patient often forms a pathogen-specific immune response, and the role of antibiotic therapy in the relief of symptoms is uncertain (23).

Taken together, chronic bronchitis and emphysema were the fourth leading cause of death in the United States in 2002, and in 2004, the total cost to the United States was more than $37 billion (24). In spite of these dramatic numbers, the frequency of this illness may be underestimated because many affected patients have minimal symptoms and do not seek medical attention until the disease has far advanced. Exacerbations are more commonly managed out of the hospital than in the hospital. Using insurance company and Medicare data from 1994, one study estimated that there were 280,000 hospital admissions for exacerbations of chronic bronchitis, most involving patients over the age of 65, compared with 10 million outpatient visits, a ratio of more than 30:1 for outpatient versus inpatient management (25). Exacerbations lead to both short-term and medium-term disability, with many patients requiring several months to return to a baseline level of function after such an episode.

IV. Overview of Pneumonia Pathogenesis

Pneumonia occurs when a patient's host defenses are overwhelmed by an infectious pathogen. Thus, if the patient has an ineffective immune response for any reason, pneumonia can result after exposure of the lower respiratory tract to a potential pathogen. Host impairments can occur for a variety of reasons, including an underlying chronic medical disease (congestive heart failure, diabetes, renal failure, chronic obstructive lung disease, or malnutrition), anatomic abnormalities (endobronchial obstruction or bronchiectasis), acute illness–associated immune dysfunction (as can occur with sepsis or acute lung injury), or therapy-induced dysfunction of the immune system (corticosteroids or endotracheal intubation). On the other hand, some commonly used therapies may actually reduce the mortality risk of pneumonia, including angiotensin-converting enzyme (ACE) inhibitors and statins (26). Admission hyperglycemia may increase mortality risk in CAP, but it is unclear if therapy can reduce this risk (27).

Pneumonia can still occur in patients who have an adequate immune system, if the host defense system is overwhelmed by a large inoculum of microorganisms, which can occur in the setting of massive aspiration of gastric contents. Patients with impaired gastrointestinal or neurologic function may also aspirate, and this process involves failure to protect the lower respiratory tract from the entry of oropharyngeal secretions, which are often overgrown with potentially pathogenic gram-negative bacteria in hospitalized patients (28). In patients outside the hospital, a normal immune system can also be overcome by a particularly virulent organism, to which the patient has no preexisting immunity (such as certain bacteria or viruses) or to which the patient has an inability to form an adequate acute immune response. The epidemic spread of severe acute respiratory syndrome (SARS), due to a virulent virus, is one example of this phenomenon.

Although bacteria can enter the lung via several routes, aspiration from a previously colonized oropharynx is the most common mechanism for pneumonia (28). Although most pneumonias result from microaspiration, some patients can also aspirate large volumes of bacteria if they have impaired neurologic protection of the upper airway (stroke or seizure), or if they have intestinal illnesses that predispose to vomiting. Other routes of entry include inhalation, which applies primarily to viruses, *L. pneumophila* and *M. tuberculosis*; hematogenous dissemination from extrapulmonary sites of infection (right-sided endocarditis); and direct extension from contiguous sites of infection (e.g., liver abscess).

With this overview in mind, certain pathogens are more likely to occur in certain hosts. Previously healthy individuals often develop infection with virulent pathogens such as viruses, *L. pneumophila*, *M. pneumoniae*, *C. pneumoniae*, and *S. pneumoniae* (pneumococcus). On the other hand, chronically ill patients can be infected by these organisms, but also by organisms that commonly colonize the oropharynx (primarily enteric gram-negatives), but only cause infection when immune responses are inadequate. These organisms include enteric gram-negative bacteria (*E. coli, K. pneumoniae, P. aeruginosa, Acinetobacter* spp.), as well as fungi.

Recent investigations have focused on the heterogeneity of the immune response and its genetic determinants, in order to explain why the same pathogen leads to infection of different severity in different individuals. Severe forms of pneumonia can occur when the infection is not contained (inadequate immune response) or, alternatively, if the inflammatory response to infection is unable to be localized to the site of infection (excessive immune response), and it "spills over" into the systemic circulation (sepsis) or to the rest of the lung (acute respiratory distress syndrome). The normal lung immune response to infection is generally "compartmentalized," and thus most patients with unilateral pneumonia, have an inflammatory response that is limited to the site of infection. In patients with localized pneumonia, tumor necrosis factor alpha (TNFα), interleukin (IL)-6 and IL-8 levels are increased in the pneumonic lung and generally not increased in the uninvolved lung or in the serum (29). However, patients with severe pneumonia do not always localize the immune response and can have increased serum levels of TNFα and IL-6, possibly because of genetic polymorphisms in the immune response. Certain patients can have specific inherited patterns of response, making them more prone than others to severe forms of pneumonia and even mortality from this illness (30). For example, CAP severity is increased with genetic changes in the IL-10–1082 locus, which are often present along with changes in the TNFα-308 locus (30,31). Currently, there are a large number of genes that have been identified as being able to affect the severity and outcome of CAP, but the ability to use this information to impact patient management does not currently exist.

V. Current Challenges in Managing Respiratory Tract Infections

A. Drug-Resistance and the Limited Availability of New Therapies

The major management issue in all respiratory infections is the narrowing of therapeutic options as the responsible bacterial pathogens become increasingly resistant to available antimicrobial therapies, and the prospect of new drug development declines. In CAP, the organisms of concern are drug-resistant pneumococcus (DRSP) and community-acquired methicillin-resistant *S. aureus* (CA-MRSA), while for nosocomial pneumonia, the concerning pathogens are *P. aeruginosa, Acinetobacter* spp. and MRSA (hospital acquired).

In CAP, concern about DRSP has led to guideline recommendations that the most active agent available be used. However, at current levels of pneumococcal resistance, most therapies are still effective, and clinically relevant resistance only seems to occur with minimum inhibitory concentrations (MICs) for penicillin of at least 4 mg/L, a finding that is rare. In addition, this degree of in vitro resistance only seems to have an impact on mortality for patients who survive the first four days of illness, implying that early mortality is not modifiable by therapy (32). More recently, the rates of penicillin resistance in the pneumococcus have stabilized, while macrolide resistant pneumococcus is increasing. In North America, most macrolide resistance in the pneumococcus is still low level (efflux) and not high level (ribosomal), making macrolide therapy a viable option for uncomplicated patients (3,33). Reliable empiric therapy for suspected DRSP includes cefotaxime and ceftriaxone, as well as the antipneumococcal fluoroquinolones (gemifloxacin, levofloxacin 750 mg/day, and moxifloxacin). Although fluoroquinolone-resistant pneumococcus is uncommon, up to 20% of sensitive organisms do contain first-step mutations, and if a second mutation occurs, fluoroquinolone resistance may become a more important consideration (33).

In patients with nosocomial pneumonia, MRSA is becoming more common, accounting for over half of the *S. aureus* infections, and the infecting gram-negatives are now often resistant to agents that in the past were reliable. For *Acinetobacter* infection, carbapenems are no longer always effective, and some hospitals have had to utilize older agents such as colistin and polymyxin. The prospect of new antibiotics for these pathogens is uncertain, because new agents are not being developed and those that have become available, such as tigecycline, are not reliable as monotherapy for *Acinetobacter* pneumonia (34). Among patients with nosocomial pneumonia, *P. aeruginosa* remains a challenging pathogen, and dual therapy is usually necessary as empiric therapy as no single agent can reliably cover this pathogen and it provides a greater likelihood of successful initial therapy (4).

While a logical solution to this rising tide of resistant pathogens would be the development of new antibiotics, the reality is that very few new agents are being developed, as most drug development is now focused on chronic illnesses, such as hypertension and diabetes, and not on acute infection. From 1983 to 2002, there has been a decline in the FDA approval of new antibiotics by over 50%, a situation described as "bad bugs, no drugs" (35). In addition, most new agents are simply refinements of older drugs, and antibiotics with new mechanisms of action are not generally being developed. This has led to a focus on optimizing existing options by focusing on proper dosing, novel dosing regimens (single daily dosing for concentration-dependent killing agents and prolonged infusions for time-dependent killing agents), the reevaluation of aerosolized antibiotic therapies and of older agents (polymyxins and colistin). The problem of new drug development for respiratory infections has been further complicated by the FDA's position that acute exacerbations of chronic bronchitis (AECB) and acute sinusitis are conditions that may not need antibiotics. This has led to some agents having these indications removed from their label and a ramping up of the standards needed for new agents to be approved for these indications. Particularly for AECB, the FDA is insisting on placebo-controlled trials of antibiotics, a prospect that has limited drug development because of the difficulty for investigators and patients to participate in such trials.

B. The Need to Minimize the Overuse of Antibiotics

The problem of antibiotic resistance has been created by the overuse of antibiotics, including therapy for colonization and not infection; use for viral infections; use of a broader agent than is needed; use of therapy for a longer time than is needed; and use of too low a dose of antibiotic. All of these behaviors can further propagate the problem of resistance and have led to programs of "antimicrobial stewardship" that emphasize the proper use of antibiotics. In general, such programs urge that antibiotics only be used when necessary and for no longer than is needed to eradicate the infection (36). The issue of using too broad a spectrum of therapy is relevant for the treatment of HCAP, where we now understand that, contrary to guideline recommendations, not all of these patients are at risk for infection with MDR pathogens and that certain subsets of patients can receive a more narrow and focused therapy (4,5). In addition, in the therapy of VAP, the concept of "de-escalation" has emerged, emphasizing that as clinical and microbiologic data become available, the initial broad-spectrum empiric therapy regimen can be narrowed and focused and often the duration of therapy reduced (4,37). Antimicrobial stewardship programs emphasize these principles and the use of prospective audit and feedback, as well as dose optimization, rather than the restriction of access to specific agents (36).

In the future, it is likely that there will be an additional focus on the avoidance of antibiotics for viral respiratory infection and the shortening of the duration of therapy for CAP and HAP. To facilitate this process, it is likely that we will turn to serial measurements of biologic markers, the most promising of which are C-reactive protein and serum procalcitonin (PCT). PCT is a liver-synthesized acute phase reactant that rises with bacterial infection and not with viral illness. Measurements acutely and during the course of illness have been able to successfully guide the withholding of antibiotics and the shortening of the duration of therapy for patients with CAP, AECB, and acute bronchitis (38,39). More investigations are needed, but the promising findings have emerged with the use of highly sensitive immunoassay, the Kryptor assay, and not with the luminescent assay (38). The most impressive findings have been with CAP, where PCT-guided therapy led to the safe withholding of antibiotics in 15% of patients with radiographic pneumonia and to a shortening of therapy duration by more than 50% in patients who were given antibiotics (39). The role of PCT in HAP and VAP is less certain, but currently de-escalation is possible in these patients provided that respiratory tract cultures are obtained prior to the initiation of therapy. One large study suggested that de-escalation was possible in over 70% of patients, and that it made no difference whether the cultures that guided management were quantitative lavage samples or simple endotracheal aspirates (40).

C. The Availability of Guidelines for Respiratory Infections: Valuable, but How Should They Be Implemented?

Since the early 1990s, numerous professional societies throughout the world have published national guidelines for the management of CAP, HAP, AECB and sinusitis. Recently, data have been collected to show an outcomes benefit to the use of CAP and HAP guidelines, but it still remains uncertain how to best implement these guidelines in any given clinical setting.

CAP guidelines have been available since 1993, and since 1998 have specifically focused on how to manage pneumonia when there is concern about DRSP. Guidelines include more than just recommendations about antibiotic choice, but also include management advice about when to admit patients to the hospital, when to use the intensive care unit, how long to continue therapy, how to approach a pathogen-specific diagnosis, how to evaluate the response to therapy and how to prevent infection through immunization and other strategies. In studies of CAP, the use of guidelines can reduce mortality compared with when guideline-recommended therapies are not used, and in patients with severe pneumonia, guideline adherence has been associated with a reduced duration of mechanical ventilation (41,42). Guidelines can also lead to improved adherence to standards of care and may reduce the length of hospital stay, but in both of these instances, the magnitude of benefit varies with the intensity of plan for implementation of the guideline (43,44). In general, simply developing a guideline and making it available to physicians is of little value. However, if a "high-intensity" implementation strategy is employed, using real-time reminders to doctors, doctor audit and feedback, and intensive educational efforts, the likelihood that doctors will follow recommended processes of care is enhanced compared with programs without such a high-intensity implementation process (43). In another study, investigators showed that hospitalized CAP patients became clinically stable at a similar time in each of three time periods. However, in the time period when a guideline was added, along with prospective intervention to identify variations from recommended care, the time from stability to switch to oral therapy and the time to discharge were reduced compared with the periods when no guideline was used, or when a guideline without an implementation plan was used (44). Thus, even if the ideas in a guideline are valuable, the guideline itself will not improve outcome, unless it is coupled with a plan to be sure it is utilized.

In studies of VAP, several studies have shown that the use of a protocol-specified therapy regimen, using multiple empiric antimicrobial agents, selected by a knowledge of local pathogens, can lead to a greater likelihood of correct initial therapy compared with when no such protocol was available (45,46). In addition, the use of such a protocol can reduce the duration of therapy and in some instances reduce mortality, provided that it is coupled with a plan for de-escalation. Once again, the essential components for benefit are both the protocol itself, as well as the plan for implementation.

D. Performance Measures and Public Reporting for Pneumonia Management and Prevention

A recent development in pneumonia management in the United States has been the development of publicly reported performance measures for hospitalized patients, intended to assure a minimum standard of care. For patients with CAP, Medicare has developed a set of "core measures" that are collected for every hospital and reported on the Hospital Compare Web site, with the implication that hospitals with the best performance are providing the highest level of care (Table 2). The core measures include timely administration of antibiotics, measurement of oxygenation, selection of the correct antibiotics in the hospital and in the ICU, collection of blood cultures in seriously

Table 2 Community-Acquired Pneumonia Core Measures

- First dose of antibiotics within 6 hr of arrival at hospital
  - Exempt if diagnostic uncertainty when first evaluated
- Oxygenation assessment within 24 hr of admission
- Correct antibiotic choice for admitted patients (HCAP patients exempt)
  - Non-ICU
  - ICU
    Includes no monotherapy with any agent, such as fluoroquinolones
- Blood cultures within 24 hr for all patients admitted to ICU
  - Blood cultures before antibiotics for those drawn in ED
- Smoking cessation advice
- Evaluation of need and offering of pneumococcal and influenza vaccines to all appropriate candidates

---

ill patients prior to antibiotic administration, provision of smoking cessation advice, and offering of pneumococcal and influenza vaccines to at-risk individuals (3).

Although this approach may have been well intended, it has led to a variety of adverse, unintended consequences, best illustrated by the previous standard of requiring all patients to receive their first dose of antibiotics within four hours of arrival to the hospital, a standard that has now been modified to extend to six hours. Although retrospectively collected data have shown a lower mortality for patients given therapy within four hours compared with those given therapy later, the explanation may not be timely administration alone (47). In fact, delay in therapy may be a surrogate marker of patients with diagnostic uncertainty and of patients with impaired host responses who have indistinct clinical presentations and thus are not easily recognized as having pneumonia (48). In addition, when hospitals have increased the number of patients getting early antibiotics in an effort to comply with core measures, there have been some data to suggest that there are more patients who do not actually have pneumonia but are given antibiotic therapy (49). In addition, some of the patients given this timely therapy and who do not have pneumonia have developed antibiotic complications such as antibiotic-associated colitis (50). One other unexpected consequence of the well-intentioned effort at CAP prevention through vaccination has recently been identified with the use of the 7-valent conjugate vaccine in children. Initially, this vaccine led to "herd immunity" in the older caregivers of vaccinated children, with a decline in the frequency of infection by vaccinated strains (51). However, more recently, in the children who have been vaccinated, there has been an emergence of "replacement strains," with infection being caused by pneumococcal strains that are not included in the vaccine. What is particularly concerning is that the use of the vaccine has led to vaccinated patients having a higher frequency of necrotizing pneumonia than prior to the widespread use of vaccination, with most of the necrotizing pneumonias being caused by nonvaccine strains (51). Thus, even our best preventive efforts may be thwarted by bacterial adaptation.

Although there are no public reporting requirements for VAP, there has been a belief that VAP is largely preventable and that it may be a medical error that might not be reimbursed by Medicare. This belief has been largely fueled by the Institute for Healthcare Improvement (IHI), which has stated on its Web site that "zero VAP" is an appropriate and achievable goal, largely through the use of "ventilator bundles." A ventilator bundle is a series of interventions done daily on all ventilated patients, including intestinal bleed prophylaxis, deep venous thrombosis prophylaxis, head of the bed elevation, daily interruption of sedation, and daily weaning trials (52). While the use of bundles may prevent some episodes of pneumonia, it is unlikely to eliminate the problem, and statements that zero VAP is achievable may actually discourage future research and investigation in the area. Zero VAP is not likely in most hospitals where patients with nonmodifiable, disease-related impairments in host defense are commonly treated. In addition, the exact rate of VAP is difficult to estimate because of imprecision in the definition of a case. Finally, the reports of zero VAP are at best questionable, since most studies show a decline in the rate of pneumonia, with no documented decline in the consequences of VAP such as antibiotic use, duration of mechanical ventilation, length of stay, and mortality. The concern is that many hospitals with ostensibly good results of bundles have not eliminated VAP, but have simply renamed it as another process, and that if a zero VAP mentality prevails, hospitals may be reluctant to treat certain high-risk populations.

E. A New Interest in Adjunctive Therapy Approaches for Severe Pneumonia

The mainstay of therapy for respiratory infections has been antibiotics, but now there is interest in several adjunctive therapies, particularly for patients with severe pneumonia. Activated protein C (APC or drotrecogin alpha) has been approved for use in patients with severe sepsis, and in the pivotal PROWESS study, 35.6% of all patients had CAP, and an additional cohort had nosocomial pneumonia (53). APC had a survival benefit for CAP, but not nosocomial pneumonia patients, particularly for those with an APACHE II score more than 25, a pneumonia severity index (PSI) class of IV or higher and a CURB-65 score of 3 or more. In addition, the benefit was greatest to those receiving inadequate therapy (53). Other biologically active agents such as recombinant tissue factor pathway inhibitor are of potential value and are being studied in patients with severe CAP.

Another adjunctive therapy for patients with severe CAP may be systemic corticosteroid therapy. One small prospective randomized trial showed a mortality benefit for a seven-day continuous infusion of moderate doses (240 mg/day) of hydrocortisone (54). While the study was too small to establish the value of this therapy, retrospective analysis has shown that when patients with more severe forms of CAP received corticosteroids for other reasons [asthma or chronic obstructive pulmonary disease (COPD)], there was a decreased mortality compared with patients who did not receive this therapy, and there was no increased mortality in CAP in patients with COPD (55). Thus, although steroid therapy has not been proven to be necessary for patients with severe CAP, it seems safe to use, even in the face of severe infection, if needed for other purposes (56).

Inhaled antibiotics have been used as adjunctive therapy for VAP caused by MDR pathogens, with limited anecdotal success (4). There is now renewed interest in this form of therapy for patients with nosocomial tracheobronchitis during mechanical ventilation (57) and possibly to accelerate the clinical response and reduce the duration of systemic antibiotic therapy in patients with VAP. The use of this approach is being facilitated by the development of new small-particle nebulizers.

References

1. Ryu J. Classification and approach to bronchiolar diseases. Curr Opin Pulm Med 2006; 12:145–151.
2. Farr BM, Kaiser DL, Harrison BW, et al. Prediction of microbial aetiology at admission to hospital for pneumonia from presenting clinical features. Thorax 1989; 44:1031–1035.
3. Mandell LA, Wunderink RG, Anzueto A, et al. Infectious diseases society of America/American thoracic society consensus guidelines on the management of community-acquired pneumonia in adults. Clin Infect Dis 2007; 44:S27–S72.
4. Niederman MS, Craven DE, Bonten MJ, et al. Guidelines for the management of adults with hospital-acquired, ventilator-associated, and healthcare-associated pneumonia. Am J Respir Crit Care Med 2005; 171:388–416.
5. Niederman MS, Brito V. Pneumonia in the older patient. Clin Chest Med 2007; 28:751–771.
6. American Thoracic Society.Trends in pneumonia and influenza morbidity and mortality. Available at: http://www.thoracic.org. Accessed on July 10 2008.
7. American Thoracic Society, Centers for Disease Control and Prevention, Infectious Diseases Society of America.Controlling tuberculosis in the United States. Am J Respir Crit Care Med 2005; 172:1169–1227.
8. Niederman MS, McCombs JS, Unger AN, et al. The cost of treating community-acquired pneumonia. Clin Ther 1998; 20(4):820–837.

9. Fine MJ, Smith MA, Carson CA, et al. Prognosis and outcomes of patients with community-acquired pneumonia: a meta-analysis. JAMA 1996; 275:134–141.

10. Marston BJ, Plouffe JF, File TM Jr., et al. Incidence of community-acquired pneumonia requiring hospitalization. Results of a population-based active surveillance study in Ohio. The community-based pneumonia incidence study group. Arch Int Med 1997; 157:1709–1718.

11. Kaplan V, Clermont G, Griffin MF, et al. Pneumonia: still the old man's friend? Arch Intern Med 2003; 163:317–323.

12. Cook D, Walter SD, Cook RJ, et al. Incidence of and risk factors for ventilator-associated pneumonia in critically Ill patients. Ann Intern Med 1998; 129:433–440.

13. Girou E, Brun-Buisson C, Taille S, et al. Secular trends in nosocomial infections and mortality associated with noninvasive ventilation in patients with exacerbation of COPD and pulmonary edema. JAMA 2003; 290:2985–2991.

14. Kollef M, Ahrens T, Shannon W. Clinical predictors and outcomes for patients requiring tracheostomy in the intensive care unit. Crit Care Med 1999; 27:1714–1720.

15. Heyland DK, Cook DJ, Marshall J, et al. The attributable morbidity and mortality of ventilator-associated pneumonia in the critically ill patient. Am J Respir Crit Care Med 1999; 159:1249–1256.

16. Luna CM, Vujacich P, Niederman MS, et al. Impact of BAL data on the therapy and outcome of ventilator associated pneumonia. Chest 1997; 111:676–685.

17. Kollef MH, Sherman G, Ward S, et al. Inadequate antimicrobial treatment of infections: a risk factor for hospital mortality among critically Ill patients. Chest 1999; 115:462–474.

18. Rello J, Ollendorf DA, Oster G, et al. Epidemiology and outcomes of ventilator-associated pneumonia in a large US database. Chest 2002; 122:2115–2121.

19. Georges H, Leroy O, Guery B, et al. Predisposing factors for nosocomial pneumonia in patients receiving mechanical ventilation and requiring tracheotomy. Chest 2000; 118:767–774.

20. Niederman MS. Antibiotic therapy of exacerbations of chronic bronchitis. Semin Respir Infect 2000; 15:59–70.

21. American Lung Association. Trends in chronic bronchitis and emphysema: morbidity and mortality. May 2005. Available at: http://www.lungusa.org. Accessed August 10, 2008.

22. Murphy TF, Sethi A, Niederman MS. The role of bacteria in exacerbations of COPD: a constructive view. Chest 2000; 118:204–209.

23. Niederman MS. Does the presence of antibodies justify the use of antibiotics in exacerbations of chronic bronchitis? Am J Respir Crit Care Med 2004; 169:434–435.

24. National Heart, Lung, and Blood Institute Data Fact Sheet. Chronic Obstructive Pulmonary Disease, Washington DC, U.S. Government Printing Office, March 2003. (NIH Publication No. 03-5229.)

25. Niederman MS, McCombs JS, Unger AN, et al. Treatment cost of acute exacerbations of chronic bronchitis. Clin Ther 1999; 21:576–591.

26. Mortensen EM, Pugh MJ, Copeland LA. Impact of statins and angiotensin-converting enzyme inhibitors on mortality of subjects hospitalised with pneumonia. Eur Resp J 2008; 31:611–617.

27. McAlister FA, Majumdar SR, Blitz S, et al. The relationship between hyperglycemia and outcomes in 2,471 patients admitted to the hospital with community-acquired pneumonia. Diabetes Care 2005; 28:810–815.

28. Ahmed QA, Niederman MS. Respiratory infection in the chronically critically ill patient. Ventilator-associated pneumonia and tracheobronchitis. Clin Chest Med 2001; 22:71–85.

29. Dehoux MS, Boutten A, Ostinelli J, et al. Compartmentalized cytokine production within the human lung in unilateral pneumonia. Am J Respir Crit Care Me 1994;150(3):710–716.

30. Waterer GW, Wunderink RG. Genetic susceptibility to pneumonia. Clin Chest Med 2005; 26:29–38.

31. Waterer GW, Quasney MW, Cantor RM, et al. Septic shock and respiratory failure in community-acquired pneumonia have different TNF polymorphism associations. Am J Respir Crit Care Med 2001; 163:1599–1604.

32. Feikin DR, Schuchat A, Kolczak M, et al. Mortality from invasive pneumococcal pneumonia in the era of antibiotic resistance, 1995-1997. Am J Public Health 2000; 90:223–229.

33. Doern GV, Richter SS, Miller A, et al. Antimicrobial resistance among Streptococcus pneumoniae in the United States: have we begun to turn the corner on resistance to certain antimicrobial classes? Clin Infect Dis 2005; 41:139–148.

34. Schafer JJ, Goff DA, Stevenson KB, et al. Early experience with tigecycline for ventilator-associated pneumonia and bacteremia caused by multidrug-resistant *Acinetobacter baumannii*. Pharmacotherapy 2007; 27:980–987.

35. Spellberg B, Powers JH, Brass EP, et al. Trends in antimicrobial drug development: implications for the future. Clin Infect Dis 2004; 38:1279–1286.

36. Dellit TH, Owens RC, McGowan JE Jr., et al. Infectious Diseases Society of America and the Society for Healthcare Epidemiology of America guidelines for developing an institutional program to enhance antimicrobial stewardship. Clin Infect Dis 2007; 44:159–177.

37. Niederman MS. De-escalation therapy in ventilator-associated pneumonia. Curr Opin Crit Care 2006; 5:452–457.

38. Christ-Crain M, Muller B. Biomarkers in respiratory tract infections: diagnostic guides to antibiotic prescription, prognostic markers and mediators. Eur Resp J 2007; 30:556–573.

39. Christ-Crain M, Stolz D, Bingisser R, et al. Procalcitonin guidance of antibiotic therapy in community-acquired pneumonia: a randomized trial. Am J Respir Crit Care Med 2006; 174:84–93.

40. Canadian Critical Care Trials Group. A randomized trial of diagnostic techniques for ventilator-associated pneumonia. N Engl J Med 2006; 355:2619–2630.

41. Frei CR, Restrepo MI, Mortensen EM, et al. Impact of guideline-concordant empiric antibiotic therapy in community-acquired pneumonia. Am J Med 2006; 119:865–871.

42. Shorr AF, Bodi M, Rodriguez A, et al. Impact of antibiotic guideline compliance on duration of mechanical ventilation in critically ill patients with community-acquired pneumonia. Chest 2006; 130:93–100.

43. Yealy DM, Auble TF, Stone RA, et al. Effect of increasing the intensity of implementing pneumonia guidelines: a randomized, controlled trial. Ann Intern Med 2005; 143:881–894.

44. Fishbane S, Niederman MS, Daly C, et al. The impact of standardized order sets and intensive clinical case management on outcomes in community-acquired pneumonia. Arch Intern Med 2007; 167:1664–1669.

45. Soo Hoo GW, Wen YE, Nguyen TV, et al. Impact of clinical guidelines in the management of severe hospital-acquired pneumonia. Chest 2005; 128:2778–2787.

46. Micek ST, Ward S, Fraser VJ, et al. A randomized controlled trial of an antibiotic discontinuation policy for clinically suspected ventilator-associated pneumonia. Chest 2004; 125:1791–1799.

47. Houck PM, Bratzler DW, Nsa W, et al. Timing of antibiotic administration and outcomes for Medicare patients hospitalized with community-acquired pneumonia. Arch Intern Med 2004; 164:637–644.

48. Wachter RM, Flanders SA, Fee C, et al. Public reporting of antibiotic timing in patients with pneumonia: lessons from a flawed performance measure. Ann Intern Med 2008; 149:29–32.

49. Welker JA, Huston M, McCue JD. Antibiotic timing and errors in diagnosing pneumonia. Arch Intern Med 2008; 168:351–356.

50. Polgreen PM, Chen YY, Cavanaugh JE. An outbreak of severe Clostridium difficile-associated disease possibly related to inappropriate antimicrobial therapy for community-acquired pneumonia. Infect Control Hosp Epidemiol 2007; 28:212–214.

51. Bender JM, Ampofo K, Korgenski K, et al. Pneumococcal necrotizing pneumonia in Utah: does serotype matter? Clin Infect Dis 2008; 46:1346–1352.
52. Omrane R, Eid J, Perreault MM, et al. Impact of a protocol for prevention of ventilator-associated pneumonia. Ann Pharmacother 2007; 41:1390–1396.
53. Laterre PF, Garber G, Levy H, et al. Severe community-acquired pneumonia as a cause of severe sepsis: data from the PROWESS study. Crit Care Med 2005;33:952–961.
54. Confalonieri M, Urbino R, Potena A, et al. Hydrocortisone infusion for severe community-acquired pneumonia: a preliminary randomized study. Am J Respir Crit Care Med 2005; 171(3): 242–248.
55. Garcia-Vidal C, Calbo E, Pascual V, et al. Effects of systemic steroids in patients with severe community-acquired pneumonia. Eur Respir J 2007; 30(5):951–956.
56. Salluh JI, Povoa P, Soares M, et al. The role of corticosteroids in severe community-acquired pneumonia: a systematic review. Crit Care 2008; 12:R76.
57. Palmer LB, Smaldone GC, Chen JJ, et al. Aerosolized antibiotics and ventilator-associated tracheobronchitis in the intensive care unit. Crit Care Med 2008; 36:2008–2013.

2
Host Defense Against Infection in the Airways

PIETER S. HIEMSTRA
Leiden University Medical Center, Leiden, The Netherlands

I. Introduction

The epithelium of the lung is the largest surface area of the body and is exposed to gaseous compounds and numerous inhaled particles present in inhaled air that have escaped the filtering function of the nose and have not deposited in the nasopharynx. These particles include respiratory pathogens that may cause severe infections resulting in substantial morbidity and mortality. Nevertheless, the peripheral small airways and alveoli are sterile in healthy subjects and severe infections are relatively rare in such individuals. This is explained by the presence of an efficient host-defense system in the lung. A breach in this defense or aberrant functioning of the system results in infectious and inflammatory lung disease. Intense research has led to the characterization of the various elements that constitute this defense system, and has provided new insight into the pathogenesis of a variety of infectious and inflammatory lung disorders. Host defense in the lung includes the barrier function and mucociliary clearance provided by the epithelium, as well as innate and adaptive immune responses mediated by a range of cell types in the lung, including epithelial cells, phagocytes, dendritic cells (DCs), and lymphocytes. In this chapter, an overview is provided of the various elements of this defense system.

II. Epithelial Cells: Barrier Function and Mucociliary Clearance

With a surface area that equals that of half a tennis court (70–140 m^2), the epithelial surface of the lung forms the major interface between the host and the environment. The surface of the upper and lower airways and of the alveoli is lined with an epithelial layer that rests on a basement membrane (1). In the central airways of the lung, this epithelium is covered by a continuous layer of mucus that is positioned on top of an aqueous layer. In the more distal bronchi, the mucus layer is discontinuous, whereas in the small bronchioles of a healthy individual it is absent. The composition of the epithelial layer is markedly different in the various parts of the bronchial tree. Although a pseudostratified epithelium is present in the trachea, bronchi, and bronchioles, the alveoli are lined with a thin layer of type I and type II cells. Also, the composition of the pseudostratified epithelium of the conducting airways differs along the bronchial tree: mucus-producing goblet cells are present in substantial numbers in the large airways, but this cell type is relatively scarce in smaller airways from healthy individuals, which is reflected by the different distribution of the mucus layer in the differently sized airways.

The epithelium of the airways consists of a range of cell types (1,2): ciliated cells and mucus-producing goblet cells involved in mucociliary clearance (as outlined later in the chapter), basal cells that serve as progenitors, neuroendocrine cells involved in regeneration and repair, Clara cells that produce anti-inflammatory molecules such as the 10-kDa CC10 and secretory leukocyte proteinase inhibitor (SLPI), and brush cells with a function that is incompletely understood. Clara cells are most numerous in the terminal bronchiole, whereas goblet cells are more numerous in the surface epithelium of the large proximal airways. In addition to these cell types that make up the surface epithelium of the airways, submucosal glands are essential to host defense. The mucous cells of these glands produce most of the mucins, whereas the serous cells produce water, electrolytes, and a range of antimicrobial and anti-inflammatory molecules such as lysozyme, lactoferrin, and SLPI (3). Finally, the alveoli are lined with the flattened type I alveolar epithelial cells that cover the largest surface area of the alveoli and facilitate gas exchange, and the taller and more numerous surfactant-producing type II alveolar cells.

A. Mucociliary Clearance and Barrier Function

Epithelial cells form intercellular junctions and thereby restrict the movement of molecules and particles across the epithelial layer. This provides an efficient barrier and first-line defense against invading pathogens and toxic compounds that reach the epithelial surface. The epithelium of the conducting airways is equipped with an efficient mucociliary clearance mechanism that acts as an additional barrier and removes inhaled substances. Both the submucosal glands of the large airways that lie beneath the epithelium and are connected to the surface by ducts and the goblet cells of the surface epithelium contribute to the production of mucus. Mucus traps inhaled particles including respiratory pathogens, and the action of the cilia of the ciliated cells propels the mucus towards the oropharyngeal cavity, where it is often removed by swallowing. The presence of the pericellular layer on which the mucus layer is positioned and in which the cilia move is essential to allow transport of mucus (Fig. 1). The removal of mucus through this "mucociliary escalator" is further assisted by coughing.

Mucus is composed of a variety of compounds including water, electrolytes, antimicrobial peptides and proteins, as well as high-molecular-weight mucin glyco-proteins (4). Mucins are the major component of mucus and produced by the submucosal glands and the goblet cells of the surface epithelium. The secreted gel-forming mucins produced by these cells are essential for the viscoelastic properties of mucus, and MUC5AC and MUC5B are the most abundant mucins present in airway secretions. A range of endogenous stimuli increase mucin gene expression, including growth factors, proinflammatory cytokines [such as interleukin (IL)-1β, tumor necrosis factor (TNF)α, and IL-17A], Th2 cytokines (IL-4, IL-9, and IL-13), and inflammatory mediators such as neutrophil elastase (5). Inhaled substances such as microbial products and cigarette smoke are also well-characterized stimuli of mucin production. Several studies have identified the epidermal growth factor receptor (EGFR) as essential in the regulation of mucin expression. Secretion of mucus by submucosal glands and airway surface epithelial goblet cells is a tightly regulated exocytosis process that is stimulated by a range of secretagogues. These include inflammatory mediators and proteolytic enzymes produced during inflammation, nucleotides such as ATP and UTP acting through purinergic receptors, and acetylcholine.

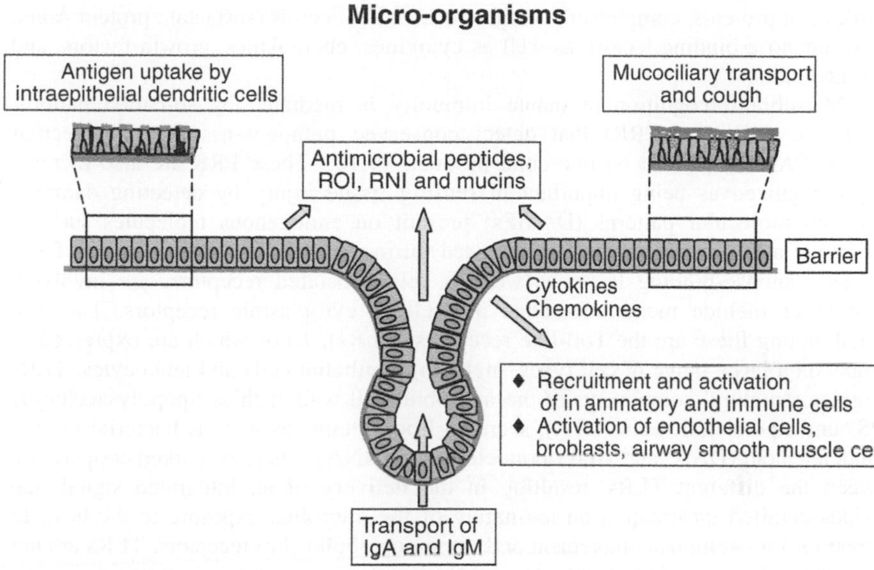

Micro-organisms

Figure 1 Central role of airway epithelial cells in host defense against infection. Microbial challenges by inhaled respiratory microorganisms are dealt with by the epithelial barrier function and mucociliary transport, production of antimicrobial molecules, and cytokines and chemokines that recruit and activate a range of structural cells as well as leukocytes. Epithelial cells are also involved in transport of secretory antibodies and in the initiation of adaptive immune responses by subepithelial and intraepithelial DCs. The extensions of some of the intraepithelial dendritic cells may reach into the lumen of the airways and thus efficiently sample substances from the airway lumen. *Abbreviations*: DCs, dendritic cells; RNI, reactive nitrogen intermediates; ROI, reactive oxygen intermediates.

The epithelium is a rich source of antimicrobial peptides, cytokines, chemokines, and other mediators (Fig. 1). These mediators of innate immunity are discussed in the following section.

III. Innate Immunity

Together with the barrier function of the epithelium and mucociliary clearance, the innate and adaptive immune systems form the major elements of host defense against infection in the lung. Compared with adaptive immunity, the specificity of the innate immune system is rather broad, and it is always active. Defense and clearance of microorganisms are the main functions of innate immunity, but it is also involved in activation and shaping the adaptive immune response (for reviews on pulmonary innate immunity, see Refs. 6–8). Innate immunity in the lung is mediated by structural cells such as epithelial cells, fibroblasts, endothelial cells, and airway smooth muscle cells, as well as by a range of leukocyte cell types. In addition, a range of soluble molecules secreted by these cells contribute to innate immunity, including antimicrobial peptides and proteins, complement components, and collectins (surfactant protein A and D and mannose-binding lectin), as well as cytokines, chemokines, growth factors, and lipid mediators.

Microbial recognition in innate immunity is mediated by so-called pattern-recognition receptors (PRR) that detect conserved pathogen-associated molecular patterns (PAMPs) present on microbial products (9,10). These PRR are also increasingly recognized as being important in sensing tissue injury by detecting damage-associated molecular patterns (DAMPs) present on endogenous molecules such as hyaluronan and fibronectin that are released during injury (11). Both secreted PRR, such as mannose-binding lectin as well as cell-associated receptors, are involved. These latter include membrane-bound as well as cytoplasmic receptors. The best studied among these are the Toll-like receptors (TLRs), 10 of which are expressed in humans on a large range of cell types, including epithelial cells and leukocytes. TLRs recognize structural components of the microbial cell wall such as lipopolysaccharide (LPS) and lipoteichoic acid (LTA), secreted lipoproteins, as well as bacterial deoxy-ribonucleic acid (DNA) and viral ribonucleic acid (RNA). There is marked cooperation between the different TLRs, resulting in the delivery of an integrated signal that provides detailed information on the nature of the microbial exposure to the host. In contrast to, for example, complement and immunoglobulin (Fc) receptors, TLRs are not involved in phagocytosis but serve to signal microbial exposure and mount an appropriate cellular response. TLRs are part of the IL-1 receptor/TLR superfamily and characterized by an intracellular Toll/interleukin-1 receptor (TIR) domain. Effective signaling by TLR4, involved in the recognition of LPS, relies on two accessory proteins: MD2 and CD14. This feature is unique for TLR4. After binding of a ligand, TLRs recruit adaptor molecules to transfer the signal. MyD88 serves as an adaptor molecule involved in intracellular signaling by all TLRs, except TLR3. The importance of TLRs to innate immunity in the lung is illustrated by the observation that subjects with a mutation in TLR4 show decreased airway responsiveness to inhaled LPS (12).

Other PRR include C-type lectins such as the mannose receptor and dectin-1 that mediate phagocytosis and cellular responses to a range of microbial products (8). Although TLRs and these C-type lectins sense microbial exposure at the cell surface or in the endosomes, other PRR are involved in the detection of pathogens that have escaped into the cytosol. Currently these are classified as nucleotide oligomerization domain (NOD)-like receptors involved in detection of bacteria, and caspase activation and recruitment domain (CARD)-helicase proteins that recognize cytosolic viral double-stranded RNA produced during viral replication (9,13).

A. Cells of the Innate Immune System
Structural Cells
Various structural cells contribute to innate immunity in the lung, including epithelial cells, fibroblasts, endothelial cells, and airway smooth muscle cells. Epithelial cells are of special importance because they form the first contact between an invading micro-organism and the host, contribute to host defense through their barrier function and mucociliary transport (as discussed earlier), and production of a range of effector molecules that directly target microorganisms such as antimicrobial peptides and proteins (Table 1), as well as cytokines, chemokines, growth factors, etc. (Fig. 1).

Table 1 Effector Molecules Involved in Host Defense Produced by Airway Epithelial Cells

---

* Mucins
* Antimicrobial peptides and proteins (β-defensins, hCAP-18/LL-37, lactoferrin, lysozyme, antimicrobial chemokines, SLPI, elafin, and PLUNC proteins)
* SP-A, SP-D
* Complement components
* ROI and RNI

Abbreviations: SLPI, secretory leukocyte proteinase inhibitor; SP, surfactant proteins; ROI, reactive oxygen intermediates; RNI, reactive nitrogen intermediates; PLUNC, palate, lung and nasal epithelium associated.

Monocytes and Macrophages

Monocytes are produced in the bone marrow and mature into macrophages after migration to the tissues. Local conditions are essential for the development of macrophages with a distinct phenotype. The alveolar macrophage is the best-studied macrophage type in the lung. Macrophages display a range of functions relevant to host defense. They are involved in intracellular killing of ingested microorganisms [using reactive oxygen and nitrogen intermediates (ROIs, RNIs), antimicrobial peptides and proteins, and enzymes] as well as extracellular killing. They can present antigen to T cells, although not as efficiently as DCs. In addition, they release a large range of mediators that cause tissue injury, contribute to tissue repair, and signal to immune and other cells. Thus they contribute to the important role of the innate immune system in shaping adaptive immune responses.

Throughout the body, various subsets of macrophages have been identified that display different functional activities. This is illustrated by the distinct phenotype of alveolar macrophages that are immunosuppressive and poor at antigen presentation (14,15). In line with these observations, it has been shown that the phenotype of macrophages can be modulated in vitro, resulting in subsets with different functions. Studies in mice and humans have led to the identification of a subset with a classical, proinflammatory phenotype and a subset with a nonclassical, partly anti-inflammatory phenotype (16–18). In contrast to the proinflammatory subset, the nonclassical anti-inflammatory subset is characterized by the absence of secretion of proinflammatory IL-12, but marked secretion of anti-inflammatory IL-10. In addition, these anti-inflammatory macrophages are efficient in the clearance of apoptotic cells.

Dendritic Cells

DCs are the main antigen-presenting cell type in the body and are strategically positioned at sites of potential pathogen entry, including the mucosal surface of the lung (for recent reviews, see Refs. 19–21). DCs are involved both in innate and adaptive immunity. In addition to their essential role in mounting an effective adaptive immune response against pathogens, they are a crucial element in the control of unwanted immune responses against harmless environmental compounds and particles. Microbial exposure and inflammation results in the rapid recruitment of DCs into the lung (22).

Within the lung, DCs are positioned in the epithelium and lamina propria of the airways and in the interstitium and alveolar lumen of the distal lung. The extensions of a subset of the epithelial DCs can reach the lumen of the airways and thus efficiently sample the content of the inspired air and take up large molecules that are unable to cross epithelial tight junctions (22). After taking up antigen, DCs can rapidly migrate to the draining lymph nodes, where they can activate naive T cells. Both myeloid and plasmacytoid DCs are present in the lung, but myeloid DCs are more abundant and have been best studied so far. However, there is an increasing interest in plasmacytoid DCs because of their potential involvement in the suppression of cell-mediated immune responses and the fact that they produce substantial amounts of the antiviral type I interferons (IFNs), thus playing an important role in the contribution of innate immunity to defense against viral infections (21,23). The presence and activity of DCs present in the alveolar space appears to be under the control of alveolar macrophages, thus ensuring the absence of unwanted immune responses.

Neutrophils

Neutrophils are crucial to an effective innate immune system in the lung and rapidly migrate to the lung during infection. They contribute to host defense against infection in various ways. First neutrophils are efficient in the uptake of microorganisms, that subsequently can be killed by an effective killing machinery using oxygen-dependent mechanisms, involving production of ROIs, and nonoxidative mechanisms using antimicrobial peptides and proteins and proteolytic enzymes (24,25). In addition, recent studies have identified the neutrophil extracellular trap (NET) as an additional antimicrobial mechanism operative in neutrophils (26). These NETs consist of a chromatin structure to which granule proteins are attached and are released by neutrophils as a result of cell death initiated by neutrophil activation. Thus bacteria and fungi are trapped in this structure in which the high concentration of antimicrobial granule proteins ensures efficient killing. In addition to their role as effector cells in killing invading microorganisms and tissue injury, neutrophils also release a variety of mediators that enable them to shape the immune response and control wound repair by affecting DCs, monocyte, and macrophage recruitment and function (24).

Eosinophils

Eosinophils are best known for their role in host defense against parasites and allergic inflammation. Recent studies suggest a much broader role of eosinophils in the inflammatory reaction, as well as in adaptive immunity through their direct interaction with T cells (27). Eosinophils produce and release various molecules that contribute to this activity against parasites and microorganisms as well as cause tissue injury, including eosinophil cationic protein, major basic protein, eosinophil peroxidase, and eosinophil-derived neurotoxin. In addition, eosinophils signal to other cells by the production and release of a range of cytokines, chemokines, and growth factors. The importance of this function is illustrated by the observation that eosinophils are the major source of the multifunctional cytokine transforming growth factor beta (TGFβ) in the lung.

Mast Cells

Although mast cells may be best known for their involvement in allergic reactions, they play a central role in host defense against infection (28). Mast cells are phenotypically diverse and use a variety of receptors to respond to triggers. These include the high-affinity

IgE receptor (FcεRI), complement receptors, as well as TLRs. Mast cells synthesize and release various mediators and effector molecules, including histamine, proteases, lipid mediators, cytokines, and antimicrobial peptides such as hCAP-18/LL-37. This way, mast cells contribute to inflammation and antimicrobial defense, as well as shaping the immune response by their ability to for example, polarize T-cell responses.

NK and NKT Cells

Natural killer (NK) cells, natural killer T-cells (NKT cells), and CD8 lymphocytes are killer types involved in immunity in the lung. NK and NKT cells are elements of innate immunity that share functions and other characteristics with the CD8 cells of the adaptive immune system. NK cells have been extensively described in various reviews. More recently the role of NKT cells, which form a small population of cells in the lung, is beginning to be recognized. Like NK cells, NKT cells bridge innate and adaptive immunity. NKT cells can be activated by direct contact with microbial molecules such as glycolipids presented by CD1d molecules to the invariant T-cell receptor present on these cells (hence the name invariant NKT cells). NKT cells can be also be activated indirectly by endogenous antigens, cytokines, or both. NKT cells exert their activity at least in part by producing large amounts of Th1 and Th2 cytokines. Although an increasing number of studies suggest a role of NKT cells in host defense against respiratory infection (and possibly in asthma), there are also many contradictory findings. Studies are hampered by the lack of good reagents.

B. Innate Immunity: Mediators and Effector Molecules

Cytokines, Chemokines, and Growth Factors

The efficient defense provided by epithelial cells and intraluminal macrophages deals with most microbial challenges. In the event that such a challenge is overwhelming, macrophages and epithelial cells use production of chemokines and cytokines to recruit other leukocytes to the site of infection (8,29). These mediators are produced in response to triggering of PRR by microbial compounds or tissue injury. The two major classes of chemokines are the CXC and CC chemokines. CXC chemokines are primarily involved in the attraction of neutrophils, whereas CC chemokines mediate recruitment of various cell types, including monocytes, eosinophils, and lymphocytes. Proinflammatory cytokines of the IL-1 family and TNFα are also produced as part of the innate immune response to infection. These cytokines are involved in the activation of a wide range of structural cell types and leukocyte subsets, resulting in processes such as leukocyte extravasation, production of antimicrobial substances, and tissue remodeling. In addition to these cytokines, a range of other cytokines is produced as part of the innate immune response that is not discussed in detail here. Also not discussed here are the various growth factors that are produced during infections, that mediate survival of invading leukocytes, epithelial repair following wounding, extracellular matrix production, and other elements of tissue remodeling.

Type I IFN-α/β are cytokines that are an essential component of the innate antiviral response (30). These IFNs are produced in response to triggering of membrane-bound and cytosolic PRR that act as sensors for viral exposure and initiate a range of cellular reactions in cells that express the type I IFN receptor that bring this cell to an antiviral state.

*Antimicrobial Peptides and Proteins, Reactive Oxygen
and Nitrogen Intermediates*

These endogenous antibiotics are mainly produced by epithelial cells and neutrophils in the lung and are involved in extracellular killing as well as intracellular killing of ingested microorganisms (for reviews, see Refs. 31–35). In addition, they serve an array of functions distinct from their direct antimicrobial activity. Several studies have shown their involvement in inflammation, immunity, and wound repair processes.

The main families of antimicrobial peptides present in human airway secretions are the defensins and the cathelicidins. Although various defensins can be found in airway secretions, humans only express one member of the cathelicidin family of antimicrobial peptides, hCAP-18/LL-37. Two defensin families can be distinguished on the basis of their structure (pairing of disulfide bridges): the α- and the β-defensins. The major constituent of the azurophilic granule of neutrophils are the α-defensins [or human neutrophil peptide (HNP) 1–4]. Epithelial cells are the main cellular source of the human β-defensin (hBD)1–4. Although neutrophils and epithelial cells are the main cellular sources of these defensins, other cell types such as monocytes, macrophages, DCs and T cells also contribute. hCAP-18 is the precursor of the cathelicidin peptide LL-37, which is released from hCAP-18 by proteolytic cleavage. LL-37 is a cationic 4.5-kDa peptide that is characterized by the presence of an amphipathic α-helix. Its main cellular source is the neutrophil, and following neutrophil stimulation hCAP-18 that is stored in the specific granules is processed to LL-37 by proteinase 3 derived from azurophilic granules. Also other cell types such as epithelial cells and mast cells contribute to synthesis of hCAP-18/LL-37.

In addition to antimicrobial peptides, a range of larger antimicrobial proteins is produced (8,31,36,37). These include well-known antimicrobial proteins such as lactoferrin and lysozyme, as well as cationic epithelial proteinase inhibitors (SLPI and elafin), surfactant proteins (SP)-A and SP-D, selected chemokines with antimicrobial properties, fragments from the activated complement component C3, PLUNC proteins, and peptidoglycan recognition proteins (PGLYRPs). Some of these molecules were initially identified on the basis of their antimicrobial activity and later shown to have other activities as well. Other molecules were initially discovered as a component of surfactant or a chemokine and later shown to display antimicrobial activity.

Although the antimicrobial activity of these antimicrobial peptides and proteins is usually investigated using bacteria grown in the laboratory in the free-living planktonic phase, bacteria causing infections are likely also present in biofilms. Biofilms are structured communities of bacteria that are encapsulated in a self-produced matrix and attached to a surface (38). Bacteria that are present in such biofilms are largely resistant to antibiotics and leukocyte-mediated killing and thus constitute an important clinical problem. Studies on lactoferrin (39) and the cathelicidin LL-37 (40) indicate that these antimicrobials inhibit biofilm formation at submicrobicidal concentrations, and, as shown for LL-37, may target bacteria present in biofilms (40) (Fig. 2). The relevance of these findings to host defense against bacteria present in biofilms in vivo remains to be determined.

Another group of antimicrobial molecules are the ROIs and RNIs. ROI are an essential element of innate immunity that has been well characterized in phagocytes, where they are produced as a result of the ability of the phagocyte NADPH oxidase (*PhoX*) enzymatic system to generate superoxide. Superoxide produces hydrogen peroxide that is converted to hypochlorous acid by myeloperoxidase. It is now recognized

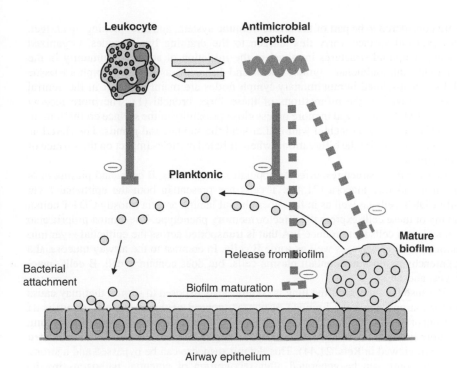

Figure 2 Role of antimicrobial peptides in host defense against bacterial infection. Antimicrobial peptides derived from epithelial cells and leukocyte subsets have direct effects on bacteria and indirect effects that are mediated via activation of leukocytes. Bacteria may be present as free-living bacteria in the planktonic phase, but many bacteria are likely present in biofilms adherent to, for example, epithelia. Phagocytes rapidly ingest and kill planktonic bacteria but are not effective against bacteria present in biofilms. Antimicrobial peptides are also active against planktonic bacteria, and some recent reports indicate that they may also affect biofilms.

that epithelial cells also express homologues of NADPH oxidase (DUOX1 and DUOX2) and generate hydrogen peroxide, which is used by lactoperoxidase from the submucosal glands to oxidize thiocyanate to generate the antimicrobial hypothiocyanate (41,42). Synthesis of nitric oxide by three different NO-synthesizing enzymes expressed in lung tissue is the essential step in production of a range of RNIs, among which especially peroxynitrite, produced by the interaction between superoxide anion and NO, is highly antimicrobial (43).

IV. Adaptive Immunity

The innate immune system protects against most microbial challenges that the lung encounters. The adaptive immune system comes into action to specifically target pathogens by a humoral and/or cell-mediated response. In contrast to the innate immune system, it requires days to weeks to mount an effective response, is specific, and builds up memory to respond quicker and stronger to subsequent challenges. The antigen-presenting

DCs are considered to be part of the innate immune system, and after picking up antigen at the epithelial surface, carry this antigen to the draining lymph nodes. Organized secondary lymphoid structures involved in the initiation of adaptive immunity in the lung include intrapulmonary lymph nodes and bronchus-associated lymphoid tissue (BALT). Encapsulated intrapulmonary lymph nodes are mainly present in the central airways, localized to the bifurcations of these large bronchi (1). The more loosely organized BALT is localized in more or less close proximity of the surface epithelium, in the outer layers of the bronchial wall and around the submucosal glands. The BALT is also mainly localized at the bifurcations, where inhaled particles impact on the surface of the epithelium.

Outside these structures, effector populations of T cells, B cells, and plasma cells reside in the airway mucosa (21,44). T cells are present in both the epithelial layer (mostly CD8 T cells) as well as in the subepithelial lamina propria (mostly CD4 T cells), and many of these cells express the effector/memory phenotype. The lamina propria also contains plasma cells that produce IgA that is transported across the epithelial layer into the lumen of the airways, as well as some B cells. In contrast to the airway mucosa, the lung parenchyma does not contain plasma cells, but does contain T cell, B cells, macrophages, and DCs.

Because the mucosa of the lung is continuously exposed to stimuli that may cause inflammation and unwanted immune responses, control of the immune response is of utmost importance to the integrity of the host. The default immune response of the lung is therefore limited, and is characterized by a low Th2 response and/or T cell–mediated tolerance (reviewed in Refs. 21,44). This default response can be bypassed and a strong immune response can be generated after recognition of potential pathogens by the aforementioned PRRs such as TLRs on DC. This recognition of microbial exposure results in the generation of activated DCs that are essential in the generation of an effective immune response directed at the elimination of respiratory pathogens.

These characteristics of pulmonary innate immunity suggest that in addition to effector T cells that are needed for an effective immune response, also induction of regulatory T cells (T_{reg}) is essential to prevent unwanted immune responses and to dampen inflammation during and after respiratory infections. There is currently a lot of interest in the role of T_{reg} in inflammatory lung diseases such as asthma, and this cell type is topic of many excellent reviews (45.46).

Various types of effector T cells are active in the lung. CD8 cells are able to cause direct cell lysis of virus-infected cells and produce cytokines to signal to other cells. T helper cells are characterized by the CD4 antigen and traditionally divided into the Th1 and Th2 subsets. Recently a third subset has been identified that is characterized by the production of IL-17 (47). These Th17 cells play an important role in host defense against infection, and IL-17 is now recognized as an important regulator of epithelial cell function.

V. Concluding Remarks

Host defense against infection is a wide and still expanding area of active research and much progress has been made in the last decades in this area. It relies on an effective innate immune system together with the barrier function and mucociliary clearance provided by the epithelium of the airways and alveoli. The adaptive immune system serves as an essential backup for overwhelming microbial exposure, threats resulting from breaches in innate immunity and the ability of respiratory pathogens to evade immune defenses. Understanding the basic concepts of this system is essential for understanding the pathogenesis and treatment of respiratory infections, as well as chronic inflammatory lung disease. This chapter serves as an introduction into this area of research, and many excellent reviews—some of which are cited in this contribution—are available for those interested in more detailed information on certain aspects of host defense.

References

1. Corrin B, Nicholson A. Pathology of the Lungs. 2nd ed. New York, NY: Churchill Livingstone, 2006.
2. Chang MM, Shih L, Wu R. Pulmonary epithelium: cell types and functions. In: Proud D, ed. The Pulmonary Epithelium in Health and Disease. Chichester, UK: Wiley, 2008:1–14.
3. Wine JJ, Joo NS. Submucosal glands and airway defense. Proc Am Thorac Soc 2004; 1(1): 47–53.
4. Thornton DJ, Rousseau K, McGuckin MA. Structure and function of the polymeric mucins in airways mucus. Annu Rev Physiol 2008; 70(1):459–486.
5. Thai P, Loukoianov A, Wachi S, et al. Regulation of airway mucin gene expression. Annu Rev Physiol 2008; 70:405–429.
6. Martin TR, Frevert CW. Innate immunity in the lungs. Proc Am Thorac Soc 2005; 2(5):403–411.
7. Zaas AK, Schwartz DA. Innate immunity and the lung: defense at the interface between host and environment. Trends Cardiovasc Med 2005; 15(6):195–202.
8. Suzuki T, Chow CW, Downey GP. Role of innate immune cells and their products in lung immunopathology. Int J Biochem Cell Biol 2008; 40(6–7):1348–1361.
9. Akira S, Uematsu S, Takeuchi O. Pathogen recognition and innate immunity. Cell 2006; 124(4): 783–801.
10. Sabroe I, Parker LC, Dower SK, et al. The role of TLR activation in inflammation. J Pathol 2008; 214(2):126–135.
11. Bianchi ME. DAMPs, PAMPs and alarmins: all we need to know about danger. J Leukoc Biol 2007; 81(1):1–5.
12. Arbour NC, Lorenz E, Schutte BC, et al. TLR4 mutations are associated with endotoxin hyporesponsiveness in humans. Nat Genet 2000; 25(2):187–191.
13. Lee MS, Kim YJ. Signaling pathways downstream of pattern-recognition receptors and their cross talk. Annu Rev Biochem 2007; 76:447–480.
14. Thepen T, Van Rooijen N, Kraal G. Alveolar macrophage elimination in vivo is associated with an increase in pulmonary immune response in mice. J Exp Med 1989; 170(2):499–509.
15. Blumenthal RL, Campbell DE, Hwang P, et al. Human alveolar macrophages induce functional inactivation in antigen-specific CD4 T cells. J Allergy Clin Immunol 2001; 107(2): 258–264.
16. Gordon S. Alternative activation of macrophages. Nat Rev Immunol 2003; 3(1):23–35.
17. Mosser DM. The many faces of macrophage activation. J Leukoc Biol 2003; 73(2):209–212.
18. Mantovani A, Sica A, Sozzani S, et al. The chemokine system in diverse forms of macrophage activation and polarization. Trends Immunol 2004; 25(12):677–686.
19. Iwasaki A. Mucosal dendritic cells. Annu Rev Immunol 2007; 25:381–418.
20. Novak N, Bieber T. 2. Dendritic cells as regulators of immunity and tolerance. J Allergy Clin Immunol 2008; 121(2 suppl):S370–S374.
21. Holt PG, Strickland DH, Wikstrom ME, et al. Regulation of immunological homeostasis in the respiratory tract. Nat Rev Immunol 2008; 8(2):142–152.
22. Jahnsen FL, Strickland DH, Thomas JA, et al. Accelerated antigen sampling and transport by airway mucosal dendritic cells following inhalation of a bacterial stimulus. J Immunol 2006; 177(9):5861–5867.

23. Cao W, Liu YJ. Innate immune functions of plasmacytoid dendritic cells. Curr Opin Immunol 2007; 19(1):24–30.

24. Nathan C. Neutrophils and immunity: challenges and opportunities. Nat Rev Immunol 2006; 6(3):173–182.

25. Borregaard N, Sorensen OE, Theilgaard-Monch K. Neutrophil granules: a library of innate immunity proteins. Trends Immunol 2007; 28(8):340–345.

26. Brinkmann V, Zychlinsky A. Beneficial suicide: why neutrophils die to make NETs. Nat Rev Micro 2007; 5(8):577–582.

27. Hogan SP, Rosenberg HF, Moqbel R, et al. Eosinophils: biological properties and role in health and disease. Clin Exp Allergy 2008; 38(5):709–750.

28. Galli SJ, Kalesnikoff J, Grimbaldeston MA, et al. Mast cells as "tunable" effector and immunoregulatory cells: recent advances. Annu Rev Immunol 2005; 23:749–786.

29. Strieter RM, Belperio JA, Keane MP. Host innate defenses in the lung: the role of cytokines. Curr Opin Infect Dis 2003; 16(3):193–198.

30. Garcia-Sastre A, Biron CA. Type 1 interferons and the virus-host relationship: a lesson in detente. Science 2006; 312(5775):879–882.

31. Rogan MP, Geraghty P, Greene CM, et al. Antimicrobial proteins and polypeptides in pulmonary innate defence. Respir Res 2006; 7:29.

32. Oppenheim JJ, Yang D. Alarmins: chemotactic activators of immune responses. Curr Opin Immunol 2005; 17(4):359–365.

33. Ganz T. Antimicrobial polypeptides. J Leukoc Biol 2004; 75(1):34–38.

34. Bals R, Hiemstra PS. Innate immunity in the lung: how epithelial cells fight against respiratory pathogens. Eur Respir J 2004; 23:327–733.

35. Hiemstra PS. The role of epithelial beta-defensins and cathelicidins in host defense of the lung. Exp Lung Res 2007; 33(10):537–542.

36. Hiemstra PS. Epithelial antimicrobial molecules. In: Proud D, ed. The Pulmonary Epithelium in Health and Disease. Chichester, UK: Wiley, 2008:187–200.

37. Wright JR. The "wisdom" of lung surfactant: balancing host defense and surface tension-reducing functions. Am J Physiol Lung Cell Mol Physiol 2006; 291(5):L847–L850.

38. Costerton JW, Stewart PS, Greenberg EP. Bacterial biofilms: a common cause of persistent infections. Science 1999; 284(5418):1318.

39. Singh PK, Parsek MR, Greenberg EP, et al. A component of innate immunity prevents bacterial biofilm development. Nature 2002; 417(6888):552–555.

40. Overhage J, Campisano A, Bains M, et al. The human host defence peptide LL-37 prevents bacterial biofilm formation. Infect Immun 2008; 76(9):4176–4182.

41. Moskwa P, Lorentzen D, Excoffon KJDA, et al. A novel host defense system of airways is defective in cystic fibrosis. Am J Respir Crit Care Med 2007; 175(2):174–183.

42. van der Vliet A. NADPH oxidases in lung biology and pathology: host defense enzymes, and more. Free Radic Biol Med 2008; 44(6):938–955.

43. Ricciardolo FL, Sterk PJ, Gaston B, et al. Nitric oxide in health and disease of the respiratory system. Physiol Rev 2004; 84(3):731–765.

44. Lefrancois L, Puddington L. Intestinal and pulmonary mucosal T cells: local heroes fight to maintain the status quo. Annu Rev Immunol 2006; 24:681–704.

45. Vignali DA, Collison LW, Workman CJ. How regulatory T cells work. Nat Rev Immunol 2008; 8(7):523–532.

46. Akdis M, Blaser K, Akdis CA. T regulatory cells in allergy: novel concepts in the pathogenesis, prevention, and treatment of allergic diseases. J Allergy Clin Immunol 2005; 116(5): 961–968.

47. Ouyang W, Kolls JK, Zheng Y. The biological functions of T helper 17 cell effector cytokines in inflammation. Immunity 2008; 28(4):454–467.

3
Mechanisms of Bacterial Pathogenesis in Respiratory Tract Infection

TIMOTHY F. MURPHY
University at Buffalo, State University of New York and Veterans Affairs Western New York Healthcare System, Buffalo, New York, U.S.A.

I. Introduction

The human airways below the vocal cords are sterile as a result of innate immune defenses. The development of pulmonary infection occurs with either a defect in host defenses, a particularly virulent pathogen, an overwhelming inoculum, or a combination of these three factors. A feature of many bacterial respiratory tract pathogens is that under usual circumstances, they colonize the upper respiratory tract without causing clinical symptoms. The development of clinical infection represents a perturbation of the symbiosis between colonizing bacteria and the host.

The application of modern methods to the study of molecular mechanisms of pathogenesis of human respiratory infection has resulted in a growing understanding of these mechanisms, particularly with regard to identifying and characterizing microbial virulence factors and elucidating how they interact with the human host. These observations have the potential to lead to the development of novel approaches to treatment and prevention of bacterial infections. Such approaches might include antimicrobial agents, immunomodulators, vaccines, and others.

Streptococcus pneumoniae is the most common cause of community-acquired pneumonia in adults and also causes exacerbations of chronic obstructive pulmonary disease (COPD) (1). Nontypeable *Haemophilus influenzae* and *Moraxella catarrhalis* are the two most common causes of exacerbations of COPD (2,3). This chapter will focus on common themes of bacterial pathogenesis in the human lower respiratory tract, using research on these three bacteria as examples (4,5). The discussion is not intended to be a comprehensive consideration of the pathogenesis of infection by these pathogens; rather, observations involving these pathogens will be used to illustrate themes and principles of pathogenesis.

The pathogenesis of respiratory tract infection will be considered by a discussion of three key elements of pathogenesis: (*i*) adherence and colonization, (*ii*) invasion of host cells, and (*iii*) induction of inflammation.

II. Adherence and Colonization
A. Interaction of Bacteria with Mucus

The first step in the pathogenesis of infection is colonization of the respiratory tract. Bacteria initially encounter mucus, which covers the human respiratory epithelium. Mucus is a complex mixture of secreted molecules, cells, and debris. Mucins are high-molecular-weight glycoproteins with O-glycoside linked carbohydrate side chains. In addition to the nonspecific "stickiness" of mucus, bacteria interact specifically with components of mucus. Purified human nasopharyngeal mucin binds outer membrane proteins P2, P5, and a third yet-to-be-identified protein of *H. influenzae* (6–8). It appears that a protein-oligosaccharide interaction is responsible for binding because asialomucin (i.e., mucin glycoprotein that lacks the carbohydrate moiety sialic acid) does not bind outer membrane proteins of *H. influenzae*.

Mucins bind bacteria and, therefore, influence bacterial adherence to the epithelium. Mucin-bacterial interactions may serve as a host defense mechanism facilitating clearance of bacteria from the respiratory tract by the mucociliary escalator. Alternatively, binding of bacteria to mucin may represent the initial step in adherence to the epithelium and colonization of the airways.

B. Bacterial Adhesins

Bacterial pathogens express surface molecules, called adhesins, that mediate specific adherence to host receptors. A common theme among human respiratory bacterial pathogens is the expression of multiple adhesins (Table 1). From an evolutionary perspective, the expression of multiple adhesin molecules and the capability to modulate expression of these adhesins supports the notion that adherence to the respiratory tract is critical for survival of the bacterium.

Microbial Genomics to Identify Adhesins

The application of microbial genomics to the study of mechanisms of bacterial pathogenesis has advanced the field considerably, including facilitating the identification of previously unrecognized adhesins. Before the availability of microbial genome sequences, virulence factors were identified individually, often by creating knockout mutants and studying their behavior in animal models and in in vitro systems. The availability of genome sequences permits the targeting of families of genes that encode molecules with recognizable structural features. For example, several choline-binding

Table 1 Adhesins and Putative Adhesins of *Streptococcus pneumoniae*, *Haemophilus influenzae*, and *Moraxella catarrhalis*

S. pneumoniae	Nontypeable H. influenzae	M. catarrhalis
Multiple choline-binding proteins	High-molecular-weight proteins 1 and 2	UspA1
Phosphoryl choline	Hemagglutinating (LKP) pili	MID/Hag
Pili (*RgrA*)	Type 4 pili	OMP CD
Glutamyl tRNA synthetase	Hia (*H. influenzae* adhesin)	McmA
SP1492 (binds mucin)	Hap (*Haemophilus* adhesin protein)	McaP
6-Phosphogluconate dehydrogenase	P5 fimbriae	MchA1, MchA2 (MhaB1, MhaB2)
	Opacity associated protein	
	Phosphoryl choline	
	Lipooligosaccharide	
	Protein E	
	P2 porin (binds mucin)	

proteins attach to phosphoryl choline moieties on bacterial cell wall teichoic acid or membrane-associated lipoteichoic acid of *S. pneumoniae*. These proteins were identified using conventional techniques such as elution from the bacterial surface with choline. Searching the pneumococcal genome for a choline-binding repeat identified a previously unrecognized family of 12 genes with choline-binding motifs. Site-specific mutagenesis revealed that several of these proteins mediate adherence to epithelial cells, nasopharyngeal colonization, or sepsis (9).

Redundancy of Adhesins

Bacterial respiratory tract pathogens express multiple adhesins on the cell surface. As noted earlier, analysis of the genome of *S. pneumoniae* revealed the presence of multiple adhesins. Nontypeable *H. influenzae* expresses at least two major types of pili and several major nonpilus adhesins (Table 1) (10–13). *M. catarrhalis* expresses several adhesins and each has specificity for various types of respiratory epithelial cell lines (14–19). The observation that these pathogens express multiple adhesins with specificity for human respiratory tract epithelial cells likely reflects the importance of adherence to the survival of the organisms.

Phosphorylcholine

Phosphorylcholine is an interesting and important molecule that appears to act as an adhesin for multiple bacterial pathogens (20). In the pneumococcus, phosphorylcholine is attached to teichoic acid molecules on the pneumococcal surface. Phosphorylcholine moieties are also present on the surface of *H. influenzae* but are part of the lipooligosaccharide (LOS) molecule in this bacterium (21). In *Neisseria* spp., phosphorylcholine is bound to pili (22). In addition to mediating adherence, phosphorylcholine is a target of host C-reactive protein (23). The presence of this moiety on the surface of a diverse group of mucosal pathogens suggests that these pathogens exploit a common mechanism of adherence.

C. Exoglycosidases

Enzymes expressed on the bacterial surface also play a role in adherence to respiratory epithelial cells. For example, the pneumococcus expresses three surface-associated glycosidases, including a neuraminidase, a β-galactosidase, and a β-*N*-acetylglucosaminidase, which sequentially cleave terminal sugars that are present on human glycoconjugates in the respiratory tract (24,25). Thus, these enzymes may expose additional receptor moieties for the pneumococcal adhesins.

D. Biofilms

In the past decade, research on the role of biofilms in human infections has raised new ways of looking at bacterial colonization of the human respiratory tract. A biofilm is a structured community of bacteria encased in a polymeric matrix attached to a surface (26). In nature, bacteria exist predominantly as biofilms rather than in the planktonic form in which they are grown in the laboratory. *S. pneumoniae*, *H. influenzae*, and *M. catarrhalis* can all grow as biofilms in vitro. *H. influenzae* forms biofilms in animal models of infections (27,28). More recently, *H. influenzae* biofilms have been detected in the middle ear of children with chronic otitis media and in the lower airways of children with cystic fibrosis (29,30). Compared with planktonic bacteria, bacteria in the form of biofilms are more resistant to antimicrobial agents and are more resistant to both innate and adaptive immune mechanisms. Thus, infections caused by biofilms are generally more difficult to eradicate. Furthermore, in some settings biofilms may evoke less potent host responses compared with planktonic bacteria (31). Colonization in the form of biofilms is more likely to be operative in the setting of infections in chronic conditions such as COPD and cystic fibrosis and less likely to be an important mechanism in acute pneumonia. The study of biofilms is an area of active research that is needed to elucidate the precise role of biofilms in human respiratory tract infection.

III. Invasion of Host Cells

The respiratory pathogens *S. pneumoniae*, nontypeable *H. influenzae*, and *M. catarrhalis* have long been thought to represent classic "extracellular" pathogens as opposed to bacteria such as *Listeria* and *Salmonella* that are well known to invade and multiply intracellularly. However, the niche in the human respiratory tract of the classic bacterial respiratory pathogens under consideration is not limited to adherence to the surface of epithelial cells. Rather, *S. pneumoniae*, nontypeable *H. influenzae*, and *M. catarrhalis* have mechanisms to invade beyond the surface of the respiratory epithelium. Indeed, several potential initial outcomes may result from the encounter between a bacterial pathogen and the human respiratory epithelium. Bacteria may colonize or infect the respiratory tract by binding to the mucus layer, adhering to epithelial cells in a planktonic or biofilm form, by invading cells, or by invading between cells (Figure 1). A pathogen may inhabit several of these niches during the course of colonization or infection.

Studies with cultures of human epithelial cells show that a small proportion of adherent *H. influenzae* enter epithelial cells in a process that involves actin filaments and microtubules (32). Organ culture studies utilizing lung epithelial cells on permeable supports have demonstrated that *H. influenzae* bacterial cells penetrate the epithelial cell layer by a process of paracytosis or passage between cells (33). In assays using primary human airway cultures, nontypeable *H. influenzae* adheres to and enters nonciliated epithelial cells (34). This invasion occurs by different mechanisms, including specific interaction between phosphoryl choline with the platelet activating factor (PAF) receptor and by the process of macropinocytosis (34,35).

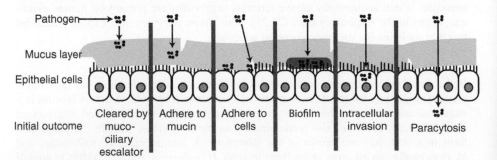

Figure 1 Schematic diagram illustrating several different potential initial outcomes of an encounter between a bacterial pathogen and the human respiratory tract mucosal surface.

In addition to these lines of evidence from in vitro studies, two lines of evidence based on in vivo studies indicate that *H. influenzae* penetrates beyond the epithelial surface. In situ hybridization and selective cultures reveal that viable nontypeable *H. influenzae* are present in macrophage-like cells in the adenoids of children (36). Analysis of bronchial biopsies from adults with COPD by in situ hybridization and immunofluorescence microscopy demonstrate that *H. influenzae* is present intracellularly, suggesting a role for intracellular infection by nontypeable *H. influenzae* in the pathogenesis of infection in the setting of COPD (37).

More recently, in vitro studies have demonstrated that *M. catarrhalis* also invades human respiratory epithelial cells, including bronchial epithelial cells, type II pneumocytes, primary small airway epithelial cells, and Chang conjunctival cells (38,39). Invasion involves cellular microfilament formation and is characterized by macropinocytosis, which leads to the formation of lamellipodia and engulfment of bacteria into macropinosomes, indicating a trigger-like uptake mechanism. The adhesin protein UspA1 and LOS are involved in the invasion process (39).

Analysis of pharyngeal lymphoid tissue from children who underwent tonsillectomy and adenoidectomy provides an in vivo correlate to these in vitro studies (40). Analysis of tissue samples by immunohistochemical studies and confocal laser scanning microscopy identified *M. catarrhalis* cells in crypts in both intraepithelial and subepithelial locations. *M. catarrhalis* also co-localized with macrophages and B cells in lymphoid follicles.

It is well known that the pneumococcus has the potential to penetrate the mucosal barrier and cause invasive disease. Based on the observations outlined above, it is now clear that the human respiratory tract niche that is occupied by *H. influenzae* and *M. catarrhalis* includes intracellular and submucosal sites. Bacteria that reside inside of cells are relatively protected from the bactericidal activity of several antibiotics and antibody mediated bactericidal activity (41). Thus, these observations have important implications in understanding mechanisms of pathogenesis and protection from infection.

IV. Induction of Inflammation
A. Innate Immunity

The healthy human respiratory tract is sterile below the vocal cords as a result of innate immune mechanisms. Innate immunity in the respiratory tract is multifaceted and redundant. The mucociliary escalator removes particles including bacteria from the airways. Airway epithelial cells play an important role in innate immunity not just as physical barriers but also as orchestrators of innate immunity. The presence of a bacterium in the respiratory tract is initially detected by the innate immune system. Host cell receptors called pattern-recognition receptors distinguish molecules that are unique to bacteria, resulting in triggering of multiple signaling pathways (42,43). Pulmonary host defenses against bacterial pathogens involve the activation of epithelial cells and macrophages, the release of proinflammatory cytokines and chemokines, and recruitment of neutrophils (44). Furthermore, the induction of neutrophil necrosis by *H. influenzae* may represent another mechanism of inflammation as neutrophils release inflammatory products as they undergo necrosis (45).

These mechanisms are central to the pathogenesis of bacterial respiratory tract infection. Inflammation is critical for innate immunity but also contributes to lung injury and disease pathogenesis. Indeed, activation of nuclear factor kappa B (NFκB) pathway signaling by bacteria induces the production of inflammatory cytokines and neutrophilic lung inflammation (46–48). NFκB regulates a large number of genes, including cytokines, chemokines, and other mediators of inflammation. In addition to NFκB, bacterial molecules activate other signaling pathways in the respiratory tract, including tumor growth factor (TGF)β, Smad, p38 mitogen-activated protein (MAP) kinase, and phosphoinositide-3-kinase (46,49–51).

B. Bacterial Ligands That Induce Inflammation in the Respiratory Tract

A key to understanding the role of inflammation in respiratory tract bacterial infection has been the identification of microbial molecules that activate signal transduction pathways. Characterization and elucidation of such microbial ligands is the focus of active investigation, which has led to much recent progress (Table 2). The following sections present a brief summary of some of the important classes of microbial ligands that trigger signal transduction pathways, with a brief consideration of examples of each.

Bacterial Lipoproteins

Bacterial lipoproteins have an amino terminal cysteine to which a glycerol molecule is covalently bound. Palmitic acid residues are bound to each of the three carbon atoms of the glycerol, resulting in a characteristic cysteine-tripalmitoyl terminal motif. Lipoproteins with this motif recognize Toll-like receptor (TLR)2 that activates transcription of NFκB. (47). Outer membrane protein P6 of *H. influenzae* is a prototype bacterial lipoprotein.

To assess the contribution of P6 to inflammatory responses Berenson et al. (52) purified P6 and other outer membrane antigens of *H. influenzae*, incubated them with human blood monocyte-derived macrophages, and measured interleukin (IL)-1β, tumor necrosis factor (TNF)α, IL-10, IL-12, and IL-8. P6 was found to be a potent and specific activator of IL-8, a critical cytokine that induces neutrophil chemotaxis in the respiratory tract. P6 induced macrophage IL-8 at concentrations as low as 10 pg/mL, a concentration that is present in the lower airways during infection. Bacterial lipoproteins are specific triggers of human macrophage inflammatory events, with IL-8 as a key effector.

Endotoxin

The outer membrane of gram-negative bacteria contains endotoxin, a potent inflammatory molecule. The endotoxin of enteric gram-negatives is lipopolysaccharide, while nonenteric gram-negative pathogens, including *H. influenzae* and *M. catarrhalis* have

Table 2 Bacterial Ligands of Respiratory Tract Pathogens That Trigger Signal Transduction Pathways in the Human Respiratory Tract

Streptococcus pneumoniae	Nontypeable *Haemophilus influenzae*	*Moraxella catarrhalis*
Lipoteichoic acid	Lipooligosaccharide	Lipooligosaccharide
Teichoic acid	Outer membrane protein P6	Peptidoglycan fragments
Peptidoglycan fragments	Peptidoglycan fragments	UspA1
Pneumolysin	P2 porin	UspA2
CpG dinucleotides	Lipoproteins	

LOS. The LOS molecule consists of lipid A, core sugars, and oligosaccharide side chains. The lipid A moiety is recognized by TLR4, and this interaction is facilitated by CD14 (53). Binding of LOS by TLR4 activates at least two intracellular signaling pathways, one mediated by MyD88-dependent and the other that relies on TRIF (54). LOS of *H. influenzae* induces human blood monocyte-derived macrophages to express IL-8 and TNFα (52). Thus, LOS is a potent inflammatory antigen that induces respiratory tract inflammation through pattern recognition receptors, particularly TLR4.

Lipoteichoic Acid
The cell wall of *S. pneumoniae* contains an abundant surface molecule called lipoteichoic acid, which consists of extended repeat carbohydrates and fatty acids that anchor the molecule to the plasma membrane. Lipoteichoic acid is an important mediator of inflammatory responses, inducing the production of a range of proinflammatory cytokines and chemokines by cells of the innate immune system (53). The major cellular recognition and signaling receptor for lipoteichoic acid is TLR2, but TLR4, and PAF receptor also influence lung inflammation induced by lipoteichoic acid (55).

Pneumococcal Peptidoglycan
The pneumococcal cell wall is a multilayered network of peptidoglycan, which is a polymer consisting of a backbone of *N*-acetylglucosamine alternating with *N*-acetylmuramic acid with pentapeptide side chains. Peptidoglycan gives the bacterial cell its shape. Purified pneumococcal cell wall induces meningeal inflammation that mimics meningitis caused by the pneumococcus (56). Soluble, fragmented cell wall results from the lysis of bacteria, and these fragments are highly inflammatory. Interestingly, pneumococcal cell wall fragments bind specifically to lipopolysaccharide-binding protein (LBP), which induces cell signaling and TNFα release (57). Although LBP has had a well-established role in LPS-induced immune responses by gram-negative bacteria, the observation that pneumococcal cell wall fragments trigger inflammation by binding LBP expands our understanding of the role of LBP in inflammation induced by the pneumococcus.

Pneumolysin
Pneumolysin is a member of cholesterol-dependent cytolysins of gram-positive bacteria and is a well-characterized virulence factor of *S. pneumoniae*. Pneumolysin has cytolytic activity and triggers a range of cell modulatory activities, including inhibition of ciliary beating, induction of cytokine synthesis, CD4 T-cell activation, and chemotaxis (58,59). Pneumolysin also triggers inflammatory responses in host macrophages by binding TLR4 (42). In addition to inducing inflammatory responses, pneumolysin is a critical virulence factor in spread of the pneumococcus from the lung to the bloodstream in invasive infection (60,61).

V. Summary and Future Directions
The application of modern approaches to the study of the pathogenesis of bacterial respiratory tract infection is elucidating molecular mechanisms of pathogenesis. Exciting progress has been made in three broad areas of pathogenesis, including (*i*) colonization and adherence, (*ii*) invasion of host cells, and (*iii*) induction of inflammation. Understanding these mechanisms presents opportunities to develop novel methods to interrupt or prevent infection, for example, by blocking adherence or invasion and

modulating inflammatory responses induced by bacterial ligands. Such molecular approaches have the potential to prevent some of the enormous global morbidity and mortality caused by respiratory bacterial infections.

References
1. Mandell LA, Wunderink RG, Anzueto A, et al. Infectious Diseases Society of America/ American Thoracic Society consensus guidelines on the management of community-acquired pneumonia in adults. Clin Infect Dis 2007; 44(suppl 2):S27–S72.
2. Sethi S, Murphy TF. Acute exacerbations of chronic bronchitis: new developments concerning microbiology and pathophysiology–impact on approaches to risk stratification and therapy. Infect Dis Clin North Am 2004; 18:861–882, ix.
3. Murphy TF, Brauer AL, Grant BJ, et al. *Moraxella catarrhalis* in chronic obstructive pulmonary disease. Burden of disease and immune response. Am J Respir Crit Care Med 2005; 172:195–199.
4. McCullers JA, Tuomanen EI. Molecular pathogenesis of pneumococcal pneumonia. Front Biosci 2001; 6:D877–D889.
5. Kadioglu A, Weiser JN, Paton JC, et al. The role of *Streptococcus pneumoniae* virulence factors in host respiratory colonization and disease. Nat Rev Microbiol 2008; 6:288–301.
6. Kubiet M, Ramphal R. Adhesion of nontypeable *Haemophilus influenzae* from blood and sputum to human tracheobronchial mucins and lactoferrin. Infect Immun 1995; 63:899–902.
7. Reddy MS, Murphy TF, Faden HS, et al. Middle ear mucin glycoprotein: purification and interaction with nontypable *Haemophilus influenzae* and *Moraxella catarrhalis*. Otolaryngol Head Neck Surg 1997; 116:175–189.
8. Reddy MS, Bernstein JM, Murphy TF, et al. Binding between outer membrane proteins of nontypeable *Haemophilus influenzae* and human nasopharyngeal mucin. Infect Immun 1996; 64:1477–1479.
9. Gosink KK, Mann ER, Guglielmo C, et al. Role of novel choline binding proteins in virulence of *Streptococcus pneumoniae*. Infect Immun 2000; 68:5690–5695.
10. St. Geme JW III. Molecular and cellular determinants of non-typeable *Haemophilus influenzae* adherence and invasion. Cell Microbiol 2002; 4:191–200.
11. Buscher AZ, Burmeister K, Barenkamp SJ, et al. Evolutionary and functional relationships among the nontypeable *Haemophilus influenzae* HMW family of adhesins. J Bacteriol 2004; 186:4209–4217.
12. Rodriguez CA, Avadhanula V, Buscher A, et al. Prevalence and distribution of adhesins in invasive non-type b encapsulated *Haemophilus influenzae*. Infect Immun 2003; 71:1635–1642.
13. Ronander E, Brant M, Janson H, et al. Identification of a novel *Haemophilus influenzae* protein important for adhesion to epithelial cells. Microbes Infect 2008; 10:87–96.
14. Plamondon P, Luke NR, Campagnari AA. Identification of a novel two-partner secretion locus in *Moraxella catarrhalis*. Infect Immun 2007; 75(6):2929–2936.
15. Bullard B, Lipski SL, Lafontaine ER. Hag directly mediates the adherence of *Moraxella catarrhalis* to human middle ear cells. Infect Immun 2005; 73:5127–5136.
16. Lipski SL, Holm MM, Lafontaine ER. Identification of a *Moraxella catarrhalis* gene that confers adherence to various human epithelial cell lines in vitro. FEMS Microbiol Lett 2007; 267:207–213.
17. Lafontaine ER, Cope LD, Aebi C, et al. The UspA1 protein and a second type of UspA2 protein mediate adherence of *Moraxella catarrhalis* to human epithelial cells in vitro. J Bacteriol 2000; 182:1364–1373.
18. Timpe JM, Holm MM, Vanlerberg SL, et al. Identification of a *Moraxella catarrhalis* outer membrane protein exhibiting both adhesin and lipolytic activities. Infect Immun 2003; 71:4341–4350.

19. Akimana C, Lafontaine ER. The *Moraxella catarrhalis* outer membrane protein CD contains two distinct domains specifying adherence to human lung cells. FEMS Microbiol Lett 2007; 271:12–19.

20. Rosenow C, Ryan P, Weiser JN, et al. Contribution of novel choline-binding proteins to adherence, colonization and immunogenicity of *Streptococcus pneumoniae*. Mol Microbiol 1997; 25:819–829.

21. Swords WE, Buscher BA, Ver Steeg Ii K, et al. Non-typeable *Haemophilus influenzae* adhere to and invade human bronchial epithelial cells via an interaction of lipooligosaccharide with the PAF receptor. Mol Microbiol 2000; 37:13–27.

22. Weiser JN, Goldberg JB, Pan N, et al. The phosphorylcholine epitope undergoes phase variation on a 43-kilodalton protein in *Pseudomonas aeruginosa* and on pili of *Neisseria meningitidis* and *Neisseria gonorrhoeae*. Infect Immun 1998; 66:4263–4267.

23. Gould JM, Weiser JN. The inhibitory effect of C-reactive protein on bacterial phosphorylcholine platelet-activating factor receptor-mediated adherence is blocked by surfactant. J Infect Dis 2002; 186:361–371.

24. Manco S, Hernon F, Yesilkaya H, et al. Pneumococcal neuraminidases A and B both have essential roles during infection of the respiratory tract and sepsis. Infect Immun 2006; 74:4014–4020.

25. King SJ, Hippe KR, Weiser JN. Deglycosylation of human glycoconjugates by the sequential activities of exoglycosidases expressed by *Streptococcus pneumoniae*. Mol Microbiol 2006; 59:961–974.

26. Costerton JW, Stewart PS, Greenberg EP. Bacterial biofilms: a common cause of persistent infections. Science 1999; 284:1318–1322.

27. Post JC. Direct evidence of bacterial biofilms in otitis media. Laryngoscope 2001; 111: 2083–2094.

28. Jurcisek JA, Bakaletz LO. Biofilms formed by nontypeable *Haemophilus influenzae* in vivo contain both dsDNA as well as type IV pilin protein. J Bacteriol 2007; 189(10):3868–3875.

29. Hall-Stoodley L., Hu FZ, Gieseke A, et al. Direct detection of bacterial biofilms on the middle-ear mucosa of children with chronic otitis media. JAMA 2006; 296:202–211.

30. Starner TD, Zhang N, Kim G, et al. *Haemophilus influenzae* forms biofilms on airway epithelia: implications in cystic fibrosis. Am J Respir Crit Care Med 2006; 174:213–220.

31. West-Barnette S, Rockel A, Swords WE. Biofilm growth increases phosphorylcholine content and decreases potency of nontypeable *Haemophilus influenzae* endotoxins. Infect Immun 2006; 74:1828–1836.

32. St. Geme JW III, Falkow S. *Haemophilus influenzae* adheres to and enters cultured human epithelial cells. Infect Immun 1990; 58:4036–4044.

33. van Schilfgaarde M, Van Alphen L, Eijk P, et al. Paracytosis of *Haemophilus influenzae* through cell layers of NCI-H292 lung epithelial cells. Infect Immun 1995; 63:4729–4737.

34. Ketterer MR, Shao JQ, Hornick DB, et al. Infection of primary human bronchial epithelial cells by *Haemophilus influenzae*: macropinocytosis as a mechanism of airway epithelial cell entry. Infect Immun 1999; 67:4161–4170.

35. Swords WE, Ketterer MR, Shao J, et al. Binding of the non-typeable *Haemophilus influenzae* lipooligosaccharide to the PAF receptor initiates host cell signalling. Cell Microbiol 2001; 3:525–536.

36. Forsgren J, Samuelson A, Ahlin A, et al. *Haemophilus influenzae* resides and multiplies intracellularly in human adenoid tissue as demonstrated by in situ hybridization and bacterial viability assay. Infect Immun 1994; 62:673–679.

37. Bandi V, Apicella MA, Mason E, et al. Nontypeable *Haemophilus influenzae* in the lower respiratory tract of patients with chronic bronchitis. Am J Respir Crit Care Med 2001; 164:2114–2119.

38. Slevogt H, Seybold J, Tiwari KN, et al. *Moraxella catarrhalis* is internalized in respiratory epithelial cells by a trigger-like mechanism and initiates a TLR2- and partly NOD1-dependent inflammatory immune response. Cell Microbiol 2007; 9:694–707.

39. Spaniol V, Heiniger N, Troller R, et al. Outer membrane protein UspA1 and lipooligosaccharide are involved in invasion of human epithelial cells by *Moraxella catarrhalis*. Microbes Infect 2008; 10:3–11.

40. Heiniger N, Spaniol V, Troller R, et al. A reservoir of *Moraxella catarrhalis* in human pharyngeal lymphoid tissue. J Infect Dis 2007; 196:1080–1087.

41. van Schilfgaarde M, Eijk P, Regelink A, et al. *Haemophilus influenzae* localized in epithelial cell layers is shielded from antibiotics and antibody-mediated bactericidal activity. Microb Pathogen 1999; 26:249–262.

42. Malley R, Henneke P, Morse SC, et al. Recognition of pneumolysin by Toll-like receptor 4 confers resistance to pneumococcal infection. Proc Natl Acad Sci U S A 2003; 100:1966–1971.

43. Ratner AJ, Aguilar JL, Shchepetov M, et al. Nod1 mediates cytoplasmic sensing of combinations of extracellular bacteria. Cell Microbiol 2007; 9:1343–1351.

44. Mizgerd JP. Acute lower respiratory tract infection. N Engl J Med 2008; 358:716–727.

45. Naylor EJ, Bakstad D, Biffen M, et al. *Haemophilus influenzae* induces neutrophil necrosis: a role in chronic obstructive pulmonary disease? Am J Respir Cell Mol Biol 2007; 37:135–143.

46. Takeuchi O, Akira S. Signaling pathways activated by microorganisms. Curr Opin Cell Biol 2007; 19:185–191.

47. Shuto T, Xu H, Wang B, et al. Activation of NF-kappa B by nontypeable *Hemophilus influenzae* is mediated by toll-like receptor 2-TAK1-dependent NIK-IKK alpha /beta-I kappa B alpha and MKK3/6-p38 MAP kinase signaling pathways in epithelial cells. Proc Natl Acad Sci U S A 2001; 98:8774–8779.

48. Slevogt H, Maqami L, Vardarowa K, et al. Differential regulation of *Moraxella catarrhalis*-induced IL-8 response by PKC isoforms. Eur Respir J. 2008; 31(4):725–735.

49. Mikami F, Lim JH, Ishinaga H, et al. The transforming growth factor-beta-Smad3/4 signaling pathway acts as a positive regulator for TLR2 induction by bacteria via a dual mechanism involving functional cooperation with NF-kappaB and MAPK phosphatase 1-dependent negative cross-talk with p38 MAPK. J Biol Chem 2006; 281:22397–22408.

50. Slevogt H, Schmeck B, Jonatat C, et al. *Moraxella catarrhalis* induces inflammatory response of bronchial epithelial cells via MAPK and NF-kappaB activation and histone deacetylase activity reduction. Am J Physiol Lung Cell Mol Physiol 2006; 290:L818–L826.

51. N'Guessan PD, Temmesfeld-Wollbruck B, Zahlten J, et al. *Moraxella catarrhalis* induces ERK- and NF-kappaB-dependent COX-2 and prostaglandin E2 in lung epithelium. Eur Respir J 2007; 30:443–451.

52. Berenson CS, Murphy TF, Wrona CT, et al. Outer membrane protein P6 of nontypeable *Haemophilus influenzae* is a potent and selective inducer of human macrophage proinflammatory cytokines. Infect Immun 2005; 73:2728–2735.

53. Hoogerwerf JJ, de Vos AF, Bresser P, et al. Lung inflammation induced by lipoteichoic acid or lipopolysaccharide in humans. Am J Respir Crit Care Med 2008; 178(1):34–41.

54. Wieland CW, Florquin S, Maris NA, et al. The MyD88-dependent, but not the MyD88-independent, pathway of TLR4 signaling is important in clearing nontypeable *Haemophilus influenzae* from the mouse lung. J Immunol 2005; 175:6042–6049.

55. Knapp S, von Aulock S, Leendertse M, et al. Lipoteichoic acid-induced lung inflammation depends on TLR2 and the concerted action of TLR4 and the platelet-activating factor receptor. J Immunol 2008; 180:3478–3484.

56. Tuomanen E, Liu H, Hengstler B, et al. The induction of meningeal inflammation by components of the pneumococcal cell wall. J Infect Dis 1985; 151:859–868.

57. Weber JR, Freyer D, Alexander C, et al. Recognition of pneumococcal peptidoglycan: an expanded, pivotal role for LPS binding protein. Immunity 2003; 19:269–279.

58. Hirst RA, Kadioglu A, O'Callaghan C, et al. The role of pneumolysin in pneumococcal pneumonia and meningitis. Clin Exp Immunol 2004; 138:195–201.
59. Kadioglu A, Coward W, Colston MJ, et al. CD4-T-lymphocyte interactions with pneumolysin and pneumococci suggest a crucial protective role in the host response to pneumococcal infection. Infect Immun 2004; 72:2689–2697.
60. Kadioglu A, Taylor S, Iannelli F, et al. Upper and lower respiratory tract infection by *Streptococcus pneumoniae* is affected by pneumolysin deficiency and differences in capsule type. Infect Immun 2002; 70:2886–2890.
61. Berry AM, Yother J, Briles DE, et al. Reduced virulence of a defined pneumolysin-negative mutant of *Streptococcus pneumoniae*. Infect Immun 1989; 57:2037–2042.

4
Acute Bronchitis

THOMAS J. KUFEL
Veterans Affairs Western New York Healthcare System and University at Buffalo,
State University of New York, Buffalo, New York, U.S.A.

I. Introduction

Acute bronchitis is an exceedingly common disorder encountered in the ambulatory care setting. It has resulted in approximately 2.5 million visits to U.S. physicians in 1998 (1), affects 44/1000 adults in the United Kingdom each year (2), and is the fifth most common reason for visits to general practitioners in Australia (3). Despite the high incidence worldwide, a uniform definition is lacking, diagnosis is not standardized, and sensitive or specific confirmatory tests are not available. Of greater concern is the continued use of antibiotics for acute bronchitis despite expert recommendations against this practice.

II. Definition

Sir William Osler's description of acute bronchitis is as informative today as it was when written in 1892.

> Acute bronchitis is a common sequence of catching cold and is often nothing more than the extension downward of an ordinary coryza .... Its association with cold is well indicated by the popular expression "cold on the chest." ... It is present also in asthma and whooping-cough.... The affection is probably microbic ... there is scarcely any fever ... The symptoms of an ordinary "cold" accompany the onset of an acute bronchitis.... The cough is rough at first, cutting and sore ... in paroxysms which rack and distress the patient extremely ... at first the cough is dry but in a few days the secretion becomes muco-purulent and abundant, and finally purulent ... a feeling of tightness and rawness beneath the sternum ... by the end of a week the fever subsides and the cough loosens. In another week or ten days convalescence is fully established.... The diagnosis of acute bronchitis is rarely difficult. (4)

Acute bronchitis is a transient, self-limiting inflammation of the trachea and major bronchi that manifests predominantly as a cough that lasts for up to three weeks (5). Additional findings can include sputum production, dyspnea, wheeze, chest discomfort, or pain. Alternative explanations such as the common cold, acute asthma, exacerbation of chronic obstructive pulmonary disease (COPD), and most importantly pneumonia must be excluded before acute bronchitis can be diagnosed. Generally, most patients with acute bronchitis are considered healthy, without complicating factors of underlying lung disease, cardiac disease, or compromised immune system. This distinction is important since the etiology, treatment, and response for those patients with complicating factors are distinctly different from that encountered by previously healthy individuals.

Recent reports indicate that, unlike Osler, clinicians have difficulty differentiating acute bronchitis from other common conditions and often have divergent views on which constellation of symptoms and signs define the presence of acute bronchitis. Oeffinger and colleagues reported that 58% of physicians diagnosed acute bronchitis only if a productive cough was present, and 60% felt the sputum should be purulent (6). However, 39% stated that the presence of a productive cough is not essential to diagnose acute bronchitis. Hueston and colleagues found that clinicians rely on few clinical factors to differentiate acute bronchitis from an upper respiratory tract infection (7). Cough and wheezing were the strongest predictors of acute bronchitis while nausea, nasal erythema, or rhinorrhea were the strongest predictors of upper respiratory tract infection. Despite the large number of clinical variables considered in this report, the logistic model explained only 37% of the differences between acute bronchitis and upper respiratory tract infection, suggesting that physicians use other factors in differentiating the two conditions. More importantly, they found that the diagnosis influenced treatment decisions. Specifically, those patients diagnosed with acute bronchitis were more likely to receive a bronchodilator (70% vs. 8%, $p < 0.001$) or an antibiotic (26% vs. 4%, $p < 0.001$).

Patients have similar difficulty in defining an episode of acute bronchitis. In a survey to describe patients' knowledge of acute bronchitis, Gonzales and coworkers found that 73% of respondents felt that chest colds and bronchitis were different illnesses, while 57% considered a productive cough a chest cold, whereas 16% referred to it as bronchitis (8). More importantly, 44% of those respondents who felt that chest colds and bronchitis were different illnesses felt that antibiotics were necessary to get better from bronchitis compared with 11% ($p = 0.0001$) with chest colds (8).

On the basis of the above-mentioned studies, it seems prudent to consider a new approach to the classification of viral respiratory tract infections such as that proposed by Hueston (7). In that classification scheme, all viral respiratory tract infections, including sinusitis and bronchitis, would be viewed as a single disease entity with anatomic specification based on the predominance of symptoms. Thus, all patients with infectious symptoms involving the sinuses, nose, pharynx, and bronchial tree would be diagnosed with an "acute respiratory infection" with either "sinus predominant," "bronchial predominant," or "generalized" if both upper and lower respiratory tract symptoms were present.

To further complicate the issue, other reports indicate that acute asthma is frequently misdiagnosed as acute bronchitis. In a study of previously normal adults three years after presentation with acute bronchitis, 19%, 21%, and 6% of the patients who returned the questionnaire fulfilled the criteria for asthma, chronic bronchitis, or both, respectively (9). Another study found that 65% of patients with at least two doctor-diagnosed episodes of acute bronchitis over the previous five years could be identified as having mild asthma (10).

III. Epidemiology

Published incidence of acute bronchitis is likely to underestimate the true incidence since most cases are treated by self-care alone and not reported to physicians. Despite this, acute bronchitis is one of the most common diagnoses among primary care providers and in emergency departments worldwide, affecting 5% of adults annually and resulting in 10 ambulatory visits per 1000 people years, with 82% of cases occurring during the autumn and winter (1–3,11). The economic impact of acute bronchitis is also significant. Data obtained from a 1997 claims database of a national Fortune 100 company revealed that acute bronchitis resulted in health-care and work-loss costs totaling $4219 per beneficiary, with 78.3% of the cost attributed to health care (12).

IV. Etiology

Viruses are generally felt to be the major cause of acute bronchitis; however, well-designed clinical trials to define its etiology are lacking or flawed. Viruses reported to cause acute bronchitis include *influenza, adenovirus, rhinovirus, coronavirus, parainfluenza virus, respiratory syncytial virus, and human metapneumovirus*. It is unclear what proportion of acute bronchitis episodes are related to infection with typical bacterial pathogens, including S*treptoccocus pneumoniae, Haemophilus influenzae, Moraxella catarrhalis,* and with the atypical bacterial pathogens *Mycoplasma pneumoniae* and *Chlamydophila* (formerly *Chlamydia) pneumonia.* This lack of clarity is related to the lack of systematic studies, the difficulty in differentiating colonization from infection for the typical pathogens, and the difficulty in interpreting serological results for the atypical pathogens. *Bordatella pertussis,* the etiologic agent of whooping cough, has emerged as an important cause of acute bronchitis in previously immunized adults whose vaccine-induced protection has waned over time. One study projected that *B. pertussis* could be responsible for cough of more than five days in nearly one million patients aged 15 years or older, yearly in the United States (13). Unfortunately, very few characteristics distinguish pertussis infection from other causes of prolonged cough illnesses. The duration of cough may be of some value in identifying a group in which *B. pertussis* should be considered. Specifically, *B. pertussis* was the cause of the cough illness in 0.79% when cough was present for less than 21 days, and in 2.5% of patients when cough was present for more than 21 days (13). Other factors suggestive of pertussis infection include adolescence and absence of fever.

V. Pathogenesis

Acute bronchitis results in hyperemic, edematous mucous membranes within the large airway. Increased bronchial secretions can follow. The severity of respiratory epithelial destruction depends on the causative organism. Traditionally, influenza virus infection results in a severe destructive response. The infectious process results in increased interleukin (IL) production and diminished mucociliary function. The severity of the attack can be exacerbated by exposure to cigarette smoke or air pollutants.

For most patients, acute bronchitis generally results in a mild, self-limiting disease. However, in one study nearly one out of every five patients returned to their family physician for a follow-up visit within the first month of being diagnosed with acute bronchitis because of continued unrelenting symptoms (2). The duration of symptoms and impact on daily activity can be extrapolated from data obtained from the untreated group in placebo-controlled trials evaluating the impact of antibiotic use in acute bronchitis. One study found that the duration of daytime cough was 6.2 ± 3.2 days, while productive cough resolved earlier in 2.2 ± 2.7 days, and patients experienced impaired activity for 2.5 ± 3.3 days (14) Another study found that 63% of untreated patients with acute bronchitis returned to usual activity within three days and 89% within seven days (15). These data indicate that acute bronchitis symptoms resolve within a week for the majority of patients; however, there is a small subset that experiences persistent symptoms that impact quality of life.

VI. Diagnostic Approach

Acute bronchitis is a clinical diagnosis based on the presence of cough with or without sputum production and the exclusion of other chronic lung or heart diseases, immuno-compromised, states and pneumonia. Cough is the prominent symptom and, in a minority of patients, can last several weeks. A variety of nonspecific symptoms may be present, including wheezing, sweating, fever, dyspnea, or burning substernal chest pain. Fever is more common with *influenza, adenovirus*, and *M. pneumoniae* infection.

In most patients the diagnosis of acute bronchitis is clinical, and the causative organism is infrequently identified even when extensive testing is undertaken (2). The utility of viral cultures, serologic assays, and sputum analyses are not known. However, considering the benign natural history, routine testing to identify the responsible organism is not recommended (5). Some historical details of recent or current community outbreaks of influenza or pertussis can be important in the diagnosis and treatment of acute bronchitis. Patients should be questioned about influenza vaccination status. Testing for influenza and pertussis is reasonable if suspected clinically.

As untreated pneumonia is not a self-limiting disease and can result in considerable morbidity and mortality, it is essential to consider pneumonia as a diagnostic possibility when evaluating patients with acute cough. It is often difficult to differentiate between acute bronchitis and pneumonia on clinical grounds alone. Pneumonia should be excluded by chest radiograph if clinical suspicion is elevated. In most circumstances, chest radiograph is not required in the absence of (*i*) heart rate more than 100 beats/min, (*ii*) respiratory rate more than 24 breaths/min, (*iii*) oral body temperature more than 38°C, and (*iv*) chest examination findings of focal consolidation, egophony, or fremitus (5) (Fig. 1).

Transient reductions in airflow and bronchial hyperresponsiveness are common in acute bronchitis (10,17). Since the reduction in airflow as a result of acute bronchitis is generally mild and typically resolves within six weeks, routine measurement is not recommended. However, differentiating asthma from acute bronchitis can be difficult in those patients with audible wheeze; thus, the diagnosis of asthma should be considered in patients whose cough fails to resolve within three weeks or in those with recurrent episodes of doctor diagnosed acute bronchitis.

A rapid, office-based diagnostic test that could reliably differentiate bacterial infection from viral infection or pneumonia from acute bronchitis may identify patients that could be monitored safely without using antibiotic therapy. Studies evaluating the C-reactive protein (CRP) test and procalcitonin assays for this purpose are promising and worthy of further investigation. However, their routine use in the clinical arena outside of an investigational study is not recommended.

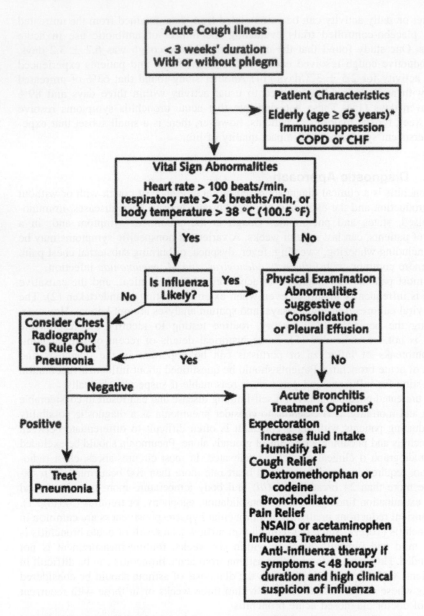

Figure 1 Proposed algorithm for evaluation and management of adults with acute cough illness. *Abbreviation*: NSAID, nonsteroidal anti-inflammatory drug. *Source*: From Ref. 16.

VII. Management

Antibiotic prescription rates for acute bronchitis exceed 50% (2,18,19) despite evidence that antibiotics do not provide any clinically meaningful benefits (20) and expert recommendation against this practice (5). A systematic review of nine trials comparing antibiotics with placebo for the treatment of acute bronchitis found that antibiotics shortened the duration of cough [weighted mean difference (WMD) 0.58 days; 95% CI, 0.01–1.16 days], shortened duration of productive cough (WMD 0.52 days; 95% CI, 0.01–1.03 days), and shortened the duration of feeling ill (WMD 0.58 days; 95% CI, 0.00–1.16 days) (20). There were no significant differences regarding the presence of night cough, activity limitations at follow-up, or in the mean duration of activity limitation. There was a nonsignificant increase in adverse effects in the antibiotic group [risk ratio (RR) 1.22; 95% CI, 0.94–1.58]. The clinical relevance of a reduction in symptoms with the use of antibiotics of less than one day compared with placebo in acute bronchitis is not known. Routine use of antibiotics for acute bronchitis is not justified on the basis of minimal clinical benefit, the concern of propagation of widespread antibiotic resistance among bacteria, cost considerations, and potential medication side effects (5). Further research is needed to determine if a subset of patients exists that may derive clinically relevant benefits from antibiotic treatment.

Studies to evaluate interventions to reduce antibiotic use in acute bronchitis have provided useful information. In patients who reported with suspected acute bronchitis to suburban general practitioners in England, Macfarlane and colleagues assessed the effectiveness of a leaflet that described the uncertain benefit of antibiotics in the treatment of acute bronchitis, the expected disease natural history, the adverse effects of medications, a list of nonantibiotic remedies, and a reminder of symptoms that might prompt them to fill their prescription (21). On the basis of this clinical judgment, patients were divided into two groups: one in which antibiotics were deemed to be indicated on the day of evaluation and another in which antibiotics were not definitely indicated on the day of presentation. Patients in the first group were instructed to take the antibiotic, while those in the second group were provided verbal information that there was no immediate need for antibiotics, but they were provided with a prescription that they were instructed to fill only if symptoms worsened. Patients in this group were randomized to receive or not receive the written leaflet described above. Eighteen percent of patients were felt to require antibiotics on the day of presentation. Forty-seven percent of those who received the written leaflet filled their prescription compared with 62% in the group that did not receive the leaflet (RR 0.76; 95% CI, 0.59–0.97, $p = 0.04$; number needed to treat 6.7). There was no difference between these groups in terms of adverse outcomes. Surprisingly, antibiotic use for acute bronchitis remained unacceptably high in the intervention group in this study.

An earlier study performed in the United States by Gonzales and coworkers demonstrated a similar reduction in antibiotic use for acute bronchitis in the intervention group (48% vs. 74%; $p = 0.003$) without an increase in return office visits (22). The intervention included household and office-based patient educational material and clinician education, practice profiling, and academic detailing. Clinician education involved a description of the patient education intervention, evidence-based management of acute bronchitis, and advice on how to say "no" to patient demands for antibiotics.

Bronchodilators are frequently prescribed for patients with acute bronchitis. However, a Cochrane review on the use of β-agonists in children and adults with acute bronchitis concluded that there is insufficient evidence to support the routine use of these agents (23), and their use is not recommended (5). Subgroup analysis of patients with evidence of airflow obstruction demonstrated an improvement in cough and dyspnea with the use of β-agonist. The use of cough suppressant medication for acute bronchitis has not been studied in placebo controlled trials. However, cough suppressants may reduce cough severity and can be offered for severe coughing (5).

In summary, acute bronchitis is a common disorder in which clinicians frequently encounter difficulty in identifying the constellation of symptoms and findings that define the disease. A simplified approach is to classify all viral respiratory tract infections as a single disease entity with anatomic specification based on the source of predominant symptoms. Acute bronchitis should not be diagnosed in patients with chronic lung or heart diseases, immunocompromised states, or pneumonia. Although antibiotic use seems to reduce the duration of some symptoms of acute bronchitis, the benefits of this statistical improvement do not justify the risk of propagation of antibiotic resistance, cost of medication, and side effects that would occur with routine antibiotic use.

References

1. Slusarcick AL, McCaig LF. National hospital ambulatory medical care Survey: 1998 outpatient department summary. Hyattsville, MD: U.S. Dept. of Health and Human Services, Center for Disease Control and Prevention, National Center for Health Statistics, 2000. [DDHS publ. no. (PHS) 2000-1250/0-0520.]
2. Macfarlane J, Holmes W, Gard P, et al. Prospective study of the incidence, aetiology and outcome of adult lower respiratory tract illness in the community. Thorax 2001; 56:109–114.
3. Meza RA. The management of acute bronchitis in general practice results from the Australian morbidity and treatment survey. Aust Fam Physician 1994; 23:1550–1553.
4. Osler W. The Principles and Practice of Medicine: Designed for the Use of Practitioners and Students of Medicine. Edinburgh: Young J. Pentland, 1982.
5. Braman SS. Chronic cough due to acute bronchitis: ACCP evidence-based clinical practice guidelines. Chest 2006; 129(1 suppl):104S–115S.
6. Oeffinger KC, Snell LM, Foster BM, et al. Diagnosis of acute bronchitis in adults: a national survey of family physicians. J Fam Pract 1997; 45:402–409.
7. Hueston WJ, Mainous AG, Dacus EN, et al. Does acute bronchitis really exist? A reconceptualization of acute viral respiratory infections. J Fam Pract 2006; 49(3):401–406.
8. Gonzales R, Wilson A, Crane LA, et al. What's in a name? Public knowledge, attitudes, and experiences with antibiotic use for acute bronchitis. Am J Med 2000; 108:83–85.
9. Jonsson JS, Gislason T, Gislason D, et al. Acute bronchitis and clinical outcome three years later: prospective cohort study. Br Med J 1998; 317(7170): 1433–1434.
10. Hallett JS, Jacobs RL. Recurrent acute bronchitis: the association with undiagnosed bronchial asthma. Ann. Allergy 1985; 55:568–570.
11. Armstrong GL, Pinner RW. Outpatient visits for infectious disease in the United States, 1980 through 1996. Arch Intern Med 1999; 159:2531–2536.
12. Birnbaum HG, Morley M, Greenberg PE, et al. Economic burden of respiratory infections in an employed population. Chest 2002; 122(2):603–611.
13. Ward JI, Cherry JD, Chang S-J, et al. Efficacy of an acellular pertussis vaccine among adolescents and adults. N Engl J Med 2005; 353(15):1555–1563.
14. Verheij TJ, Hermans J, Mulder JD. Effects of doxycycline in patients with acute cough and purulent sputum: a double blind placebo controlled trial. Br J Gen Pract 1994; 44:400–404.

15. Evans AT, Husain S, Durairaj L, et al. Azithromycin for acute bronchitis: a randomized, double-blind, controlled trial. Lancet 2002; 359:1648–1654.
16. Gonzales R, Sande MA. Uncomplicated acute bronchitis. Ann Intern Med 2000; 133(12): 981–991.
17. Boldy DAR, Skidmore SJ, Ayres JG. Acute bronchitis in the community: clinical features, infective factors, changes in pulmonary function and bronchial reactivity to histamine. Respir Med 1990; 84:377–385.
18. Hall KK, Philbrick J, Nadkarni M. Evaluation and treatment of acute bronchitis at an academic teaching clinic. Am J Med Sci 2003; 325(1):7–9.
19. McIsaac WJ, To T. Antibiotics for lower respiratory tract infections: Still too frequently prescribed? Can Fam Physician 2004; 50:569–75.
20. Fahey T, Smucny J, Glazier R. Antibiotics for acute bronchitis. Cochrane Database Syst Rev 2004; (4):CD000245.
21. Macfarlane J, Holmes W, Gard P, et al. Reducing antibiotic use for acute bronchitis in primary care: blinded, randomised controlled trial of patient information leaflet. Br Med J 2002; 324:1–6.
22. Gonzales R, Steiner JF, Lum A, et al. Decreasing antibiotic use in ambulatory practice: impact of multidimensional intervention on the treatment of uncomplicated acute bronchitis in adults. JAMA 1999; 281(16):1512–1519.
23. Smucny J, Becker L, Glazier R. Beta 2-agonists for acute bronchitis. Cochrane Database Syst Rev 2006; (4):CD001726.

5

Exacerbations of Chronic Obstructive Pulmonary Disease

HIMANSHU DESAI
University at Buffalo, State University of New York, Buffalo, New York, U.S.A.

SANJAY SETHI
Veterans Affairs Western New York Healthcare System and University at Buffalo,
State University of New York, Buffalo, New York, U.S.A.

I. Introduction

Chronic obstructive pulmonary disease (COPD) is a leading cause of morbidity and mortality globally and will continue to increase in importance as the world population continues to age (1,2). Exacerbations, characteristic of the course of COPD, are intermittent episodes of increased respiratory symptoms and worse pulmonary function that may be accompanied by fever and other constitutional symptoms. These episodes contribute significantly to the morbidity associated with COPD, and in advanced disease, they are also the most frequent cause of death (3–5). The clinical manifestations of exacerbations result from direct effects of virus and bacteria and from the host response to infection. However, not all exacerbations are infectious and air pollution and other environmental conditions that increase airway inflammation or bronchomotor tone likely account for 15% to 20% of exacerbations. Increased respiratory symptoms due to comorbid conditions such as congestive heart failure and pulmonary emboli should be clinically excluded in the evaluation of exacerbations. Several new clinical trials as well as observational studies have given us a base of evidence to refine our approach to treating exacerbations that should lead to improved outcomes for patients. A rational, stratified approach to the use of antibiotics for this condition based on these recent basic and clinical studies has been developed. Prevention of lower respiratory tract infections in COPD is possible; however, substantial research is required for such prevention to reach its full potential.

II. Definition and Severity of Exacerbations

An exacerbation of COPD is defined as an event in the natural course of the disease characterized by a change in the patient's baseline dyspnea, cough, and/or sputum and beyond normal day-to-day variations that are acute in onset and may warrant a change in regular medication in a patient with underlying COPD (6,7). This definition though inclusive of symptoms of an exacerbation, is not specific with regard to the duration of symptoms, and it lacks objective measures. Also missing in this definition is the clinical exclusion of entities that could lead to increased respiratory symptoms in a manner similar to exacerbation, such as pneumonia, congestive heart failure, upper respiratory infection, or noncompliance with medications. In clinical studies, the authors suspect an exacerbation when a patient with COPD reports a minor increase (or new onset) of two or a major increase (or new onset) of one of the following respiratory symptoms: dyspnea, cough, sputum production, sputum tenacity, or sputum purulence (8). The increase in symptoms should be of at least 24 hours' duration and should be of greater intensity than their normal day-to-day variability. Furthermore, as described earlier, clinical evaluation should exclude other clinical entities that could present in a similar manner.

Different notions of exacerbation severity have been used. Though intuitively lung function (spirometric) changes should be used to determine severity, spirometry is difficult to measure during exacerbations, and often, the change with an exacerbation is of the same magnitude as day-to-day variability in these measurements. Severity has been also measured by site of care, with hospitalized exacerbations regarded as severe, outpatient physician–treated exacerbations regarded as moderate, and self-medicated exacerbations as mild (1). This classification is prone to error as the site of care is dependent on differences among countries and health care systems as to the threshold for admission as well as patient and physician preferences. Another measure of severity suggested is the intensity of treatment with bronchodilators only indicating mild exacerbations, with either antibiotics or steroids indicating moderate exacerbations, and with both antibiotics and steroids indicating severe exacerbations. Again, this approach is beset with problems of preferences and practice approach. Another widely used determination of severity of exacerbations is the Anthonisen classification (9). This classification relies on the number of cardinal symptoms and the presence of some supporting symptoms (Table 1). Advantages of this determination of severity include its simplicity and its correlation with benefit from antibiotics, with such benefit seen only in type 1 and 2 exacerbations. Limitations include its lack of validation against objective measures of severity and its ability to predict benefit from antibiotics has not been consistent in all studies. It is evident that a better definition and objective measures of severity of exacerbations are needed. Ongoing efforts in the development of patient reported outcomes and biomarkers should provide us with such tools in the future.

Table 1 Anthonisen Classification of COPD Exacerbations Based on Cardinal Symptoms

Severity of exacerbation	Type of exacerbation	Characteristics
Severe	Type 1	Increased dyspnea, sputum volume, and sputum purulence
Moderate	Type 2	Any two of the above three cardinal symptoms
Mild	Type 3	Any one of the above three cardinal symptoms and one or more of the following minor symptoms or signs • Cough • Wheezing • Fever without an obvious source • Upper respiratory tract infection in the past 5 days • Respiratory rate increase >20% over baseline • Heart rate increase >20% over baseline

Source: From Ref. 9.

III. Epidemiology

Studies estimate that by 2020, COPD would become the third leading cause of death in the United States and worldwide. Exacerbations of COPD results in over 110,000 deaths and over 500,000 hospitalizations per year in the United States, with over $18 billion spent in direct costs annually (6,10–12). In addition to the financial burden required to care for these patients, other "costs" such as days missed from the work and severe limitations in quality of life (QOL) are important features of this condition (13). The average frequency of exacerbations reported to health care providers is one to two exacerbations annually, and this generally increases with increasing severity of airflow obstruction (14–16). As many as half the exacerbations of COPD may not be reported by the patients to their health care providers, and as a consequence remain untreated. Using daily-symptom diary cards to detect exacerbations, Donaldson et al. (17) found that patients with severe COPD [GOLD (Global initiative for chronic Obstructive Lung Disease) category III] had an annual exacerbation frequency of 3.43/yr compared with 2.68/yr in those with moderate COPD (GOLD category II). Patients who suffer a high number of exacerbations during a given period of time will continue to suffer frequent exacerbations in future (18). Therefore, the frequency of exacerbations will depend on the underlying severity of lung disease and number of prior exacerbations (19).

There are several important clinical consequences of exacerbations of COPD. Though the acute symptoms tend to subside over the course of two to three weeks, QOL takes several months to recover. Furthermore, this recovery is delayed if exacerbations recur during this recover period (20). Contrary to previous studies, recent data have shown that the frequency of exacerbations is associated with accelerated long-term decline in lung function as measured by the forced expiratory volume in one second (FEV_1). This has been shown in mild disease, in the Lung Health Study, where every lower respiratory tract illness was associated with an additional loss of 7 mL of FEV_1 (21). Patients with moderate to severe COPD who experience more frequent exacerbations also experienced a decline in FEV_1 of 40 mL/yr in contrast to a decline of 32 mL/yr among patients with infrequent exacerbations (17). Several studies reported in-hospital mortality rate from 11% to 24% (22) to 22% and 35.6% after one and two years, respectively (23,24). Soler-Cataluna et al. (5) demonstrated that severe exacerbations of COPD have an independent negative prognostic impact, with mortality increasing with the frequency of severe exacerbations and those requiring hospitalization. Patients with frequent exacerbations had a risk of death 4.3 times greater than did patients requiring no hospital management of exacerbations.

IV. Etiology

Studies estimate that 70% to 80% of COPD exacerbations are due to respiratory infections. The remaining 20% to 30% is due to environmental pollution or have an unknown etiology (25). Viral and bacterial infections cause most exacerbations, while atypical bacteria are relatively uncommon (14) (Table 2).

A. Bacterial Pathogens as a Cause of Exacerbation

Recent studies with improved study design and modern investigational tools have established that bacteria cause up to 50% of exacerbations (26). Older models proposed that increases in the concentration of bacteria (bacterial load) that chronically colonized

Table 2 Microbial Pathogens Causing COPD Exacerbations

Microbe	Role in exacerbations
Bacteria	
Haemophilus influenzae	20%–30% of exacerbations
Streptococcus pneumoniae	10%–15% of exacerbations
Moraxella catarrhalis	10%–15% of exacerbations
Pseudomonas aeruginosa	5%–10% of exacerbations, prevalent in advanced disease
Enterobacteriaceae	Isolated in advanced disease, pathogenic significance undefined
Haemophilus haemolyticus	Isolated frequently, unlikely cause
Haemophilus parainfluenzae	Isolated frequently, unlikely cause
Staphylococcus aureus	Isolated infrequently, unlikely cause
Viruses	
Rhinovirus	20%–25% of exacerbations
Parainfluenza	5%–10% of exacerbations
Influenza	5%–10% of exacerbations
Respiratory syncytial virus	5%–10% of exacerbations
Coronavirus	5%–10% of exacerbations
Adenovirus	3%–5% of exacerbations
Human metapneumovirus	3%–5% of exacerbations
Atypical bacteria	
Chlamydophila pneumoniae	3%–5% of exacerbations
Mycoplasma pneumoniae	1%–2% of exacerbations
Fungi	
Pneumocystis jiroveci	Undefined

Source: Modified from Ref. 14.

the airways accounted for exacerbations. However, a comprehensive analysis of the relationship of bacterial concentrations in sputum, new pathogen acquisition, and clinical symptoms demonstrated that change in bacterial load is an unlikely independent mechanism of exacerbation (27).

Bronchoscopy with the protected specimen brush accurately samples the microbiology of the lower airways. A pooled analysis of such studies revealed that bacteria were present in significant concentrations in the airways of 4% of healthy adults, 29% of adults with stable COPD, and 54% of adults experiencing a COPD exacerbation (28). One study demonstrated intracellular *Haemophilus influenzae* in bronchial mucosal biopsies in 87% of patients intubated for exacerbations compared with 33% with stable COPD and 0% of healthy controls (29). Nontypeable *H. influenzae*, *Moraxella catarrhalis*, and *Streptococcus pneumoniae* are the bacteria most frequently isolated bronchoscopically from patients having an exacerbation of COPD, although *Pseudomonas aeruginosa* and *Enterobacteriaceae* are also isolated (30–33).

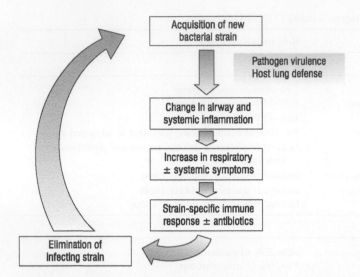

Figure 1 Model of the elements of the pathogenesis of bacterial exacerbations of COPD. *Source*: Modified from Ref. 14.

A new model of bacterial exacerbation pathogenesis has been proposed based on recent studies with newer molecular and immunological techniques (Fig. 1). Acquisition of a new strain of *H. influenzae, M. catarrhalis, S. pneumoniae*, or *P. aeruginosa* is clearly associated with the occurrence of an exacerbation (27,34–37). Whether this association extends to other bacteria isolated from sputum during exacerbations, such as *Staphylococcus aureus* and *Enterobacteriaceae*, has not been investigated. The time frame of increased risk appears to be up to four to eight weeks after acquisition of a new strain.

B. Atypical Bacteria as a Cause of Exacerbation

Considerable confusion reigns in the literature regarding the importance of *Mycoplasma pneumoniae* and *Chlamydia pneumoniae* infection in exacerbations, related to the diagnostic methods used in studies to define infection with these pathogens. These diagnostic methods include culture of respiratory secretions, detection of microbial DNA with polymerase chain reaction (PCR), and serology. Culture for these pathogens is technically difficult and of extremely low yield. The interpretation of PCR is complicated by a substantial presence of *C. pneumoniae* DNA in respiratory secretions in stable COPD (38). Serology can be reliable if the serological test used is highly specific and a minimum fourfold increase in titer between acute and convalescent sera is required to diagnose an infection. Unfortunately, several studies have chosen an unreliable diagnostic criterion of a single titer above a certain threshold (39–41). Such high titers are common in stable COPD and overdiagnose acute infection in these patients. If the focus is on studies with rigorous methodology, *M. pneumoniae* is a rare cause of exacerbation, and the incidence of *C. pneumoniae* is 4% to 5%, with coinfection with bacteria being frequent in these instances (42–44).

C. Viruses as a Cause of Exacerbation

Viruses can be detected in one-third to two-thirds of exacerbations using culture-, serology- and PCR-based methods. The most common viruses associated with exacerbations of COPD are *rhinoviruses* (45). *Influenza, parainfluenza, coronavirus,* and *adenovirus* are also common during exacerbations (44–51). *Respiratory syncytial virus* and *human metapneumovirus* were more recently associated with exacerbations (52,53). It is important to realize that the detection of viral RNA in a sputum sample by sensitive PCR-based assays does not imply virus as an etiological agent for exacerbation as viral RNA can be detected in up to 15% of sputum samples during stable COPD (45,47,51). Viral respiratory tract infections do have substantial clinical consequences in COPD, especially in moderate or severe disease where infections can precipitate emergency room visits and hospitalizations (50).

The mechanisms by which viruses induce exacerbations have been partially elucidated. Viral infection of the airway epithelial cells induces inflammation (54). This causes airway epithelial damage, muscarinic receptor stimulation, and induction of inflammatory mediators (e.g., cytokines or chemokines) (55). Airway eosinophilia is associated with viral mediated exacerbations, which highlights the importance of the host response to infection in both inflammation and symptoms (51).

D. Co-infection in Exacerbation of COPD

An antecedent viral infection is not essential for the development of bacterial exacerbations of COPD. In fact, in the few studies that have addressed this issue, exacerbations could be attributed to virus alone, to both viral and bacterial infection and to bacterial infection alone (29,51,56). Coinfection by virus and bacteria does seem to increase the severity of exacerbations. Viruses alter the expression of receptor molecules on respiratory epithelial cells allowing increased adherence and invasion by bacteria (57). Similarly, antecedent bacterial infection may increase the susceptibility to viral infection by increasing expression of host cell molecules that bind viruses (58). In hospitalized patients, a greater decrement of lung function and longer hospitalization was observed with coinfection (51). Among outpatients, coinfection was associated with more symptoms, a larger fall in FEV_1, higher bacterial loads, and more systemic inflammation (56).

E. Noninfectious Causes of Exacerbation

A variety of noninfectious stimuli can induce an acute increase in airway inflammation in COPD. Environmental pollutants, both particulate matter and nonparticulate gases, are capable of inducing inflammation in vitro and in vivo (59–61). Epidemiological studies have demonstrated increased respiratory symptoms and respiratory mortality among patients with COPD during periods of increased air pollution (62–64).

V. Pathogenesis

Recent studies have established that inflammation in the airways and parenchyma of the lung is prevalent and may be central to the pathogenesis of COPD (65). An exaggeration of this baseline airway inflammation underlies the pathogenesis of acute exacerbations (66,67). An acute increase in airway inflammation could lead to increased bronchial tone, bronchial wall edema, and mucus production. These processes could worsen ventilation-perfusion mismatch and expiratory flow limitation in an already diseased lung. Corresponding clinical manifestations would include dyspnea, cough, increased sputum production, tenacity, and purulence along with worsening gas exchange, the cardinal manifestations of an exacerbation.

Measurement of airway inflammation in exhaled breath, induced or expectorated sputum, bronchoalveolar lavage, or bronchial biopsy has shown increased airway inflammation in acute exacerbation that resolves with treatment (68–71). Increases in plasma fibrinogen, interleukin (IL)-6 and C-reactive protein, consistent with a heightened state of systemic inflammation, have been described during exacerbations (72,73).

Both pathogen and host factors are key determinants in the pathogenesis of an exacerbation. Whether acquisition and infection of the airways by a new bacterial strain or virus in a patient with COPD lead to an exacerbation is likely determined by a complex host-pathogen interaction in the airways. The balance between host defense and pathogen virulence determines the level of proliferation of the pathogen as well as its interaction with the airway mucosa, which in turn determines the increase in airway inflammation.

A. Microbial Mechanisms

Putative microbial mechanisms for respiratory bacterial pathogens include adhesion to and invasion of airway epithelial cells, inactivation of host defense mechanisms, and elicitation of inflammatory mediators from airway cells. Chin et al. demonstrated that *H. influenzae* strains isolated during exacerbations induced greater airway neutrophil recruitment than colonizing strains in a mouse pulmonary clearance model (74). Furthermore, exacerbation strains adhered in significantly higher numbers to and elicited more IL-8 from primary human airway epithelial cells. Fernaays et al. with a genomics approach found that a specific combination of genes was related to exacerbation inducing potential in *H. influenzae* strains (75). One of these genes was an IgA protease, suggesting that inactivation of host defenses is an important determinant of disease expression among bacterial strains. However, the understanding of pathogen virulence with relevance to COPD is still in its infancy, and additional observations are needed.

B. Host Mechanisms

Failure of host innate defense mechanisms in COPD leads to induction of adaptive immune responses to control and eradicate the infection. When immune responses to new strains of *M. catarrhalis* associated with COPD exacerbation and colonization were compared, a mucosal IgA response to the infecting strain was more common and vigorous with colonization, while a systemic IgG immune response was more common and vigorous with exacerbations (36). Therefore, the host immune response could dictate the clinical expression of a bacterial strain acquisition in COPD. A vigorous mucosal immune response could "exclude" the bacteria from interaction with the epithelial mucosa, resulting in less airway inflammation, and therefore favor colonization. Abe et al. demonstrated that having diminished peripheral blood mononuclear cell proliferation on exposure to a *H. influenzae* antigen, outer-membrane protein P6, was associated with a history of exacerbations with *H. influenzae* (76). This suggests that an adequate cellular response to *H. influenzae* antigens suppresses newly acquired strains of this pathogen and therefore prevents exacerbations. The degree of impairment of innate immunity, an individual's previous immunological experience with the pathogenic strain, and the nature of the adaptive immune response all impact the clinical manifestation of acquisition of a bacterial pathogen.

VI. Diagnostic Approach

Accurate diagnosis relies on clear definitions that are universally agreed upon and include objective measurements. Unfortunately, this is not the situation with acute exacerbations of COPD, with an imprecise and variable definition and the absence of objective measures (77). An exacerbation should be suspected when a patient with COPD reports an increase in respiratory symptoms that is beyond day-to-day variability and is sustained (8). Furthermore, clinical evaluation should exclude other clinical entities such as pneumonia, congestive heart failure, and upper respiratory infection.

A. Role of Chest X Ray

Chest X rays are not obtained routinely for diagnosis of exacerbations. Even when performed in exacerbations severe enough to require hospitalization, findings alter treatment in only about 10% of patients. The yield of such findings is likely to be even lower in milder episodes. Chest X ray is useful to exclude other clinical conditions such as pneumonia, congestive heart failure, or pneumothorax when these are clinically suspected. Therefore, a thorough physical examination with careful attention to the lungs is essential in determining if a chest X ray is indicated. Symptoms such as hemoptysis and pleuritic chest pain and physical signs such as high fever, elevated jugular venous pressure, lung consolidation, bibasilar rales, and pedal edema should prompt a chest X ray. Exacerbations that do not respond appropriately to treatment should also prompt a chest X ray for evaluation of alternative diagnosis.

B. Role of Sputum Culture

Sputum cultures are unreliable at identifying bacterial infection in patients with COPD exacerbations. Gram's stain and culture of expectorated sputum often yield similar results during exacerbations and stable disease (46) and cannot distinguish between true pathogens and colonizing flora. Molecular-typing studies to identify new bacterial strains are not available for routine clinical use. The most common pathogens (*H. influenzae, M. catarrhalis,* and *S. pneumoniae*) are fastidious, which increases the likelihood of false-negative results if the sputum is not promptly processed. In one study that collected sequential sputum cultures from patients with stable COPD, molecular typing revealed that apparently identical bacterial strains of *H. influenzae* were intermittently recovered, suggesting that false-negative culture results were common (78). On the basis of these limitations, the 2006 GOLD guidelines and the 2001 clinical practice guidelines from the American College of Physicians concluded that sputum cultures should not be performed during most exacerbations of COPD (1,79). Special circumstances where sputum cultures could be useful include treatment failures, recurrent exacerbations, and suspicion of *Pseudomonas* infection.

VII. Management

Traditionally, the aims of treatment of an exacerbation are the recovery to baseline clinical status over two to three weeks and the prevention of complications. Though these goals are undoubtedly important, several other important goals of treatment, both clinical and biological, should be considered. Among these clinical goals are rapid resolution of symptoms, prevention of early relapse, lengthening the "exacerbation free interval" or "time to next exacerbation," improvement in QOL measures, and improvement in exercise tolerance. Nonclinical goals of treatment include bacteriologic eradication, resolution of airway inflammation, resolution of systemic inflammation, prevention of FEV_1 decline, and others. Practical application of these biological goals awaits the development of simple, rapid, and reliable measurement tools for inflammation and infection.

Optimal therapy for an exacerbation is multipronged and depends, in part, on the site of therapy. The decision to treat in the outpatient or hospital setting remains based on clinical assessment with inconsistent guidelines (6,7,80). In general, the presence of respiratory failure, worsening of underlying comorbidity, failure to respond to outpatient management, or an uncertain diagnosis has been incorporated in recommendations to consider hospitalization.

A. Antimicrobial Treatment

Though antibiotics are widely used in the treatment of exacerbations, until recently, there was a paucity of well-designed, randomized controlled trials on which to base optimal therapy with these agents (7,81–83). Though better evidence now exists to guide the use of these agents in exacerbations, there are still considerable gaps in knowledge and further research is needed.

Antibiotics are beneficial in the treatment of moderate and severe exacerbations, especially when sputum purulence is one of the presenting symptoms (84). Observational studies have identified advanced age, severity of airflow obstruction, recurrent exacerbations, and comorbid cardiac disease as predictive factors for poor clinical outcomes following an exacerbation (85). The authors and others advocate a stratified approach to antibiotic choice on the basis of these risk factors (82,86). Though not prospectively validated, such a stratification approach addresses judicious use of antibiotics as well as concerns of antibiotic resistance and optimizing clinical outcome. The approach employing these principles is shown in Figure 2.

B. Nonantimicrobial Treatment

Bronchodilators

Inhaled β-agonists and anticholinergic agents have been documented to decrease obstruction during exacerbations of COPD. Systematic reviews have suggested that both short-acting β-agonists and anticholinergic-inhaled bronchodilators have comparable effects on spirometry and a greater effect than parenterally administered bronchodilators (87). It is reasonable to consider the addition of a second agent from a different class to a patient's regimen if there is suboptimal response to a single regimen (80). The evidence base for the addition of a methylxanthine to inhaled bronchodilators is contradictory. It is clear, however, that the high incidence of adverse reactions makes it difficult to recommend its routine use (80,88).

Corticosteroids

Systemic corticosteroid therapy improves lung function and treatment success, and reduces the length of hospital stay (89–91). The optimal dose of systemic corticosteroids for treating a COPD exacerbation is unknown. High doses of systemic corticosteroids

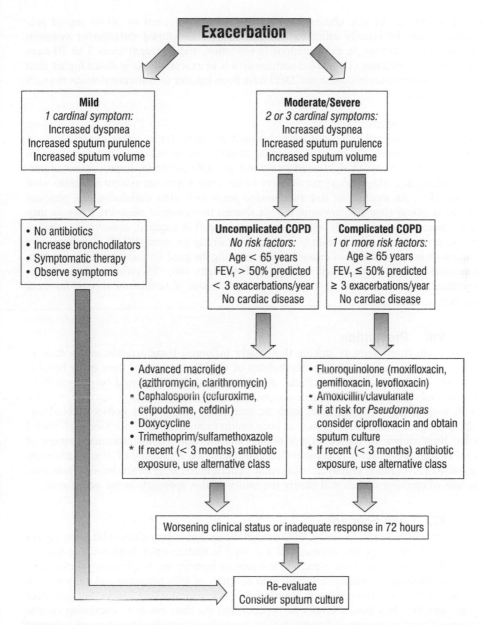

Figure 2 Algorithm for antibiotic treatment of acute exacerbations of COPD. *Source*: Modified from Ref. 14.

increase the risk of side effects. Lower doses (e.g., equivalent of 30–40 mg of prednisone) may be equally effective and safer (1). The optimal duration of systemic
glucocorticoid therapy in exacerbations is unknown, and in recent trials 7 to 10 days
appears to be adequate (1). Inhaled corticosteroids in exacerbations at doses higher than
used for maintenance treatment in COPD have been inferior to systemic steroids in small
clinical trials.

Other Therapies

Oxygen is considered a cornerstone of hospital treatment for an acute exacerbation of
COPD (80). Among the multiple potential benefits are reduction of pulmonary vaso-
constriction, decrease in right heart strain and possible ischemia, improvement of cardiac output, and adequate oxygen delivery to the central nervous system and other vital
organs (92). An analysis of five randomized controlled trials concluded that pharma-
cological mucus clearance strategies did not shorten the course of treatment although they
may improve symptoms (92). When ventilatory support is required, noninvasive positive
pressure ventilation, usually with bilevel positive airway pressure (BPAP), has been very
successful in the treatment of exacerbations, reducing the need for endotracheal intubation,
infectious complications, length of stay, and mortality (80). Therefore, unless specific
contraindications exist, this should be the preferred mode of ventilatory support for these
patients.

VIII. Prevention

Though direct evidence is lacking that yearly influenza immunization and a dose of
pneumococcal vaccine reduce exacerbations of COPD, because of their other benefits
and low incidence of adverse effects, all patients with COPD should be offered these
vaccinations. In patients with airflow obstruction of at least moderate severity, therapy
with long-acting bronchodilators such as tiotropium and inhaled corticosteroid/long-
acting β-agonist combinations such as budesonide/formoterol and fluticasone/salmeterol
have been shown to reduce exacerbations. Current optimal maintenance therapy of
COPD with these agents in combination can reduce the frequency of exacerbations by
about 40%. Antibiotic prophylaxis has some benefit in reducing exacerbations; however,
results of ongoing studies will clarify the utility of this approach in the near future.

IX. Case Scenario

A 74-year old male patient with COPD presents to an ambulatory clinic with three days of
increased dyspnea, sputum volume, and a change in sputum color from white to yellow-
green. He denies fever, chills, pleuritic chest pain, or hemoptysis. A spirometry performed a
year ago showed an obstructive pattern with an FEV_1 of 45% predicted and a forced vital
capacity (FVC) of 66% predicted. He has a 35-pack-year smoking history but quit three
years ago. He does have a history of hypertension but does not have coexisting cardiac
disease. Over the last year, he has had three exacerbations that were treated on an outpatient
basis; the last episode was four months ago. During the last episode, following treatment
with amoxicillin-clavulanate, he experienced an urticarial rash. For his COPD, he had been
prescribed regular inhaled salmeterol and ipratropium bromide.

On examination, the patient is not in acute distress and is afebrile. On lung
examination, breath sounds are diminished with scattered coarse rales; however, there

are no signs of consolidation. Heart sounds are distant; however, no murmur is heard. Pulse oximetry reveals an oxygen saturation of 92% on room air.

Several important management issues arise with this patient.

1. *Does he need further diagnostic work-up?* His symptoms are classical for an exacerbation and physical exam is not revealing of an alternative explanation for his symptoms such as congestive heart failure or pneumonia. Therefore, a chest X ray is unlikely to yield an alternative diagnosis and is not indicated. Though he has frequent exacerbations, he is not a clinical failure. He does not have very severe airflow obstruction or concomitant bronchiectasis, has not received multiple courses of antibiotics, and has not experienced a recent hospitalization. Therefore, he is at low risk for *Pseudomonas* infection. For these reasons a sputum culture is not indicated either.

2. *Is antibiotic therapy indicated, and which antibiotic should be prescribed?* As shown in Figure 2, a stratification approach to antibiotic choice should be applied. The patient has all three of the cardinal symptoms of exacerbation; therefore, antibiotic treatment is indicated. For several reasons, the patient is a complicated patient with exacerbation, including his age, the severity of his underlying COPD and a history of frequent exacerbations. Therefore, antibiotic choices include either a fluoroquinolone or amoxicillin-clavulanate. Because of a major penicillin allergy, a respiratory fluoroquinolone would be an appropriate choice. As his last antibiotic exposure was more than three months before presentation, it does not affect current antibiotic choice. For reasons stated above, he is at low risk for *Pseudomonas* infection, therefore empiric coverage for that pathogen is not indicated.

3. *What other treatment of the exacerbation should be provided?* A temporary intensification of his short-acting bronchodilator regime is indicated. The decision regarding prescriptions of a short course of oral corticosteroids needs to be individualized in such patients, as such treatment has been clearly shown to be beneficial only in patients with exacerbations severe enough to be hospitalized or requiring emergency room evaluation. In view of his underlying severe airflow obstruction and frequent exacerbations, it would be reasonable to prescribe 40 mg prednisone for 7 to 10 days in this patient.

4. *Are there preventative measures to reduce exacerbations in such a patient that should be addressed?* This patient has severe underlying COPD and experiences frequent exacerbations. His immunizations should be updated once he recovers from the exacerbation. Maintenance therapy for his COPD is suboptimal, and consideration should be given to adding long-acting bronchodilators and/or inhaled corticosteroids.

References

1. GOLD. Global strategy for the diagnosis, management, and prevention of chronic obstructive pulmonary disease. December 19, 2008; Available at: http://www.goldcopd.com.
2. Mannino DM, Buist AS. Global burden of COPD: risk factors, prevalence, and future trends. Lancet 2007; 370(9589):765–773.
3. Burrows B, Earle RH. Course and prognosis of chronic obstructive lung disease. A prospective study of 200 patients. N Engl J Med 1969; 280(8):397–404.

4. Calverley PM, Anderson JA, Celli B, et al. Salmeterol and fluticasone propionate and survival in chronic obstructive pulmonary disease. N Engl J Med 2007; 356(8):775–789.
5. Soler-Cataluna JJ, Martínez-García MA, Román Sánchez P, et al. Severe acute exacerbations and mortality in patients with chronic obstructive pulmonary disease. Thorax 2005; 60 (11):925–931.
6. Celli BR, MacNee W. Standards for the diagnosis and treatment of patients with COPD: a summary of the ATS/ERS position paper. Eur Respir J 2004; 23(6):932–946.
7. Fabbri L, Pauwels RA, Hurd SS. Global strategy for the diagnosis, management, and prevention of chronic obstructive pulmonary disease: GOLD Executive Summary updated 2003. COPD 2004; 1(1):105–141; discussion 103–104.
8. Sethi S, Evans N, Grant BJ, et al. New strains of bacteria and exacerbations of chronic obstructive pulmonary disease. N Engl J Med 2002; 347(7):465–471.
9. Anthonisen NR, Manfreda J, Warren CPW, et al. Antibiotic therapy in exacerbations of chronic obstructive pulmonary disease. Ann Intern Med 1987; 106(2):196–204.
10. Mannino DM, Homa DM, Akinbami LJ, et al. Chronic obstructive pulmonary disease surveillance–United States, 1971–2000. MMWR Surveill Summ 2002; 51(6):1–16.
11. Miravitlles M, Murio C, Guerrero T, et al. Pharmacoeconomic evaluation of acute exacerbations of chronic bronchitis and COPD. Chest 2002; 121(5):1449–1455.
12. National Heart Lung and Blood Institute. Chronic Obstructive Pulmonary Disease Data Fact Sheet. Bethesda, MD: NHLBI, 2003:5229.
13. Miravitlles M, Ferrer M, Pont A, et al. Effect of exacerbations on quality of life in patients with chronic obstructive pulmonary disease: a 2 year follow up study. Thorax 2004; 59 (5):387–395.
14. Sethi S, Murphy TF. Infection in the pathogenesis and course of chronic obstructive pulmonary disease. N Engl J Med 2008; 359(22):2355–2365.
15. Burge PS, Calverley PM, Jones PW, et al. Randomised, double blind, placebo controlled study of fluticasone propionate in patients with moderate to severe chronic obstructive pulmonary disease: the ISOLDE trial. BMJ 2000; 320(7245):1297–1303.
16. Paggiaro PL, Dahle R, Bakran I, et al. Multicentre randomised placebo-controlled trial of inhaled fluticasone propionate in patients with chronic obstructive pulmonary disease. International COPD Study Group. Lancet 1998; 351(9105):773–780.
17. Donaldson GC, Seemungal TA, Bhowmik A, et al. Relationship between exacerbation frequency and lung function decline in chronic obstructive pulmonary disease. Thorax 2002; 57 (10):847–852.
18. Gompertz S, Bayley DL, Hill SL, et al. Relationship between airway inflammation and the frequency of exacerbations in patients with smoking related COPD. Thorax 2001; 56(1):36–41.
19. Miravitlles M, Guerrero T, Mayordomo C, et al. Factors associated with increased risk of exacerbation and hospital admission in a cohort of ambulatory COPD patients: a multiple logistic regression analysis. The EOLO Study Group. Respiration 2000; 67(5):495–501.
20. Spencer S, Jones PW. Time course of recovery of health status following an infective exacerbation of chronic bronchitis. Thorax 2003; 58(7):589–593.
21. Kanner RE, Anthonisen NR, Connett JE. Lower respiratory illnesses promote FEV(1) decline in current smokers but not ex-smokers with mild chronic obstructive pulmonary disease: results from the lung health study. Am J Respir Crit Care Med 2001; 164(3):358–364.
22. Connors AF, Jr., Dawson NV, Thomas C, et al. Outcomes following acute exacerbation of severe chronic obstructive lung disease. The SUPPORT investigators (Study to Understand Prognoses and Preferences for Outcomes and Risks of Treatments). Am J Respir Crit Care Med 1996; 154(4 pt 1):959–967.
23. Almagro P, Calbo E, Ochoa de Echagüen A, et al. Mortality after hospitalization for COPD. Chest 2002; 121(5):1441–1448.

24. Groenewegen KH, Schols AM, Wouters EF. Mortality and mortality-related factors after hospitalization for acute exacerbation of COPD. Chest 2003; 124(2):459–467.
25. Sapey E, Stockley RA. COPD exacerbations. 2: aetiology. Thorax 2006; 61(3):250–258.
26. Sethi S, Murphy TF. Bacterial infection in chronic obstructive pulmonary disease in 2000: a state-of-the-art review. Clin Microbiol Rev 2001; 14(2):336–363.
27. Sethi S, Sethi R, Eschberger K, et al. Airway bacterial concentrations and exacerbations of chronic obstructive pulmonary disease. Am J Respir Crit Care Med, 2007.
28. Rosell A, Monsó E, Soler N, et al. Microbiologic determinants of exacerbation in chronic obstructive pulmonary disease. Arch Intern Med 2005; 165(8):891–897.
29. Bandi V, Apicella MA, Mason E, et al. Nontypeable Haemophilus influenzae in the lower respiratory tract of patients with chronic bronchitis. Am J Respir Crit Care Med 2001; 164 (11):2114–2119.
30. Bartlett JG. Diagnostic accuracy of transtracheal aspiration bacteriologic studies. Am Rev Respir Dis 1977; 115(5):777–782.
31. Fagon JY, Chastre J, Trouillet JL, et al. Characterization of distal bronchial microflora during acute exacerbation of chronic bronchitis. Use of the protected specimen brush technique in 54 mechanically ventilated patients. Am Rev Respir Dis 1990; 142(5):1004–1008.
32. Monso E, Ruiz J, Rosell A, et al. Bacterial infection in chronic obstructive pulmonary disease. A study of stable and exacerbated outpatients using the protected specimen brush. Am J Respir Crit Care Med 1995; 152(4 pt 1):1316–1320.
33. Soler N, Torres A, Ewig S, et al. Bronchial microbial patterns in severe exacerbations of chronic obstructive pulmonary disease (COPD) requiring mechanical ventilation. Am J Respir Crit Care Med 1998; 157(5 pt 1):1498–1505.
34. Sethi S, Evans, N, Grant, BJB, et al. Acquisition of a new bacterial strain and occurrence of exacerbations of chronic obstructive pulmonary disease. N Engl J Med 2002; 347(7):465–471.
35. Murphy TF, Brauer AL, Sethi S, et al. Haemophilus haemolyticus: a human respiratory tract commensal to be distinguished from Haemophilus influenzae. J Infect Dis 2007; 195(1):81–89.
36. Murphy TF, Brauer AL, Grant DJ, et al. Moraxella catarrhalis in chronic obstructive pulmonary disease: burden of disease and immune response. Am J Respir Crit Care Med 2005; 172(2):195–199.
37. Murphy TF, Brauer AL, Eschberger K, et al. Pseudomonas aeruginosa in chronic obstructive pulmonary disease. Am J Respir Crit Care Med 2008; 177(8):853–860.
38. Blasi F, Damato S, Cosentini R, et al. Chlamydia pneumoniae and chronic bronchitis: association with severity and bacterial clearance following treatment. Thorax 2002; 57(8): 672–676.
39. Mogulkoc N, Karakurt S, Isalska B, et al. Acute purulent exacerbation of chronic obstructive pulmonary disease and Chlamydia pneumoniae infection. Am J Respir Crit Care Med 1999; 160(1):349–353.
40. Miyashita N, Niki Y, Nakajima M, et al. Chlamydia pneumoniae infection in patients with diffuse panbronchiolitis and COPD. Chest 1998; 114(4):969–971.
41. Karnak D, Beng-sun S, Beder S, et al. Chlamydia pneumoniae infection and acute exacerbation of chronic obstructive pulmonary disease (COPD). Respir Med 2001; 95(10):811–816.
42. Beaty CD, Grayston JT, Wang SP, et al. Chlamydia pneumoniae, strain TWAR, infection in patients with chronic obstructive pulmonary disease. Am Rev Respir Dis 1991; 144(6):1408–1410.
43. Blasi F, Legnani D, Lombardo VM, et al. Chlamydia pneumoniae infection in acute exacerbations of COPD. Eur Respir J 1993; 6(1):19–22.
44. Smith CB, Golden CA, Kanner RE, et al. Association of viral and Mycoplasma pneumoniae infections with acute respiratory illness in patients with chronic obstructive pulmonary diseases. Am Rev Respir Dis 1980; 121(2):225–232.

45. Seemungal T, Harper-Owen R, Bhowmik A, et al. Respiratory viruses, symptoms, and inflammatory markers in acute exacerbations and stable chronic obstructive pulmonary disease. Am J Respir Crit Care Med 2001; 164(9):1618–1623.
46. Gump DW, Phillips CA, Forsyth BR, et al. Role of infection in chronic bronchitis. Am Rev Respir Dis 1976; 113(4):465–474.
47. Rohde G, Wiethege A, Borg I, et al. Respiratory viruses in exacerbations of chronic obstructive pulmonary disease requiring hospitalisation: a case-control study. Thorax 2003; 58(1):37–42.
48. Tan WC, Xiang X, Qiu D, et al. Epidemiology of respiratory viruses in patients hospitalized with near-fatal asthma, acute exacerbations of asthma, or chronic obstructive pulmonary disease. Am J Med 2003; 115(4):272–277.
49. McNamara MJ, Phillips IA, Williams OB. Viral and Mycoplasma pneumoniae infections in exacerbations of chronic lung disease. Am Rev Respir Dis 1969; 100(1):19–24.
50. Greenberg SB, Allen M, Wilson J, et al. Respiratory viral infections in adults with and without chronic obstructive pulmonary disease. Am J Respir Crit Care Med 2000; 162(1):167–173.
51. Papi A, Bellettato CM, Braccioni F, et al. Infections and airway inflammation in chronic obstructive pulmonary disease severe exacerbations. Am J Respir Crit Care Med 2006; 173 (10):1114–1121.
52. Falsey AR, Hennessey PA, Formica MA, et al. Respiratory syncytial virus infection in elderly and high-risk adults. N Engl J Med 2005; 352(17):1749–1759.
53. Hamelin ME, Côté S, Laforge J, et al. Human metapneumovirus infection in adults with community-acquired pneumonia and exacerbation of chronic obstructive pulmonary disease. Clin Infect Dis 2005; 41(4):498–502.
54. Papadopoulos NG, Bates PJ, Bardin PG, et al. Rhinoviruses infect the lower airways. J Infect Dis 2000; 181(6):1875–1884.
55. Mallia P, Johnston SL. How viral infections cause exacerbation of airway diseases. Chest 2006; 130(4):1203–1210.
56. Wilkinson TM, Hurst JR, Perera WR, et al. Effect of interactions between lower airway bacterial and rhinoviral infection in exacerbations of COPD. Chest 2006; 129(2):317–324.
57. Avadhanula V, Rodriguez CA, Devincenzo JP, et al. Respiratory viruses augment the adhesion of bacterial pathogens to respiratory epithelium in a viral species- and cell type-dependent manner. J Virol 2006; 80(4):1629–1636.
58. Sajjan US, Jia Y, Newcomb DC, et al. H. influenzae potentiates airway epithelial cell responses to rhinovirus by increasing ICAM-1 and TLR3 expression. FASEB J 2006; 20 (12):2121–2123.
59. Ohtoshi T, Takizawa H, Okazaki H, et al. Diesel exhaust particles stimulate human airway epithelial cells to produce cytokines relevant to airway inflammation in vitro. J Allergy Clin Immunol 1998; 101(6 pt 1):778–785.
60. Devalia JL, Rusznak C, Herdman MJ, et al. Effect of nitrogen dioxide and sulphur dioxide on airway response of mild asthmatic patients to allergen inhalation. Lancet 1994; 344 (8938):1668–1671.
61. Rudell B, Blomberg A, Helleday R, et al. Bronchoalveolar inflammation after exposure to diesel exhaust: comparison between unfiltered and particle trap filtered exhaust. Occup Environ Med 1999; 56(8):527–534.
62. Garcia-Aymerich J, Tobías A, Antó JM, et al. Air pollution and mortality in a cohort of patients with chronic obstructive pulmonary disease: a time series analysis. J Epidemiol Community Health 2000; 54(1):73–74.
63. Sunyer J, Sáez M, Murillo C, Castellsague J, et al. Air pollution and emergency room admissions for chronic obstructive pulmonary disease: a 5-year study. Am J Epidemiol 1993; 137(7):701–705.

64. Sunyer J, Schwartz J, Tobías A, et al. Patients with chronic obstructive pulmonary disease are at increased risk of death associated with urban particle air pollution: a case-crossover analysis. Am J Epidemiol 2000; 151(1):50–56.

65. Saetta M, Turato G, Maestrelli P, et al. Cellular and structural bases of chronic obstructive pulmonary disease. Am J Respir Crit Care Med 2001; 163(6):1304–1309.

66. White AJ, Gompertz S, Stockley RA. Chronic obstructive pulmonary disease. 6: The aetiology of exacerbations of chronic obstructive pulmonary disease. Thorax 2003; 58(1):73–80.

67. Sethi S. New developments in the pathogenesis of acute exacerbations of chronic obstructive pulmonary disease. Curr Opin Infect Dis 2004; 17(2):113–119.

68. Sethi S, Muscarella K, Evans N, et al. Airway inflammation and etiology of acute exacerbations of chronic bronchitis. Chest 2000; 118(6):1557–1565.

69. Gompertz S, O'Brien C, Bayley DL, et al. Changes in bronchial inflammation during acute exacerbations of chronic bronchitis. Eur Respir J 2001; 17(6):1112–1119.

70. Stockley RA. The role of proteinases in the pathogenesis of chronic bronchitis. Am J Respir Crit Care Med 1994; 150(6 pt 2):S109–S113.

71. Wouters EF. Chronic obstructive pulmonary disease. 5: systemic effects of COPD. Thorax 2002; 57(12):1067–1070.

72. Wedzicha JA, Seemungal TA, MacCallum PK, et al. Acute exacerbations of chronic obstructive pulmonary disease are accompanied by elevations of plasma fibrinogen and serum IL-6 levels. Thromb Haemost 2000; 84(2):210–215.

73. Dev D, Wallace E, Sankaran R, et al. Value of C-reactive protein measurements in exacerbations of chronic obstructive pulmonary disease. Respir Med 1998; 92(4):664–667.

74. Chin CL, Manzel LJ, Lehman EE, et al. Haemophilus influenzae from patients with chronic obstructive pulmonary disease exacerbation induce more inflammation than colonizers. Am J Respir Crit Care Med 2005; 172(1):85–91.

75. Fernaays MM, Lesse AJ, Sethi S, et al. Differential genome contents of nontypeable Haemophilus influenzae strains from adults with chronic obstructive pulmonary disease. Infect Immun 2006; 74(6):3366–3374.

76. Abe Y, Murphy TF, Sethi S, et al. Lymphocyte proliferative response to P6 of Haemophilus influenzae is associated with relative protection from exacerbations of chronic obstructive pulmonary disease. Am J Respir Crit Care Med 2002; 165(7):967–971.

77. Rodriguez-Roisin R. Toward a consensus definition for COPD exacerbations. Chest 2000; 117(5 suppl 2):398S–401S.

78. Murphy TF, Brauer AL, Schiffmacher AT, et al. Persistent colonization by Haemophilus influenzae in chronic obstructive pulmonary disease. Am J Respir Crit Care Med 2004; 170 (3):266–272.

79. Snow V, Lascher S, Mottur-Pilson C. Evidence base for management of acute exacerbations of chronic obstructive pulmonary disease. Ann Intern Med 2001; 134(7):595–599.

80. Carrera M, Sala E, Cosío BG, et al. [Hospital treatment of chronic obstructive pulmonary disease exacerbations: an evidence-based review]. Arch Bronconeumol 2005; 41(4):220–229.

81. Bach PB, Brown C, Gelfand SE, et al. Management of acute exacerbations of chronic obstructive pulmonary disease: a summary and appraisal of published evidence. Ann Intern Med 2001; 134(7):600–620.

82. Balter MS, La Forge J, Low DE, et al. Canadian guidelines for the management of acute exacerbations of chronic bronchitis. Can Respir J 2003; 10(suppl B):3B–32B.

83. Murphy TF, Sethi S. Chronic obstructive pulmonary disease: role of bacteria and guide to antibacterial selection in the older patient. Drugs Aging 2002; 19(10):761–775.

84. Ram FS, Rodriguez-Roisin R, Granados-Navarrete A, et al. Antibiotics for exacerbations of chronic obstructive pulmonary disease. Cochrane Database Syst Rev 2006; (2):CD004403.

85. Miravitlles M, Murio C, Guerrero T. Factors associated with relapse after ambulatory treatment of acute exacerbations of chronic bronchitis. DAFNE Study Group. Eur Respir J 2001; 17(5):928–933.
86. Global Initiative for Obstructive Lung Disease. Available at: www.goldcopd.com.
87. McCrory DC, Brown CD. Anticholinergic bronchodilators versus beta2-sympathomimetic agents for acute exacerbations of chronic obstructive pulmonary disease. Cochrane Database Syst Rev 2003; 1:CD003900.
88. MacNee W. Acute exacerbations of COPD. Swiss Med Wkly 2003; 133(17–18):247–257.
89. Albert RK, Martin TR, Lewis SW. Controlled clinical trial of methylprednisolone in patients with chronic bronchitis and acute respiratory insufficiency. Ann Intern Med 1980; 92(6):753–758.
90. Niewoehner DE, Erbland ML, Deupree RH, et al. Effect of systemic glucocorticoids on exacerbations of chronic obstructive pulmonary disease. Department of Veterans Affairs Cooperative Study Group. N Engl J Med 1999; 340(25):1941–1947.
91. Quon BS, Gan WQ, Sin DD. Contemporary management of acute exacerbations of COPD: a systematic review and metaanalysis. Chest 2008; 133(3):756–766.
92. McCrory DC, Brown C, Gelfand SE, et al. Management of acute exacerbations of COPD: a summary and appraisal of published evidence. Chest 2001; 119(4):1190–1209.

6
Bronchiectasis

PAUL KING
Monash Medical Centre/Monash University, Clayton, Melbourne, Victoria, Australia

I. Introduction

Bronchiectasis is defined as permanent dilatation of the bronchi and is a radiologic or pathologic diagnosis. Cylindrical or tubular bronchiectasis is characterized by dilated airways alone, varicose bronchiectasis by focal narrowed areas along dilated airways, and cystic bronchiectasis by progressive dilatation of the airways that end in cysts or saccules.

Bronchiectasis in the pre-antibiotic era predominantly affected young patients and was associated with a high mortality rate (1). The introduction of antibiotics led to a dramatic improvement in outcome, and it was generally assumed that bronchiectasis would no longer be a significant condition. However, the recent usage of high-resolution computerized tomography (HRCT) scanning had made the diagnosis of bronchiectasis considerably easier, and there has been a renewed awareness of this disease.

The prevalence of bronchiectasis is not well defined. There are reports of high rates of bronchiectasis in indigenous populations, including Australian aborigines (2) and Alaskan natives (3). A recent study by Weycker et al. estimated that there were at least 110,000 adult subjects with bronchiectasis in the United States (4). Tsang and Tipoe (5) reported that bronchiectasis remained a major health issue in Asia, with a hospital admission rate of 16.4 per 100,000 people in Hong Kong (and the actual outpatient rate in the population would be expected to be much higher). Two recent studies have reported that 29% to 50% of subjects with chronic obstructive pulmonary disease (COPD) have associated bronchiectasis on CT scanning (6,7). These data suggest that bronchiectasis remains a major health issue.

II. Pathology and Pathophysiology

The most definitive study of the pathology of bronchiectasis was performed over 50 years ago by Whitwell, who examined 200 consecutive operative lung samples (8). He described chronic inflammation of the bronchial wall with loss of the elastin layer and in more advanced cases destruction of muscle and cartilage, and in nearly all cases there was evidence of parenchymal damage. Most cases could be classified as follicular bronchiectasis with lymphoid follicles and interstitial pneumonia. The lymphoid follicles were associated with airway obstruction and loss of elastic tissue. Studies have demonstrated a mononuclear bronchial wall infiltrate with the predominant cell being the T lymphocyte (9,10). Other investigators have established that the pulmonary arteries thrombose and may recanalize, but the vascular supply to the affected area was derived mainly from the hypertrophy of bronchial arteries and their anastomoses with pulmonary arteries (11,12).

Bronchiectasis is the end result of a variety of different pathologic causes. There are no well-accepted animal models of bronchiectasis, nor have there been any studies performed on patients in the early stages of bronchiectasis. As a consequence, the pathophysiologic processes involved are still not well defined.

The dominant feature of bronchiectasis is airway inflammation, which in nearly all cases is due to infection with microorganisms that are generally bacterial. In addition to infection, factors that appear to be important in the pathogenesis of bronchiectasis include airway obstruction or impairment of host defense (9,13). Persistent nonclearing infection results in airway inflammation with host damage. A reinforcing cycle results with inflammation producing airway damage, impaired mucociliary clearance, and further infection, which then completes the cycle by causing more inflammation. This is often referred to as the "vicious cycle hypothesis" (14).

The mucosal inflammation in bronchiectasis is characterized by a complex interaction between the effects of pathogenic microorganisms and the host defense (15). Recent studies have suggested there is an excessive airway response that persisted despite control of infection (16,17).

Bacteria have been demonstrated to have a number of direct effects on the airway. A primary feature of the vicious cycle model is the ability of pathogens to impair mucociliary function resulting in airway colonization (14). *Pseudomonas aeruginosa* (18) and more recently *Haemophilus influenzae* (19) have been shown to be capable of producing biofilms on airway epithelium. *P. aeruginosa* may cause direct damage to the airway epithelium (20).

Exaggerated neutrophil responses are thought to be important, with the production of mediators that include reactive oxygen species, elastase, and matrix metalloproteinase (15). Dysregulation of cytokine networks and lymphocyte, macrophage, and epithelial cell responses have all been implicated in the pathophysiology of bronchiectasis (16,21).

III. Etiology of Bronchiectasis

There are a large number of factors and conditions that have been associated with bronchiectasis, but most commonly, the condition is idiopathic (5,22–24). In addition most factors are associative rather than being a definitive cause of the condition (Table 1).

A. Cystic Fibrosis and Noncystic Fibrosis Bronchiectasis

Bronchiectasis is generally classified into cystic fibrosis (CF) and non-CF bronchiectasis. Unless specified, literature on bronchiectasis in adults generally refers to the non-CF form. This is still some controversy about this distinction. CF arises from a mutation in the cystic fibrosis transmembrane conductance regulator (CFTR) gene, which is responsible for the movement of sodium and chloride through the apical membrane of airway epithelial cells. There are over 1000 recognized mutations of the CFTR gene, and it has been recognized recently that CF may present atypically in adults. The expression may also be modified by the presence of a 5T mutation (25). The prevalence of undiagnosed CF in adults with bronchiectasis is not known although recent work suggests that it is low (26,27).

Table 1 Conditions Associated with Bronchiectasis

Postinfection complications
Bacteria (mycobacterial), whooping cough, viral
Mucociliary clearance defects
Primary ciliary dyskinesia, Young's syndrome
Mechanical bronchial obstruction
Luminal foreign body, stenosis, tumor, lymph node
Immune disorder
Include hypogammaglobulinemia, HIV,
ABPA, post-lung transplant
Aspiration
Chronic inflammatory conditions
Rheumatoid arthritis, inflammatory bowel disease
Miscellaneous
COPD, α-1-antitrypsin deficiency

Abbreviation: ABPA, allergic bronchopulmonary aspergillosis.

B. Mucociliary Clearance

Mucociliary clearance is a first-line defense against pathogenic microorganisms and compromise may result in bronchiectasis. Apart from CF, other mucociliary defects are primary ciliary dyskinesia syndrome and Young's syndrome. Primary ciliary dyskinesia is characterized by immotile cilia that contribute to retaining of secretions and microbial pathogens. Approximately half of the patients with primary ciliary dyskinesia have Kartagener's syndrome (bronchiectasis, sinusitis, and situs inversus) (22). Young's syndrome is characterized by obstructive azoospermia, and the defect in mucociliary clearance appears to arise from tenacious, poorly cleared mucous (28,29). Family history and infertility are associated factors that suggest there may be a primary mucociliary disorder. Such subjects should all be screened for CF. Mucociliary disorders are hard to diagnose as infection damages ciliary function independently and the electron microscopy of cilia is highly specialized and not routinely available.

C. Postinfectious Complications

The factor most commonly associated with bronchiectasis is childhood infection. The implication is often that an episode of lower respiratory infection of short duration results in bronchiectasis. There is a high incidence of bronchiectasis in populations with poor health and recurrent infection such as the indigenous Australian and Alaskan Indians; however, there are other factors that complicate this association. Firstly, the attribution of bronchiectasis generally relies on long-term retrospective recall that may result in over-ascription to infective causes. Patients with primary disorders of their immune function or respiratory tract are more likely to experience significant or recurrent infections, for example, subjects with CF are prone to severe infections in early childhood. The infections that have been most commonly associated with bronchiectasis, whooping cough, measles, and pneumonia are extremely common, with the seroprevalence of whooping cough or pertussis estimated to be greater than 50% (30) and measles more than 90% in unvaccinated adults in Westernized countries. It is also generally not known whether patients have had low-grade bronchiectasis that was present before any recognized infective episode.

Mycobacterial infections [mainly *Mycobacterium tuberculosis* and *Mycobacterium avium* complex (MAC)] may result in bronchiectasis. MAC infections have a particular clinicopathologic subtype that affects older women usually in the right middle lobe and lingula. This clinical phenotype is sometimes referred to as the "Lady Windermere syndrome." MAC may cause bronchial obstruction and lung nodules with slowly progressive lung destruction (31).

D. Immune Disorders

There are an increasing number of immune deficiencies associated with bronchiectasis. Obstructive and ciliary disorders may be considered to be primary disorders of immune defense as airway clearance mechanisms contribute an important component of innate or barrier immunity. Other disorders that result in bronchiectasis are HIV infection (32), hypogammaglobulinemia, and a variety of rare immune deficiency disorders that include transporter associated with antigen processing (TAP) deficiency (33), ataxia-telangectasia (34), hyperimmunoglobulinemia E (35), and major histocompatibility complex 1 (MHC-I) deficiency. Hypogammaglobulinemia can be classified into subjects with low levels of immunoglobulin G (IgG), such as common variable immune deficiency and Bruton's disease, and other forms such as IgA deficiency and IgG subclass deficiency. Subjects with low levels of total IgG are likely to benefit from replacement therapy. The role of IgG subclass deficiency is controversial in the pathogenesis of bronchiectasis (36).

Subjects with allergic bronchopulmonary aspergillosis (ABPA) may have bronchiectasis. Possible etiologic mechanisms include obstruction arising from fungal plugs, immune reaction to the fungus in the airway wall, and eosinophilic inflammation of the peribronchial tissues. The syndrome bronchiolitis obliterans arising as a complication of lung transplantation in its advanced stages is effectively a form of bronchiectasis.

E. Mechanical Bronchial Obstruction

Obstruction of the bronchi is an important mechanism of developing bronchiectasis both in terms of a primary cause and as a secondary cause in association with excessive secretions and poor mucociliary clearance. Primary airway obstruction is associated with localized bronchiectasis and anecdotally is very common in the context of bronchogenic carcinoma.

F. Aspiration

Reflux of stomach contents with aspiration may be an important etiologic factor in bronchiectasis, although this is difficult to prove with clinical studies. Aspiration associated with bronchiectasis has been reported to have a higher-than-expected incidence of *Helicobacter pylori* seroprevalence (37). However another study found no association between *H. pylori* and bronchiectasis (38). A retrospective study of 100,000 subjects of subjects with esophagitis and stricture found an increased incidence of bronchiectasis (odds ratio of 1.26) (39).

G. Rheumatic and Chronic Inflammatory Conditions

Certain chronic inflammatory diseases, particularly rheumatoid arthritis and inflammatory bowel disease (40), are important etiologic factors. Bronchiectasis has been described as preceding arthritis as well as occurring in the course of rheumatoid arthritis.

In rheumatoid arthritis clinics the incidence of bronchiectasis has been described to be 1% to 3%, and several studies report the prevalence of bronchiectasis on HRCT in such patients being up to 30% (41,42). The immunosuppressant medications that such patients are on may also be a risk factor for the development of bronchiectasis (43).

H. α-1-Antitrypsin Deficiency

The primary manifestation of α-1-antitrypsin deficiency is COPD. A recent study of a cohort of subjects with this condition found that over 90% have evidence of bronchiectasis with clinically significant disease in 27% (44).

IV. Clinical Features of Bronchiectasis

Over the past 30 to 40 years there have been relatively few published studies about the clinical features of bronchiectasis (23,24,45–48). The main findings from these studies are that disease is more common in females and most commonly presents in the sixth decade of life (Table 2). The dominant symptom is a chronic cough with purulent sputum. Sputum volume is correlated with quality of life and decline in respiratory function (24,49). This symptom is present in over 90% of subjects and has been present for many years in most subjects. Subjects often suffer significant social embarrassment from their cough. Chest pain is present in 20% to 30%. Hemoptysis has a similar frequency to chest pain but is a dramatic symptom and will often cause patients to seek immediate medical advice. Rarely patients present with large volume hemoptysis [defined as >200 mL/hr (50)]; such patients need immediate referral to an emergency department. Two symptoms that are very common in subjects with bronchiectasis are rhinosinusitis and fatigue. The incidence of rhinosinusitis may be as high as 60% to 70% and ranges in severity from a mild postnasal drip to fulminant pansinusitis. Most subjects with bronchiectasis will have demonstrable abnormalities on CT scanning of their

Table 2 Clinical, Spirometric, and Microbiologic Findings in Bronchiectasis

	Mean	Range
Clinical features		
Age (yr)	57	52–60
Female sex (%)	65	62–69
Productive cough (%)	95	91–98
Daily sputum (%)	73	69–76
Rhinosinusitis (%)	66	58–72
Dyspnea (%)	75	72–82
Crackles (%)	75	70–86
Spirometry		
FEV_1 (% predicted)	65	49–75
BD effect $\geq$ 15% (%)	32	24–40
Microbiology		
Haemophilus influenzae	44	23–70
Pseudomonas aeruginosa	19	10–31
No growth	30	21–39

Source: From Refs. 5, 23, 24, 45–48, and 55–61.

nose and sinuses (ranging from mild mucosal thickening to purulent pansinusitis). Chronic fatigue is a prominent symptom and may be present in up to 60% to 70% of patients and be associated with weight loss presumably related to systemic inflammation (5,24).

The main finding on examination is the presence of crackles that are present in over 60% of patients and are most commonly bilateral and basal. Wheeze is present in about 20% of patients. Clubbing, often thought of as a classical feature of bronchiectasis, is rarely reported.

There is a great variety in the symptoms and clinical course of subjects with bronchiectasis. Tsang and Tipoe have described four different stereotypes of bronchiectasis: (i) rapidly progressive, (ii) slowly progressive, (iii) indolent disease, and (iv) predominantly hemoptysis (5).

V. Radiology in the Diagnosis of Bronchiectasis

Chest X rays usually have nonspecific findings of increased lung markings (51). HRCT is the standard test now used to diagnose bronchiectasis. The HRCT criteria for diagnosing bronchiectasis have been well established (52). The most specific criteria are (i) internal diameter of bronchus wider than its adjacent artery, (ii) failure of the bronchi to taper, and (iii) bronchi detectable in the outer 1 to 2 cm of lung fields (Fig. 1). These criteria have been based on the comparison of HRCT and pathology examination of subsequently resected lung samples (52). Other less-specific features are bronchial wall thickening, crowding of the bronchi, and mucus impaction. Bronchial wall thickening appears to indicate airway inflammation and is associated with increased decline in lung function (53). The most common pattern on CT scanning is tubular bronchiectasis, which is multilobar. HRCT is rapidly advancing and virtual bronchoscopy is now becoming available.

VI. Spirometry

Bronchiectasis is characterized by mild to moderate airflow obstruction (23,24,45,46). The mechanism for airflow obstruction in bronchiectasis may arise primarily from inflammation in the small airways (54). A reduced forced vital capacity (FVC) may indicate that the airways are obstructed with mucus, they collapse with forced exhalation, or there is consolidation in the lung. Airway hyperresponsiveness may be associated with bronchiectasis. One study found this to be present in 40% of subjects with bronchiectasis (55) and two other studies found that 30% to 69% of patients had a 20% decrease in FEV_1 after histamine challenge (56,57). Whether this hyperresponsiveness represents asthma or is secondary to the effects of chronic bronchial inflammation is unknown.

VII. Microbiology

A number of pathogens have been isolated from the sputum of subjects with bronchiectasis. The frequency of isolates varies significantly between different locations, and an accurate profile of the local microbiologic flora is very important in guiding management.

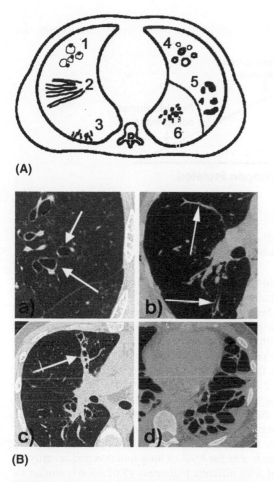

Figure 1 CT scan features of bronchiectasis (**A**) demonstrates CT features of bronchiectasis (1) bronchial dilatation, (2) non-tapering bronchi, (3) bronchi in outer 1 to 2 cm of lung, (4) bronchial thickening, (5) mucoid impaction, and (6) crowding of bronchi. (**B**) Scan of (a) bronchial dilatation, (b) nontapering bronchi, (c) varicose bronchiectasis, and (d) cystic bronchiectasis.

Recent studies have assessed the microbiologic profile in bronchiectasis (23,24,45,58–61). The most common pathogens isolated are *H. influenzae* followed by *P. aeruginosa*. Other important pathogens include *Moxarella catarrhalis*, *Streptococcus pneumoniae*, and *Aspergillus* species (principally *A. fumigatus*). *H. influenzae* in adults is nearly always the nonencapsulated form and this is designated as nontypeable *H. influenzae* (NTHi) (as opposed to type b). Yields of *H. influenzae* can be increased by the use of enriched media and bronchoscopic sampling. Both NTHi and *P. aeruginosa* have many different strains and cultures may show multiple subtypes in individual patients. *Staphylococcus aureus* is relatively uncommon, and its repeated isolation should lead to consideration of undiagnosed cystic fibrosis. A consistent finding of the studies is that about

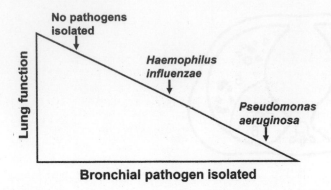

Figure 2 Relation between bronchial pathogens and lung function. As lung function declines there is a change in commonly isolated pathogens from sputum.

30% of sputum samples will show no growth. This may be partly a reflection of the fact the sputum samples are often suboptimal, but even when using bronchoscopy specimens 30% of specimens show no growth (58). There has been considerable recent interest in non-tuberculous mycobacteria (NTM) principally MAC. The reported prevalence has varied between studies, with one study reporting NTM as being uncommon (62) while another identified 10% of subjects being culture positive (63). There are no data that define the role of viruses in acute exacerbations and in the chronic phase of bronchiectasis, although viral infection has been shown to have a role in COPD (64).

There is likely to be increasing emphasis on more sophisticated microbiologic techniques, including enzyme-linked immunosorbent assay (ELISA) and polymerase chain reaction (PCR) to characterize the microbiologic flora in bronchiectasis. Ideally specimens should be obtained using bronchoscopy, including bronchoalveolar lavage and biopsy.

Another feature of bronchiectasis is that the level of lung function and severity of bronchiectasis is apparently associated with different pathogens (5,61,65–67) similar to CF (Fig. 2). Subjects with well-preserved lung function commonly will have no pathogens isolated; *H. influenzae* is most commonly present in subjects with mildly or moderately impaired lung function, while *P. aeruginosa* and other resistant gram-negative organisms are most prevalent in severe disease.

VIII. Treatment

Patients with bronchiectasis will generally need prolonged or lifelong medical support, particularly for the management of exacerbations. The development of a management plan may be of significant benefit to patients (68). A large number of options are available for the treatment of non-CF bronchiectasis, including antibiotics, physiotherapy, bronchodilators, surgery, inhaled corticosteroids, and vaccination. There have been few clinical trials of treatments in this condition, and those that have been done usually have had less than 20 patients. There is, therefore, a lack of good supporting evidence for specific therapies in bronchiectasis.

A. Antibiotics

Antibiotics are used principally to treat acute exacerbations but also to reduce chronic bacterial load and improve chronic symptoms. Antibiotic selection in bronchiectasis is complex due to the wide range of pathogens involved, the presence of resistant organisms, and the damaged lung architecture. Biofilms protect some pathogens such as *P. aeruginosa* from antibiotics. Many patients are colonized simultaneously with multiple pathogens. Bacteria may live in extracellular or intracellular components of the lung. Some bacteria are predominantly extracellular (e.g., *Staphylococcus* and *Streptococcus*), some live predominantly intracellularly (e.g., *Chlamydia* and *Legionella*), and some can be found in both extra and intracellular components (e.g., *H. influenzae*). Intracellular pathogens are protected from many antibiotics with poor cellular penetration such as β-lactams. Giving a β-lactam with an antibiotic with good intracellular penetration (e.g., tetracycline/macrolide/quinolone) may cover a broad spectrum of pathogens (69). Subjects with bronchiectasis usually receive longer courses of treatment for acute exacerbations than other subjects, although there is no proper evidence to support this practice. Microbiologic sputum analysis should be done regularly, and patients should probably have bronchoscopy samples taken at some stage.

There is debate about whether antibiotics should only be used for exacerbations or be used more regularly to control the chronic inflammation associated with bacterial infection. The main concern about the regular use of antibiotics is the development of resistance. The use of oral quinolones to treat *Pseudomonas* infections is often associated with resistance after one to two courses of treatment (70). There is some evidence to show that regular treatment with antibiotics either continuously or on a monthly basis produces some benefits, including reduction in symptoms, reduction in sputum purulence and enzyme content, reduction in colonizing microbial load in sputum, and reduction in lung inflammation and better lung function (71).

Route of administration is also important with sicker patients generally treated intravenously. In trials of nebulized antibiotics, four have assessed nebulized tobramycin and shown that some patients significantly improved and pathogen clearance occurred in many subjects (72). Further work is needed to define which patients will benefit most from nebulized tobramycin. Aerolized gentamicin administered for three days decreased sputum production and desaturation, while improving lung function (73).

Recent studies in patients with CF have demonstrated that treatment with inhaled antibiotics (e.g., colistin), which may be given in combination with oral ciprofloxacin, can eradicate early *Pseudomonas* infection. This may have significant benefit for patients (74). One small trail has assessed the use of colistin in bronchiectasis with promising results (75). It is theoretically possible that bacterial eradication therapy may have a role in the treatment of bronchiectasis not only in controlling *Pseudomonas* infection but also potentially earlier in the course of the disease for other pathogens such as *H. influenzae*.

B. Anti-inflammatory Treatment

Oral corticosteroids appear to slow progression of lung disease in CF but have major side effects (76). There are no randomized trials to recommend the use of oral steroids in bronchiectasis. There may be some benefit from the use of inhaled corticosteroids (ICS) in bronchiectasis with decreased sputum, and this may be a marker of airway inflammation (77) Macrolides have immunomodulatory properties, including inhibiting virulence factors, biofilm formation, and inflammatory mediator release, and have been shown to have significant benefit in CF. There is preliminary evidence of benefit in bronchiectasis with decreased sputum volume and improved lung function and symptom control (77).

C. Bronchopulmonary Hygiene and Pulmonary Rehabilitation

Optimizing sputum clearance may be beneficial in subjects with bronchiectasis. The patient may also be less likely to have sputum production occurring unexpectedly and causing social embarrassment and interrupting sleep. Traditional chest percussion and tipping methods have been replaced to a large extent by mechanical chest vibration or oral devices applying positive end-expiratory pressure that are better tolerated. Despite use for many years and a number of uncontrolled trials, a review found very little hard evidence to support chest physiotherapy and postural drainage (78). However, it is extremely difficult to design a randomized trial for chest physiotherapy. Dry powder mannitol improves tracheobronchial clearance; hypertonic saline has not been specifically tested in bronchiectasis but improves clearance in normal controls, CF, and chronic bronchitis (79). A randomized trial demonstrated that pulmonary rehabilitation improved exercise tolerance in bronchiectasis (80).

D. Bronchodilator Treatment

As a significant proportion of patients with bronchiectasis have airway reversibility, bronchodilators may be useful. Long-acting β-2-agonists have been used for subjects with bronchiectasis, but a Cochrane review concluded that there were no randomized trials to support their use at this stage (81). There are no good data to support the use of anticholinergic therapy in bronchiectasis. Good quality studies are needed in this area.

E. Surgery

There are no randomized trials of the use of surgery. In selected patients with localized bronchiectasis that cause intolerable symptoms despite medical therapy, surgery should be considered (76). Studies report that 80% of patients improve after surgery with low mortality and morbidity (82,83). Double lung transplantation has been carried out in patients with CF and has a 75% survival rate at one year and 48% at five years (84). Patients with non-CF bronchiectasis have also undergone lung transplant, but statistics are not available. Surgery may be required for the treatment of empyema.

F. Management of Hemoptysis

Torrential life-threatening hemoptysis can occur in bronchiectasis and requires an appropriate management plan. This complication may be associated with the hypertrophy of the bronchial arteries that occurs in this condition. Patients should be positioned to lie on the side where bleeding is suspected and the site of bleeding determined using bronchoscopy or CT angiogram (85). If interventional radiology is available, bronchial artery embolization may be performed (86).

G. Other Management Issues

Vaccination is commonly recommended for subjects with COPD. Inactivated influenza vaccines may reduce exacerbations in COPD (87) and pneumococcal vaccine may be useful. There appears to be minimal literature that reviews subjects with bronchiectasis, but it is logical to assume that they would also benefit. Smoking is associated with worse lung function (88), and all subjects should be encouraged to stop smoking. Reflux should be treated appropriately. Noninvasive ventilation (NIV) may be beneficial for acute hypercapnic respiratory failure in CF (89) and bronchiectasis (90), although its role in chronic respiratory failure is not well defined. Subjects with hypogammaglobulinemia should receive regular Ig replacement therapy. Augmentation therapy in subjects with α-1-antitrypsin deficiency should also be considered. Management of chronic rhinosinusitis may be optimized by referral to an otolaryngeal surgeon.

H. Severe Bronchiectasis

Subjects with severely impaired lung function should have an oxygen assessment and echocardiography to look for evidence of pulmonary hypertension or right-heart failure. Consideration should be given to admitting the patient regularly for a "tune-up" as occurs in cystic fibrosis. NIV with chest physiotherapy may prevent sputum retention. Early referral to a lung transplantation center should be considered.

IX. Differential Diagnosis

Bronchiectasis may be confused with other airway diseases particularly asthma and COPD. The clinical feature that distinguishes bronchiectasis from other lung conditions is the production of large amounts of purulent sputum. In other ways, the three conditions of bronchiectasis, COPD, and asthma have considerable overlap, and some patients clearly suffer from all three conditions. With the current sensitivity of HRCT scanning, bronchiectasis is increasingly being regarded as a form of chronic bronchitis.

X. Prognosis

The outcome in bronchiectasis has substantially improved, but it is still a cause of excess mortality with mortality rate reported to be 13% (death arising directly from bronchiectasis) over a five-year follow-up period (91). The general impression is that patients with bronchiectasis gradually become worse over time (5). A study of 101 nonsmoking patients who were followed up for eight years demonstrated that subjects had persistent symptoms with worse dyspnea and sputum production and an excess decline in FEV_1 of 49 mL/yr (or ~1% predicted). A significant association was found between the volume of sputum and decline in FEV_1 (24). Another recent prospective study that followed up subjects for two years found a similar excess decline in FEV_1 as well (53 mL/yr) (65). A longitudinal study with 5.7 years of follow-up found that children with bronchiectasis had a fall of 1.9% in percentage predicted FEV_1 (using best annual data) per year (92). The presence of *Pseudomonas* is associated with more sputum, more extensive bronchiectasis on HRCT, more hospitalizations, and worse quality of life (65,93).

XI. Clinical Scenarios

A. Case 1

An 18-year-old woman presented for assessment of ongoing productive cough, nasal discharge, and shortness of breath. She described respiratory symptoms since early childhood with purulent sputum production and chest infections requiring antibiotics several times a year. A CT scan demonstrated widespread bronchiectasis and pan-sinusitis. There was no identifiable etiologic factor. Lung function tests showed severe airflow obstruction with an FEV_1 of 48% predicted. The patient was treated aggressively with antibiotics, chest physiotherapy, and bronchodilators over a three-month period. This produced a marked improvement in her symptoms and lung function (FEV_1 improved to 91% predicted). She was followed up over the next three years and had a fluctuating course.

Teaching Points

- Patients often have a productive cough for a number of years before a diagnosis of bronchiectasis is made.
- Sinus involvement is common in those with childhood-onset symptoms.
- There is often no identifiable etiology.
- Subjects tend to have fluctuating severity of disease.

B. Case 2

A 75-year-old man presented for assessment of a three-year history of productive cough. He had been previously well and was a lifelong nonsmoker. He described the insidious onset of a cough with small amounts of discolored sputum that persisted. The cough caused mild discomfort and significant social embarrassment. He had been previously diagnosed as having asthma and been treated with bronchodilators and inhaled corticosteroids with no obvious benefit. An HRCT scan demonstrated mild bibasal bronchiectasis. There was no identifiable etiologic cause, and he had normal lung function.

Teaching Points

- The onset of a productive cough and the development of bronchiectasis may occur in the healthy elderly.
- Bronchiectasis should be distinguished from other airway diseases such as asthma.
- The diagnostic test required is an HRCT scan.

XII. Conclusion

The use of HRCT has made it apparent that bronchiectasis remains a common disease and a major health problem. The pathophysiology of this condition is not well under-stood, but it is likely that the role of previously unrecognized immune dysfunction will have increasing importance. Rather than being a discrete entity, bronchiectasis is the result of a variety of different mechanisms, and it may be more appropriate to consider it as a syndrome (e.g., like glomerulonephritis) characterized by chronic airway infection and bronchial damage.

Bronchiectasis is heterogeneous in its clinical features, but most patients appear to gradually become worse over time. It has considerable overlap with other chronic airway diseases. Treatment regimes are not well defined and further research is particularly needed to improve patient management.

Acknowledgment

The author would like to thank Associate Professor Peter Holmes for his help in this work.

References

1. Perry KMA, King DS. Bronchiectasis, a study of prognosis based on a follow-up of 400 cases. Am Rev Tuber 1940; 1940(41):153.
2. Chang AB, Grimwood K, Mulholland EK, et al. Bronchiectasis in indigenous children in remote Australian communities. Med J Aust 2002; 177(4):200–204.
3. Singleton R, Morris A, Redding G, et al. Bronchiectasis in Alaska Native children: causes and clinical courses. Pediatr Pulmonol 2000; 29(3):182–187.
4. Weycker D, Edelsberg J, Oster G, et al. Prevalence and economic burden of bronchiectasis. Clinical Pulm Medicine 2005; 4(12):205–209.
5. Tsang KW, Tipoe GL. Bronchiectasis: not an orphan disease in the East. Int J Tuberc Lung Dis 2004; 8(6):691–702.
6. O'Brien C, Guest PJ, Hill SL, et al. Physiological and radiological characterisation of patients diagnosed with chronic obstructive pulmonary disease in primary care. Thorax 2000; 55(8): 635–642.
7. Patel IS, Vlahos I, Wilkinson TM, et al. Bronchiectasis, exacerbation indices and inflammation in chronic obstructive pulmonary disease. Am J Respir Crit Care Med 2004; 170:400–407.
8. Whitwell F. A study of the pathology and pathogenesis of bronchiectasis. Thorax 1952; 7:213–219.
9. Lapa e Silva JR, Guerreiro D, Noble B, et al. Immunopathology of experimental bronchiectasis. Am J Respir Cell Mol Biol 1989; 1(4):297–304.
10. Eller J, Lapa e Silva JR, Poulter LW, et al. Cells and cytokines in chronic bronchial infection. Ann N Y Acad Sci 1994; 725:331–345.
11. Liebow AA, Hales MR, Lindsberg GE. Enlargement of the bronchial arteries and their anastomoses with pulmonary arteries in bronchiectasis. Am J Pathol 1949; 25:211–230.
12. Marchand P, Gilroy JC, Wilson VH. An anatomical study of the bronchial vascular system and its variation in disease. Thorax 1950; 5:207–215.
13. Tannenberg J, Pinner M. Atelectasis and bronchiectasis: an experimental study concerning their relationship. J Thorac Surg 1942; 11:571–582.
14. Cole PJ. Inflammation: a two-edged sword–the model of bronchiectasis. Eur J Respir Dis Suppl 1986; 147:6–15.
15. Fuschillo S, De Felice A, Balzano G. Mucosal inflammation in idiopathic bronchiectasis: cellular and molecular mechanisms. Eur Respir J 2008; 31(2):396–406.
16. Aldallal N, McNaughton EE, Manzel LJ, et al. Inflammatory response in airway epithelial cells isolated from patients with cystic fibrosis. Am J Respir Crit Care Med 2002; 166(9): 1248–1256.
17. Chmiel JF, Davis PB. State of the art: why do the lungs of patients with cystic fibrosis become infected and why can't they clear the infection? Respir Res 2003; 4:8.
18. Meluleni GJ, Grout M, Evans DJ, et al. Mucoid Pseudomonas aeruginosa growing in a biofilm in vitro are killed by opsonic antibodies to the mucoid exopolysaccharide capsule but not by antibodies produced during chronic lung infection in cystic fibrosis patients. J Immunol 1995; 155(4):2029–2038.
19. Starner TD, Zhang N, Kim G, et al. Haemophilus influenzae forms biofilms on airway epithelia: implications in cystic fibrosis. Am J Respir Crit Care Med 2006; 174(2):213–220.
20. Amitani R, Wilson R, Rutman A, et al. Effects of human neutrophil elastase and *Pseudomonas aeruginosa* proteinases on human respiratory epithelium. Am J Respir Cell Mol Biol 1991; 4(1):26–32.
21. King PT, Hutchinson PE, Johnson PD, et al. Adaptive immunity to nontypeable Haemophilus influenzae. Am J Respir Crit Care Med 2003; 167(4):587–592.

22. Barker AF. Bronchiectasis. N Engl J Med 2002; 346(18):1383–1393.
23. Pasteur MC, Helliwell SM, Houghton SJ, et al. An investigation into causative factors in patients with bronchiectasis. Am J Respir Crit Care Med 2000; 162(4 pt 1):1277–1284.
24. King PT, Holdsworth SR, Freezer NJ, et al. Outcome in adult bronchiectasis. J COPD 2005; 2 (1):27–34.
25. Griesenbach U, Geddes DM, Alton EW. The pathogenic consequences of a single mutated CFTR gene. Thorax 1999; 54(suppl 2):S19–S23.
26. King PT, Freezer NJ, Holmes PW, et al. Role of CFTR mutations in adult bronchiectasis. Thorax 2004; 59(4):357–358.
27. Divac A, Nikolic A, Mitic-Milikic M, et al. CFTR mutations and polymorphisms in adults with disseminated bronchiectasis: a controversial issue. Thorax 2005; 60(1):85.
28. Greenstone MA, Rutman A, Hendry WF, et al. Ciliary function in Young's syndrome. Thorax 1988; 43(2):153–154.
29. Friedman KJ, Teichtahl H, De Kretser DM, et al. Screening Young syndrome patients for CFTR mutations. Am J Respir Crit Care Med 1995; 152(4 pt 1):1353–1357.
30. Garcia-Corbeira P, Dal-Re R, Aguilar L, et al. Seroepidemiology of Bordetella pertussis infections in the Spanish population: a cross-sectional study. Vaccine 2000; 18(21):2173–2176.
31. Prince DS, Peterson DD, Steiner RM, et al. Infections with Mycobacterium avium complex in patients without predisposing conditions. N Engl J Med 1989; 321:896–898.
32. Zar HJ. Chronic lung disease in human immunodeficiency virus (HIV) infected children. Pediatr Pulmonol 2008; 43(1):1–10.
33. Zimmer J, Andres E, Hentges F. Transporter associated with antigen processing deficiency: an additional condition associated with bronchiectasis. Intern Med J 2007; 37(3):208–209; author reply 9–10.
34. Bott L, Lebreton J, Thumerelle C, et al. Lung disease in ataxia-telangiectasia. Acta Paediatr 2007; 96(7):1021–1024.
35. L'Huillier JP, Thoreux PH, Delaval P, et al. The hyperimmunoglobulinaemia E and recurrent infections syndrome in an adult. Thorax 1990; 45(9):707–708.
36. Hill SL, Mitchell JL, Burnett D, Stockley RA. IgG subclasses in the serum and sputum from patients with bronchiectasis. Thorax 1998; 53(6):463–468.
37. Tsang KW, Lam SK, Lam WK, et al. High seroprevalence of Helicobacter pylori in active bronchiectasis. Am J Respir Crit Care Med 1998; 158(4):1047–1051.
38. Angrill J, Sanchez N, Agusti C, et al. Does Helicobacter pylori have a pathogenic role in bronchiectasis? Respir Med 2006; 100(7):1202–1207.
39. el-Serag HB, Sonnenberg A. Comorbid occurrence of laryngeal or pulmonary disease with esophagitis in United States military veterans. Gastroenterology 1997; 113(3):755–760.
40. Black H, Mendoza M, Murin S. Thoracic manifestations of inflammatory bowel disease. Chest 2007; 131(2):524–532.
41. Cortet B, Flipo RM, Remy-Jardin M, et al. Use of high resolution computed tomography of the lungs in patients with rheumatoid arthritis. Ann Rheum Dis 1995; 54(10):815–819.
42. Hassan WU, Keaney NP, Holland CD, et al. High resolution computed tomography of the lung in lifelong non-smoking patients with rheumatoid arthritis. Ann Rheum Dis 1995; 54(4): 308–310.
43. King P. Churgh-Strauss syndrome and bronchiectasis. Respir Med Extra 2007; 3:26–28.
44. Parr DG, Guest PG, Reynolds JH, et al. Prevalence and impact of bronchiectasis in alpha1-antitrypsin deficiency. Am J Respir Crit Care Med 2007; 176(12):1215–1221.
45. Nicotra MB, Rivera M, Dale AM, et al. Clinical, pathophysiologic, and microbiologic characterization of bronchiectasis in an aging cohort. Chest 1995; 108(4):955–961.
46. O'Donnell AE, Barker AF, Ilowite JS, et al. Treatment of idiopathic bronchiectasis with aerosolized recombinant human DNase I. rhDNase Study Group. Chest 1998; 113(5):1329–1334.

47. Smith IE, Jurriaans E, Diederich S, et al. Chronic sputum production: correlations between clinical features and findings on high resolution computed tomographic scanning of the chest. Thorax 1996; 51(9):914–918.
48. Mackay IS, Cole PJ. Rhinisitis, sinusitis and associated chest disease. In: Mackay IS, Bull TR, eds. Rhinology, Scott-Brown's Otolaryntology. 5th ed. London: Butterworths, 1987:61–90.
49. Martinez-Garcia MA, Perpina-Tordera M, Roman-Sanchez P, et al. Quality-of-life determinants in patients with clinically stable bronchiectasis. Chest 2005; 128(2):739–745.
50. Mal H, Rullon I, Mellot F, et al. Immediate and long-term results of bronchial artery embolization for life-threatening hemoptysis. Chest 1999; 115(4):996–1001.
51. Currie DC, Cooke JC, Morgan AD, et al. Interpretation of bronchograms and chest radiographs in patients with chronic sputum production. Thorax 1987; 42(4):278–284.
52. McGuinness G, Naidich DP. CT of airways disease and bronchiectasis. Radiol Clin North Am 2002; 40(1):1–19.
53. Sheehan RE, Wells AU, Copley SJ, et al. A comparison of serial computed tomography and functional change in bronchiectasis. Eur Respir J 2002; 20(3):581–857.
54. Roberts HR, Wells AU, Milne DG, et al. Airflow obstruction in bronchiectasis: correlation between computed tomography features and pulmonary function tests. Thorax 2000; 55(3):198–204.
55. Murphy MB, Reen DJ, Fitzgerald MX. Atopy, immunological changes, and respiratory function in bronchiectasis. Thorax 1984; 39(3):179–184.
56. Pang J, Chan HS, Sung JY. Prevalence of asthma, atopy, and bronchial hyperreactivity in bronchiectasis: a controlled study. Thorax 1989; 44(11):948–951.
57. Bahous J, Cartier A, Pineau L, et al. Pulmonary function tests and airway responsiveness to methacholine in chronic bronchiectasis of the adult. Bull Eur Physiopathol Respir 1984; 20(4):375–380.
58. Angrill J, Agusti C, de Celis R, et al. Bacterial colonisation in patients with bronchiectasis: microbiological pattern and risk factors. Thorax 2002; 57(1):15–19.
59. Pang JA, Cheng A, Chan HS, et al. The bacteriology of bronchiectasis in Hong Kong investigated by protected catheter brush and bronchoalveolar lavage. Am Rev Respir Dis 1989; 139(1):14–17.
60. Roberts DE, Cole P. Use of selective media in bacteriological investigation of patients with chronic suppurative respiratory infection. Lancet 1980; 1(8172):796–797.
61. King PT, Holdsworth SR, Freezer NJ, et al. Microbiologic follow-up study in adult bronchiectasis. Respir Med 2007; 101(8):1633–1638.
62. Wickremasinghe M, Ozerovitch LJ, Davies G, et al. Non-tuberculous mycobacteria in patients with bronchiectasis. Thorax 2005; 60(12):1045–1051.
63. Fowler SJ, French J, Screaton NJ, et al. Nontuberculous mycobacteria in bronchiectasis: Prevalence and patient characteristics. Eur Respir J 2006; 28(6):1204–1210.
64. Seemungal T, Harper-Owen R, Bhowmik A, et al. Respiratory viruses, symptoms, and inflammatory markers in acute exacerbations and stable chronic obstructive pulmonary disease. Am J Respir Crit Care Med 2001; 164(9):1618–1623.
65. Martinez-Garcia MA, Soler-Cataluna JJ, Perpina-Tordera M, et al. Factors associated with lung function decline in adult patients with stable non-cystic fibrosis bronchiectasis. Chest 2007; 132(5):1565–1572.
66. Wilson CB, Jones PW, O'Leary CJ, et al. Effect of sputum bacteriology on the quality of life of patients with bronchiectasis. Eur Respir J 1997; 10(8):1754–1760.
67. Angrill J, Agusti C, De Celis R, et al. Bronchial inflammation and colonization in patients with clinically stable bronchiectasis. Am J Respir Crit Care Med 2001; 164(9):1628–1632.
68. Lavery K, O'Neill B, Elborn JS, et al. Self-management in bronchiectasis: the patients' perspective. Eur Respir J 2007; 29(3):541–547.

69. Ahren IL, Karlsson E, Forsgren A, et al. Comparison of the antibacterial activities of
     ampicillin, ciprofloxacin, clarithromycin, telithromycin and quinupristin/dalfopristin against
     intracellular non-typeable Haemophilus influenzae. J Antimicrob Chemother 2002; 50(6):
     903–906.
70. Rayner CF, Tillotson G, Cole PJ, et al. Efficacy and safety of long-term ciprofloxacin in the
     management of severe bronchiectasis. J Antimicrob Chemother 1994; 34(1):149–156.
71. Evans DJ, Bara AI, Greenstone M. Prolonged antibiotics for purulent bronchiectasis.
     Cochrane Database Syst Rev 2003; (4):CD001392.
72. Lobue PA. Inhaled tobramycin: not just for cystic fibrosis anymore? Chest 2005; 127(4):
     1098–1101.
73. Lin HC, Cheng HF, Wang CH, et al. Inhaled gentamicin reduces airway neutrophil activity
     and mucus secretion in bronchiectasis. Am J Respir Crit Care Med 1997; 155(6):2024–2029.
74. Ratjen F. Treatment of early Pseudomonas aeruginosa infection in patients with cystic fib-
     rosis. Curr Opin Pulm Med 2006; 12(6):428–432.
75. Steinfort DP, Steinfort C. Effect of long-term nebulized colistin on lung function and quality
     of life in patients with chronic bronchial sepsis. Intern Med J 2007; 37(7):495–498.
76. Rosen MJ. Chronic cough due to bronchiectasis: ACCP evidence-based clinical practice
     guidelines. Chest 2006; 129(1 suppl):122S–131S.
77. King P. Is there a role for inhaled corticosteroids and macrolide therapy in bronchiectasis?
     Drugs 2007; 67(7):965–974.
78. Jones AP, Rowe BH. Bronchopulmonary hygiene physical therapy for chronic obstructive
     pulmonary disease and bronchiectasis. Cochrane Database Syst Rev 2000; (2):CD000045.
79. Wills P, Greenstone M. Inhaled hyperosmolar agents for bronchiectasis. Cochrane Database
     Syst Rev 2001; (2):CD002996.
80. Newall C, Stockley RA, Hill SL. Exercise training and inspiratory muscle training in patients
     with bronchiectasis. Thorax 2005; 60(11):943–948.
81. Sheikh A, Nolan D, Greenstone M. Long-acting beta-2-agonists for bronchiectasis. Cochrane
     Database Syst Rev 2001; (4):CD002155.
82. Agasthian T, Deschamps C, Trastek VF, et al. Surgical management of bronchiectasis. Ann
     Thorac Surg 1996; 62(4):976–978; discussion 9–80.
83. Balkanli K, Genc O, Dakak M, et al. Surgical management of bronchiectasis: analysis and
     short-term results in 238 patients. Eur J Cardiothorac Surg 2003; 24(5):699–702.
84. Yankaskas JR, Mallory GB Jr. Lung transplantation in cystic fibrosis: consensus conference
     statement. Chest 1998; 113(1):217–226.
85. McGuinness G, Beacher JR, Harkin TJ, et al. Hemoptysis: prospective high-resolution
     CT/bronchoscopic correlation. Chest 1994; 105(4):1155–1162.
86. Ashour M, Al-Kattan K, Rafay MA, et al. Current surgical therapy for bronchiectasis. World
     J Surg 1999; 23(11):1096–1104.
87. Poole PJ, Chacko E, Wood-Baker RW, et al. Influenza vaccine for patients with chronic
     obstructive pulmonary disease. Cochrane Database Syst Rev 2000; (4):CD002733.
88. King PT, Holdsworth SR, Freezer NJ, et al. Characterisation of the onset and presenting
     clinical features of adult bronchiectasis. Respir Med 2006; 100(12):2183–2189.
89. Holland AE, Denehy L, Ntoumenopoulos G, et al. Non-invasive ventilation assists chest phys-
     iotherapy in adults with acute exacerbations of cystic fibrosis. Thorax 2003; 58(10):880–884.
90. Non-invasive ventilation in acute respiratory failure. Thorax 2002; 57(3):192–211.
91. Keistinen T, Saynajakangas O, Tuuponen T, et al. Bronchiectasis: an orphan disease with a
     poorly-understood prognosis. Eur Respir J 1997; 10(12):2784–2787.
92. Twiss J, Stewart AW, Byrnes CA. Longitudinal pulmonary function of childhood bron-
     chiectasis and comparison with cystic fibrosis. Thorax 2006; 61(5):414–418.
93. Wilson CB, Jones PW, O'Leary CJ, et al. Validation of the St. George's Respiratory
     Questionnaire in bronchiectasis. Am J Respir Crit Care Med 1997; 156(2 pt 1):536–541.

7
Exacerbations of Cystic Fibrosis

RUXANA T. SADIKOT
Department of Veterans Affairs, Jesse Brown VA Hospital, and University of Illinois at Chicago, Chicago, Illinois, U.S.A.

I. Introduction

Cystic fibrosis (CF) is the most common autosomal recessive disease in Caucasians caused by mutation in the CF transmembrane conductance regulator gene (1–3). The spectrum of clinical presentation in CF is vast and depends on which organs are affected. Since the discovery of the CFTR gene in 1989, a broad spectrum of CF phenotypes has been associated with specific CFTR gene mutations (1). CF is characterized by chronic lung infection and inflammation, with periods of acute exacerbation causing severe and irreversible lung tissue damage. Although our understanding of the pathophysiology of CF has increased, pulmonary infections remain the major cause of morbidity and mortality in patients with CF.

Recurrent pulmonary exacerbations have a significant impact on quality of life, lead to frequent hospitalizations, and reduce respiratory function that is a likely contributor to long-term respiratory decline and increased mortality (4–8). The propensity of CF patients to frequent infections is related to the inability of these patients to adequately clear secretions. Thickened secretions caused by improper regulation of airway surface liquid lead to the accumulation of mucus in the airway and defective mucociliary clearance (9,10). Retained mucus plugs provide a niche for bacterial colonization and persistence. Frequent bacterial infections of the airway lead to persistent inflammatory response (11). Data from the CF registry in United States indicate that pulmonary exacerbations are the cause for hospitalization in 4% to 78% of children and 2% to 85% on adults with CF (12). Thus treatment of chronic bacterial infections is an integral component of management of patients with cystic fibrosis.

II. Definition

Despite the significance of acute exacerbations in the course of CF, there is a lack of consensus in the definition of these exacerbations (13,14). Most definitions combine patient symptomatology, laboratory data, and clinician evaluation. Criteria published by the Cystic Fibrosis Foundation Microbiology and Infectious Disease Consensus Conference in 1994 include the presence of at least three of 11 new findings or changes in clinical status when compared with the most recent baseline visit (Table 1). These criteria are most commonly used for the diagnosis of pulmonary exacerbation in patients with CF (15).

Table 1 Diagnostic Criteria for Pulmonary Exacerbation of Cystic Fibrosis

Increased cough or dyspnea
Increased amount (or change in appearance of) sputum
Decreased exercise tolerance
School or work absenteeism
Fever (38°C for 4 hr in a 24-hr period)
Weight loss (1 kg or 5% of body weight)
Increased respiratory rate or work of breathing
New wheeze or crackles
Decrease in FEV_1 or FVC of 10%
Decrease in oxygen saturation of 10% (compared with baseline within the past 3 mo)
New chest X ray findings

Abbreviations: FEV_1, forced expiratory volume in one second; FVC, forced vital capacity.

Clinical trials have defined an acute exacerbation of pulmonary symptoms on the basis of the above criteria and CF-related pulmonary symptoms that are severe enough to warrant hospital admission or use of intravenous antibiotics. These definitions of a pulmonary exacerbation have revolved around the clinician's decision to treat a constellation of symptoms, but a treatment decision-defined outcome is often problematic. Within the United States, practice patterns are heterogeneous with regard to the treatment decision for an exacerbation (16). Another problem is variation in the symptoms included in the definition in clinical studies such as the Pulmozyme study (17) and the inhaled tobramycin study (18).

Rosenfeld et al. used a multivariate modeling approach to identify patients with acute exacerbation. Patient history, physical findings, and pulmonary function tests were used to develop a diagnostic algorithm. Symptoms rather than physical findings or laboratory values were found to be more predictive of an exacerbation (19). Smith et al. found that the most predictive symptoms of exacerbation include increased cough, change in sputum (volume or consistency), decreased appetite, or weight (20). An increase in respiratory rate and change is respiratory examination has also found to be predictive of an exacerbation (13). The distinction between a mild and severe exacerbation is often arbitrary and depends on the treating physician. The spectrum of severity of an exacerbation can vary from requiring intravenous antibiotics to necessitating admission to the intensive care with ventilatory support.

III. Epidemiology

Acute pulmonary exacerbations in CF increase with worsening lung function and progression of disease. The frequency of exacerbation also increases with age. Data from CF registry showed that 20% to 30% of patients who are 18 years or older get two to three exacerbations annually, whereas 10% of younger patients, experience more than two exacerbations annually (12). Patients with progressive worsening of lung function also experience more frequent exacerbations. Among patients with a forced expiratory volume in one second (FEV_1) less than 30%, the mean frequency of exacerbation is two or more per year (12,15).

The annual rate of exacerbation has shown to predict five-year survival (4) with a worsening of survival in patients who have more than two exacerbations annually.

Patients requiring frequent intravenous antibiotics also show a rapid decline in lung function (21). Annual rates of hospitalization for patients with CF who are followed up in specialized CF centers in the USA ranges from 4% to 78% among children (median ~35%) and from zero to 85% (median ~45%) among adults. Most hospital admissions are for treatment of infective respiratory exacerbations, particularly the treatment of *Pseudomonas aeruginosa* infection. Exacerbations are also associated with increased mortality (4), poor quality of life, and increased health care costs (5–7).

IV. Etiology

Pulmonary exacerbations can be caused by viral or bacterial infections and in rare cases by other pathogens such as fungi. Viral infections are often associated with worsening of respiratory symptoms in CF. In 13% to 52% of patients with an increase in respiratory lower tract symptoms, a viral pathogen is detected, with a greater incidence in younger patients (22,23). A virus was detected in 40% of children with exacerbation, compared with only 9% in those who were clinically stable. Viruses that can cause acute infections include respiratory syncytial virus (RSV), influenza, parainfluenza, adenovirus, and picornavirus. Viral infections as cause of infective exacerbation are less frequent in adult patients (24). Colonization of the airway with fungi such as aspergillus also occurs in a significant number of patients with CF. In some cases fungal infection may contribute to an acute exacerbation; however, the exact incidence of such exacerbations is not known.

Among adults with CF, bacterial infection is the most common cause of exacerbations. Bacterial pathogens that are recognized traditionally in CF airway disease include *P. aeruginosa, Staphylococcus aureus, Haemophilus influenzae,* and the *Burkholderia cepacia* complex (25). Other bacteria, including *Stenotrophomonas maltophilia* and *Achromobacter (Alcaligenes) xylosoxidans, Achromobacter,* certain *Ralstonia* species, and the recently described genus *Pandoraea* are also associated with exacerbations of CF, but their role as pathogens in progression of CF lung disease is not clearly established (26–29).

The etiology of the exacerbation depends on the chronicity of the disease. Early airway infections in CF are most frequently caused by *S. aureus* and *H. influenzae,* with *S. aureus* often being the first organism to be cultured from young children with CF. Although *H. influenzae* is also commonly isolated from lower airway cultures in the first year of life, its role in the progression of CF lung disease is not well defined. *P. aeruginosa* is by far the most significant pathogen in CF. By the age of 18 years, approximately 80% of individuals with CF have *P. aeruginosa* infection (15). Acquisition of *Pseudomonas,* particularly organisms producing mucoid exopolysaccharide, is associated with clinical deterioration. Bacterial pathogens that are identified later in the course of the disease include *B. cepacia* complex, *S. maltophilia,* and *A. xylosoxidans.* In recent years acquisition of methicillin resistant *S. aureus* (MRSA) is also seen in the later stages of CF (Fig. 1).

At the time of the initial infection, most isolates of *Pseudomonas* are sensitive to multiple classes of antibiotics, but over time, antibiotic resistance can develop. Infection with multiple antibiotic-resistant *P. aeruginosa* (MARPA) is increasingly recognized in CF and has caused much concern. CF patients who have lower FEV_1, CF-related diabetes, and those who receive long-term inhaled tobramycin appear to have increased risk for MARPA infection. Likewise, more frequent hospitalizations and courses of

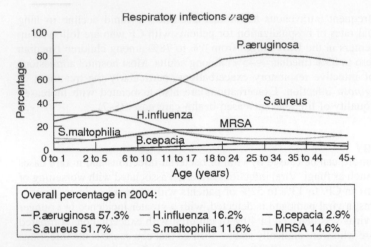

Figure 1 Prevalence of selected respiratory pathogens in respiratory cultures of cystic fibrosis patients by age. *Source*: From Ref. 12.

intravenous antibiotics, as well as more frequent exacerbations, increased the risk for MARPA over time among patients with CF. The risk of acquiring MARPA is high in centers with a high prevalence of resistant *Pseudomonas* (30). The results from this recent study emphasize the need for awareness of the potential detrimental effects of CF-related diabetes, close monitoring of the effects of prolonged antibiotic courses, and continued attention to infection-control measures in patients with CF. In contrast to *P. aeruginosa*, adult CF patients infected with *B. cepacia* seem to maintain the same strain of *B. cepacia* during exacerbations. In a recent investigation where 36 adult CF patients were followed, exacerbations were not caused by acquisition of a new *B. cepacia* species or strain (31). However, infection with *B. cepacia* complex is one of the most serious infections as there can be rapid progression to necrotizing pneumonia and death (14).

V. Pathogenesis
A. Microbial Factors
CF lung disease is characterized by persistent bacterial infection that is usually acquired in childhood and maintained throughout the patient's life. In many cases, these infections are polymicrobial and are difficult to eradicate. Infection is usually restricted to the airway lumen and persists despite intensive antimicrobial therapies. Clinical data suggest that the disease is typically initiated following viral infection or aspiration and that throughout adult life, the disease progresses with discrete acute exacerbations, also potentially linked to viral and bacterial infections with the latter being more common in adults. Chronic infections are caused by one or more of the pathogens that include *S. aureus, P. aeruginosa, B. cepacia* complex, nontypeable *H. influenzae, S. maltophilia*, and *A. xylosoidans. P. aeruginosa* is by far the commonest and most significant pathogen in patients with CF.

The microbiology of CF-associated *P. aeruginosa* infection differs in children compared with adults. Infants become infected with several strains of largely nonmucoid, environmental *Pseudomonas*. In early life, no strain emerges as a dominant one, and the *Pseudomonas* strains can be eradicated, at least temporarily, with antibiotic therapy (32–34). In adults, infection with *Pseudomonas* becomes chronic (i.e., secretions cannot be sterilized with antibiotic therapy), the bacteria are mucoid, and they form biofilms (35,36). In this environment, a single *P. aeruginosa* clone often predominates in the airway secretions of each patient. Longitudinal studies of stable adult patients with CF have reported that most patients with CF harbor a single clone or subclones of *P. aeruginosa* in their airways.

An enormous amount of work has been done to explain why *P. aeruginosa* (and not other opportunistic pathogens) is the major cause of pulmonary disease in CF. Although there is still no simple explanation, there is a wealth of information to help understand the host-pathogen interactions of *P. aeruginosa* in both the normal and the CF lung (37). The lack of normal CFTR chloride channel in the airway epithelium leads to defects in sodium and water transport, resulting in dehydrated airway secretions and mucus plugging (38). The contamination of these mucus plugs by the ubiquitous *P. aeruginosa* and its rapid adaptation to the milieu of the airway result in initially intermittent, then chronic infection. CFTR has been proposed to function as a receptor that increases clearance of *P. aeruginosa*; therefore, lack of CFTR could directly impair host defense against this organism (39,40). The ability of *P. aeruginosa* to form biofilms is another factor that allows it to predominate in the CF airways. Alginate production or mucoidy is another prominent feature of *P. aeruginosa* encountered in patients with CF (41,42). Conversion to a mucoid strain, which is capable of biofilm formation, has been associated with establishment of chronic infection. *P. aeruginosa* can induce apoptosis of a variety of cell types, including bronchial epithelial cells. The role of epithelial cell apoptosis in the pathogenesis of *P. aeruginosa* lung infection is currently not well defined. In one model system, apoptosis induced by the interaction of CD95 and CD95 ligand was found to be critical for the clearance of *P. aeruginosa* from murine lungs through the internalization of apoptotic cells containing ingested bacteria (43). Cannon and colleagues showed that there is defective apoptosis in patients with CF, which may lead to persistence of infection (44). Though several potential mechanisms have been described by which *Pseudomonas* thrives in the CF lung, the reason for its dominance in CF lung is still not clear.

B. Host Factors

Although most patients with CF have infective exacerbations, risk factors associated with more frequent exacerbations have been examined in a few studies. Block et al. examined characteristics of 249 adult and adolescent patients and found that patients who experience exacerbations are more likely to be younger, female, using inhaled steroids, have a lower FEV_1, and a history of multiple previous exacerbations (45). In contrast, in a recent study, Jarad et al. followed up 341 patients with exacerbations defined as an episode requiring intravenous antibiotics and found that age, gender, and body mass index did not influence the number of exacerbations, whereas *P. aeruginosa* in sputum, reduced FEV_1 and CF-related diabetes mellitus did so (46).

Defective mucus clearance is a key component of CF lung disease and is directly related to impaired CFTR function. Host mechanisms predisposing to infections that have been suggested include impaired mucociliary clearance related to low airway surface liquid volume (10,47), increased availability of cell surface receptors (48), the presence of severe hypoxia within mucous plugs (49) that may attract organisms capable of anaerobic survival, and decreased mucin secretion in the CF airway leaving the airway epithelium open and more susceptible to bacterial infections. Persistent inflammation and increased levels of oxidative stress are other factors that result in pulmonary damage contributing to the development of chronic lung disease in cystic fibrosis. Defects in CFTR gene alone do not explain the heterogeneity observed in CF pulmonary disease severity. Modifier genes have been implicated for this heterogeneity. Possible candidate genes that may modulate the response to infection include those related to proinflammatory cytokines and to innate immunity. A European study showed that tumor necrosis factor alpha (TNFα) polymorphisms were associated with the severity of CF lung disease in Czech and Belgian patients. TNFα is a key molecule for host defense and thus associated polymorphisms may explain the propensity to infections in CF (50). Advances in molecular genetics will provide valuable clues to the host factors in CF that predispose these individuals to infection.

VI. Diagnostic Approach

The diagnosis of pulmonary exacerbation is based on symptoms that include increased cough, sputum production, dyspnea, and a decline in lung function from baseline. As described above several criteria have been applied to the clinical diagnosis of CF exacerbation. Radiologic imaging may aid in identifying a new infiltrate in the chest although have not been systematically examined in large studies. In a small study Shah et al. prospectively evaluated nineteen symptomatic (exacerbation) and eight asymptomatic (stable) adult CF patients to determine the role of HRCT in the diagnosis of exacerbation and correlated HRCT with clinical parameters (51). Bronchiectasis, peribronchial thickening, mucus plugging, centrilobular nodules, and mosaic perfusion were identified in both groups of patients. Air-fluid levels in bronchiectatic cavities were identified in two patients and were the only finding limited to exacerbation.

Spirometric measurements may show an acute deterioration in lung function during an exacerbation and the findings may reverse with treatment (52). The confirmation of microbial etiology relies on the most recent sputum cultures obtained during the time of exacerbation. Bronchoalveolar lavage (BAL) fluid is the gold standard for detection of pathogens in the lower airways in CF. Negative culture results during pulmonary exacerbation and inflammation in the absence of pathogens do not exclude a microbial source of infection. In the routine setting, patients do not undergo a bronchoscopic diagnosis; however, if there is no clinical improvement with the initiation of antibiotics then BAL should be performed.

Most patients with CF have repeated sputum examination and are often colonized with one of the traditional CF pathogens. However, occasionally a new pathogen is identified or patients may show increased number of bacterial counts in the sputum or lavage during an exacerbation. In a recent study Harris et al. used a culture independent molecular approach using ribosomal ribonucleic acis (rRNA) sequence analysis to assess the bacterial composition of BAL fluid from 28 children with CF (53). Using these molecular markers 13 patients were found to have bacteria that were not routinely cultured. Although molecular techniques are not currently used in the diagnosis of CF exacerbation, they may provide a broader perspective than routine cultures in the future.

Further studies are needed to evaluate their role in the diagnosis of exacerbations. Finding the specific etiologic agent can guide the management of the exacerbation.

VII. Management

Considerable research has translated into improved patient care in CF, reflected by a continuing trend in improvement of life expectancy in these patients. Management of exacerbations includes a search for any treatable identifiable trigger factors, including viral or bacterial infections. In many cases triggers include uncontrolled sinus disease, gastro-esophageal reflux disease, and in some cases bronchopulmonary aspergillosis. Non-infectious factors such as pneumothorax, thromboembolism, and arrhythmias should be excluded. In general management of an acute infective exacerbation requires identification of triggers and appropriate antimicrobial agent with methods to aid airway clearance. Patients with exacerbation may present with respiratory failure requiring ventilatory support.

A. Antimicrobial Treatment

Initial antibiotic therapy for a CF exacerbation is usually determined on the basis of the antibiotic susceptibility of isolates recovered from that patient's most recent sputum culture (34,54). *P. aeruginosa* is the most common pathogen in CF exacerbations and is usually treated with a combination of aminoglycoside with another antipseudomonal agent such as a third generation cepahalosporin, carbapenem, carboxypenicillins, ure-idopenicillins, or fluoroquinolones. Monotherapy with inhaled tobramycin has been studied and is effective in initial infections (55). However, when inhaled tobramycin is used for three months continuously, the majority of patients with tobramycin-susceptible *P. aeruginosa* demonstrate a rise in *Pseudomonas* tobramycin-minimal inhibitory concentrations. Combination therapy reduces the risk of emergence of resistance and is preferred in sicker patients who are admitted to the intensive care unit. Early *Pseudomonal* infections are also susceptible to other antipseudomonal agents such as fluoroquinolones and penicillin, but as with tobramycin, resistance emerges with persistent infection. MARPA occur in up to 11% of patients, and these patients are difficult to treat (32). If the pulmonary pathogen is unknown, an antipseudomonal antibiotic is combined with an antistaphylococcal antibiotic.

Patients who have infections with *B. cepacia* complex may also be difficult to manage as many of these organisms are resistant to multiple antibiotics, including aminoglycosides and polymyxin. Antibiotics to which this species may be susceptible include carbapenems (such as meropenem), quinolones (ciprofloxacin), piperacillin, ceftazidime, trimethoprim sulfamethoxazole, and minocycline (56,57). Selection of antibiotics should be directed by the results of susceptibility tests. Some strains exhibit resistance to all antibiotics tested, in which case combination therapy is used to lower bacterial burden. Isolation of *S. maltopihilia* from the sputum during an exacerbation requires treatment with either trimethoprim sulfamethoxazole, doxycycline, or ticarcillin clavulanate, depending on the isolate's susceptibility. These organisms also have a high potential for resistance. Other agents to which they may be susceptible include minocycline and chloramphenicol. Other pathogens that have been isolated from patients with CF exacerbation include *A. (Alcaligenes) xylosoxydans* and *Acinetobacter baumannii*. The latter pathogen is often nosocomially acquired and may show resistance to multiple antibiotics. Recently infections with other species such as *Pandoraea (P. apista,*

P. pulmonicolla, P. pnomenusa, and *P. sputorum*), *Ralstonia* (*R. picketti, R. man-nitolilytica, R. paucula, and R. gilardi*), and *Inquilinus limosus* have also been identified in CF exacerbation (29).

The duration of a course of intravenous therapy to treat exacerbations varies between 14 and 21 days (53). The optimal duration of intravenous therapy is not clearly defined. Response to therapy as reflected by clinical symptoms, spirometry, and oxygenation before and after treatment may guide the duration of therapy in individual cases. A recent metanalysis and systematic review concluded that there is a need for multicenter randomized controlled trials to define the optimum duration of therapy in patients with CF exacerbation (58). Patients who have bronchopulmonary aspergillosis or other fungal infections should be treated with antifungal agents such as itraconazole, voriconazole, or amphotericin depending on the severity of infection.

B. Adjunctive Treatment
Physiotherapy and Bronchodilators
Mucociliary clearance is critical to maintain sterility of the airways. Since it is impaired in patients with CF, regular physiotherapy is an integral component of management of these patients. Mucolytics are prescribed in stable CF to maintain airway clearance, however, their role in exacerbations is not established (59,60). Chest physiotherapy with high-frequency chest wall oscillation with a vest, flutter device, or manual percussion is often helpful to loosen and clear the thick airway secretions. During an exacerbation, CF patients who have bronchospasm may benefit from use of nebulized bronchodilators, β-agonists, and anticholinergics.

Anti-inflammatory Agents
The role of steroids in the treatment of CF exacerbation is not clearly established. In a recent study, addition of oral corticosteroids to standard exacerbation therapy did not result in a statistically significant effect on lung function or sputum markers of inflammation (61). However, this study was not adequately powered to conclusively determine the role of steroids in exacerbations. Larger studies are needed before steroids can be routinely recommended.

Ventilatory Support
CF patients who present with acute or acute on chronic respiratory failure may need to be admitted to the intensive care unit and mechanically ventilated. As these patients have problems with clearance, they may need intubation. Noninvasive ventilation has been used in patients with chronic respiratory failure. Noninvasive ventilation, when used in addition to oxygen, may improve gas exchange during sleep to a greater extent than oxygen therapy alone in moderate to severe disease. These benefits of noninvasive ventilation have largely been demonstrated in single treatment sessions with small numbers of participants. The impact of this therapy on exacerbations and disease progression is not clear (62).

VIII. Prevention
The significant improvement in the outcomes of patients with CF is related to improved management of suppurative lung infections that contribute to 90% of mortality in these patients. Prevention of recurrent exacerbations is also important for maintenance of lung

function. In addition, exacerbations have a negative impact on quality of life and significantly increase health care costs.

Impaired clearance of abnormally viscous airway secretions has long been recognized as a major contributor of recurrent pulmonary infections in CF. Patients with significant pulmonary disease should receive physiotherapy with manual percussion or with devices such as oscillating vest or a flutter valve at least twice daily to help clear airway secretions (63). The role of exercise training programs on airway clearance has been investigated. Patients who received exercise training have an improved aerobic performance and quality of life (64,65). Because much of the increased viscosity of airway secretions in CF is due to DNA from neutrophils, recombinant human DNase (dornase alfa) is often used to decrease the sputum viscosity. Daily use of inhaled dornase alfa has been shown to improve FEV_1 and reduce the number of exacerbations (17). There is no evidence to support the use of N-acetylcysteine in the long-term prevention of exacerbations (66). Recently two studies investigated the role of hypertonic saline in prevention of CF exacerbations (67,68). CF patients who were treated with 7% hypertonic saline two to four times per day had significantly fewer exacerbations and demonstrated improvement in lung function. These patients also had significantly fewer days lost of school and usual activities compared to the control patients (67,68).

The use of nebulized antibiotics (tobramycin and colistin) in patients who are colonized with *P. aeruginosa* helps with short-term eradication and prevention of acute exacerbation (33,34). The potential long-term consequences of nebulized antipseudomonal antibiotics need further studies. Other inhaled antibiotics that have been demonstrated to be potentially beneficial with chronic use include colistimethate and aztreonam (17). Chronic oral antipseudomonal antibiotics are rarely used because of concerns for developing resistance. Prophylactic use of macrolides has been examined in randomized controlled trials and has demonstrated to reduce the frequency of exacerbations (69). Azithromycin administered in a dose of 500 mg three times a week (dose lowered to 250 mg for patients weighing <40 kg) for six months improves lung function and quality of life and reduces systemic markers of inflammation in CF (70). These benefits of macrolides are attributed to their anti-inflammatory effects. Additionally, macrolides also inhibit the qurom sensing molecules produced by *P. aeruginosa* (37) and hence may prevent formation of biofilms in CF airways. However, there is paucity of data to define the long-term effects and potential adverse effects of macrolides in CF.

The use of anti-inflammatory medications such as oral and inhaled steroids and nonsteroidal anti-inflammatory agents has been examined in CF. Nonsteroidal anti-inflammatory agents have shown to prevent pulmonary deterioration (71), and in one study ibuprofen tended to reduce hospital admissions (72). However, CF patients often have adverse effects with ibuprofen and are not able to tolerate the medication because of gastrointestinal side effects (73). Long-term use of oral steroids is limited in CF because of adverse effects (74). The role of inhaled steroids for long-term use is also not established except in those patients who have asthma (66).

Supportive treatment such as nutritional supplementation is recommended in all patients with CF. Several studies suggest stabilization of lung function in patients receiving nutritional supplements although the effects on prevention of exacerbation have not been carefully examined. The effects of influenza vaccination on the severity

Table 2 Strategies to Prevent pulmonary Pxacerbation in Patients with Cystic Fibrosis

Mucolytics	Dornase alfa (2.5 mg nebulized daily)
Airway clearance	Hypertonic saline 7% 2–4 times daily
Chest physiotherapy	Oscillating vest, flutter valve, or manual percussion
Antibiotics	Nebulized tobramycin 300 mg b.i.d. in alternating months or aztreonam
	Oral azithromycin 500 mg once daily 3 times/wk
Exercise	3–4 times/wk as tolerated
Vaccination	Influenza vaccine once a year, pneumovax every 5 yr
General	Avoid smoking, nutritional support, manage sinus disease, and monitor FEV_1

Abbreviation: FEV_1, forced expiratory volume in one second.

and number of exacerbations has not been evaluated however most centers provide vaccination for influenza and pneumococcus to patients with CF. Antipseudomonal vaccines have been investigated in patients with CF however, to date no effective vaccine has been developed. The respiratory management of patients with CF to prevent exacerbation is summarized in Table 2.

In summary, the median survival of patients with CF has improved dramatically in the past decade. This is related to significant advances in the understanding of the pathogenesis of the disease and better management and prevention of pulmonary infection. Strategies to reduce the frequency and severity of exacerbations are vital to ensure continued improvement in clinical outcomes of these patients.

IX. Case Scenarios

A. Case One

A 19-year-old male patient with CF G524/Δ508 presented with worsening shortness of breath, cough, hemoptysis (blood-tinged sputum), and fever of four days duration. He was known to be colonized with *P. aeruginosa* previously. His medication included oral pancreatic enzyme supplementation for pancreatic insufficiency, nebulized dornase alfa, inhaled hypertonic saline, and nutritional supplements. He was very meticulous with bronchial hygiene and used a flutter valve on a regular basis to clear his secretions. He exercised on a regular basis and was not on prophylactic antibiotics. On admission he was febrile with a temperature of 101.3°F. Oxygen saturation was 95% on room air. Chest examination showed bilateral crackles and wheezes in the lower lung fields.

Chest X-ray and CT scan demonstrated bilateral bronchiectasis in the middle and lower lobes with no focal infiltrates or pneumonia. Spirometry showed an FEV_1 50% of predicted (previous FEV_1 was 70%). He was treated with nebulized bronchodilators (albuterol and atrovent), nebulized tobramycin, and oral levofloxacin. Sputum grew *P. aeruginosa* that was sensitive to the antibiotics he was on, and he responded well to the treatment with his FEV_1 returning to baseline after seven days. This patient represents a case of CFexacerbation with bronchospasm with *P. aeruginosa* infection that was sensitive to antibiotics. In most patients who maintain airway clearance and who are not on prophylactic antibiotics, initial exacerbations are responsive to treatment with normalization of lung function and spirometry. It is the recurrence of these episodes that leads to worsening of lung function and a progressive decline in lung function.

B. Case Two

A 26-year-old female patient with CF with pancreatic insufficiency and asthma presented with increased sputum production and worsening dyspnea. Her wheezing had worsened over the past week, she needed to use albuterol more frequently, and her peak expiratory flow rate had decreased to 150–200 L/min from 350–450 L/min. She had also been producing brownish sputum for the past week. Her medication included inhaled steroids, long-acting β-agonists, and pancreatic enzyme supplementation. She was unable to tolerate hypertonic saline.

On examination, she was afebrile with diffuse crackles and wheezes bilaterally in the lower lung fields. Chest X ray and CT scan showed bronchiecatsis in both lungs with a suggestion of mucus plugs in some the bronchi. Sputum cultures were sent and treatment with inhaled tobramycin and intravenous levofloxacin was initiated. There was no improvement in her symptoms with antibiotics and nebulized bronchodilators. Her sputum grew *P. aeruginosa*, *S. maltophilia*, and *A. fumigatus*. Itraconazole, trimethoprim sulfamethoxazole and a tapering course of prednisone was added to her treatment regimen. Her Eerum immunoglobulin G was elevated at 210 IU/mL and serum precipitins for aspergillus were detected. She was treated for 12 months with itraconazole, and her lung function returned to baseline.

This case illustrates that patients with CF can develop infections with other pathogens such as *Aspergillus*. In this case the exacerbation was precipitated by multiple pathogens. In such circumstances, a regimen of multiple antimicrobials may be needed to treat the exacerbation. Patients with fungal infections may respond to antifungal therapy, and in some cases may need prolonged courses of such treatment.

C. Case Three

A 20-year-old male patient with CF and sinus disease presented with rhinorrhea, worsening shortness of breath, fever, and productive cough for four to five days. His FEV_1 was decreased to 60% of predicted (previously 80%). On examination he was febrile with a temperature of 102.4°F, had some tenderness over his right maxillary sinus, and had bilateral crackles over both the lower lung fields. There was a mucoid discharge from the right nasal cavity with a polypoid mass.

Sputum grew *P. aeruginosa* and *A. xylosoxydans*. He was previously colonized with *P. aeruginosa* that was resistant to flouroquinolones. He was treated with inhaled tobramycin and intravenous ceftazidime. Despite antibiotics he continued to feel unwell and remained febrile. A CT scan of the sinuses showed a nonenhancing mass involving the right maxillary sinus and extending into his nasal cavity consistent with an antrochoanal polyp. His ceftazidime was changed to meropenem and ENT was consulted. He underwent endoscopic sinus surgery with amputation of the polyp. His fever responded, and he continued to feel better with improvement in spirometry.

This case demonstrates that often CF exacerbations can be precipitated by sinus disease that may need appropriate treatment. Many patients with CF have upper respiratory tract problems such as rhinitis, sinusitis, and nasopharyngeal problems. Careful evaluation of the upper respiratory tract is important in all patients with CF.

References

1. Riordan JR, Rommens JM, Kerem B, et al. Identification of the cystic fibrosis gene: cloning and characterization of complementary DNA. Science 1989; 245:1066–1073.
2. Rich DP, Anderson MP, Gregory RJ, et al. Expression of cystic fibrosis transmembrane conductance regulator corrects defective chloride channel regulation in cystic fibrosis airway epithelial cells. Nature 1990; 347:358–363.
3. Stutts MJ, Canessa CM, Olsen JC, et al. CFTR as a cAMP-dependent regulator of sodium channels. Science 1995; 269:847 850.
4. Liou TG, Adler FR, Fitzsimmons SC, et al. Predictive 5-year survivorship model of cystic fibrosis. Am J Epidemiol 2001; 153:345–352.
5. Dobbin CJ, Bartlett D, Melehan K, et al. The effect of infective exacerbations on sleep and neurobehavioral function in cystic fibrosis. Am J Respir Crit Care Med 2005; 172:99–104.
6. Lieu TA, Ray GT, Farmer G, et al. The cost of medical care for patients with cystic fibrosis in a health maintenance organization. Pediatrics 1999; 103:e72.
7. Robson M, Abbott J, Webb K, et al. A cost description of an adult cystic fibrosis unit and cost analyses of different categories of patients. Thorax 1992; 47:684–689.
8. Britto MT, Kotagal UR, Hornung RW, et al. Impact of recent pulmonary exacerbations on quality of life in patients with cystic fibrosis. Chest 2002; 121:64–72.
9. Matsui H, Randell SH, Peretti SW, et al. Coordinated clearance of periciliary liquid and mucus from airway surfaces. J Clin Invest. 1998; 102:1125–1131.
10. Matsui H, Grubb BR, Tarran R. Evidence for periciliary liquid layer depletion, not abnormal ion composition, in the pathogenesis of cystic fibrosis airways disease. Cell 1998; 95:1005–1015.
11. Brennan AL, Geddes DM. Cystic fibrosis. Curr Opin Infect Dis 2002; 15:175–182.
12. Cystic Fibrosis Foundation. Patient Registry 2004 Annual Data Report. 1–2. Bethesda, MD: Cystic Fibrosis Foundation, 2005.
13. Ferkol T, Rosenfeld M, Milla CE. Cystic fibrosis pulmonary exacerbations. J Pediatr 2006; 148:259–264.
14. Goss CH, Burns TL. Exacerbations in cystic fibrosis. 1: Epidemiology and pathogenesis. Thorax 2007; 62(4):360–367.
15. Cystic Fibrosis Foundation. Microbiology and infectious disease in cystic fibrosis: V (Section 1). Bethesda, MD: Cystic Fibrosis Foundation, 1994.
16. Johnson C, Butler SM, Konstan MW, et al. Factors influencing outcomes in cystic fibrosis: a center-based analysis. Chest 2003; 123:20–27.
17. Fuchs HJ, Borowitz DS, Christiansen DH, et al. Effect of aerosolized recombinant human DNase on exacerbations of respiratory symptoms and on pulmonary function in patients with cystic fibrosis. The Pulmozyme Study Group. N Engl J Med 1994; 331:637–642.
18. Ramsey BW, Boat TF. Outcome measures for clinical trials in cystic fibrosis. Summary of a Cystic Fibrosis Foundation consensus conference. J Pediatr 1994; 124:177–192.
19. Rosenfeld M, Emerson J, Williams-Warren J, et al. Defining a pulmonary exacerbation in cystic fibrosis. J Pediatr 2001; 139(3):359–365.
20. Smith JA, Owen EC, Jones AM, et al. Objective measurement of cough during pulmonary exacerbations in adults with cystic fibrosis. Thorax 2006; 61(5):425–429.
21. Emerson J, Rosenfeld M, McNamara S, et al. Pseudomonas aeruginosa and other predictors of mortality and morbidity in young children with cystic fibrosis. Pediatr Pulmonol 2002; 34:91–100.
22. Armstrong D, Grimwood K, Carlin JB, et al. Severe viral respiratory infections in infants with cystic fibrosis. Pediatr Pulmonol 1998; 26(6):371–379.
23. van Ewijk BE, van der Zalm MM, Wolfs TF, et al. Viral respiratory infections in cystic fibrosis. J Cyst Fibros. 2005; 4(suppl 2):31–36.
24. Wat D, Gelder C, Hibbitts S, et al. The role of respiratory viruses in cystic fibrosis. J Cyst Fibros 2008; 7(4):320–328.

25. Gibson RL, Burns JL, Ramsey BW. Pathophysiology and management of pulmonary infections in cystic fibrosis. Am J Respir Crit Care Med 2003; 168:918–951.
26. Goss CH, Otto K, Aitken ML, et al. Detecting Stenotrophomonas maltophilia does not reduce survival of patients with cystic fibrosis. Am J Respir Crit Care Med 2002; 166:356–361.
27. Goss CH, Mayer-Hamblett N, Aitken ML, et al. Association between Stenotrophomonas maltophilia and lung function in cystic fibrosis. Thorax 2004; 59:955–959.
28. Tan K, Conway SP, Brownlee KG, et al. Alcaligenes infection in cystic fibrosis. Pediatr Pulmonol 2002; 34:101–104.
29. Davies JC, Rubin BK. Emerging and unusual gram-negative infections in cystic fibrosis. Semin Respir Crit Care Med 2007; 28(3):312–321.
30. Merlo CA, Boyle MP, Diener-West M, et al. Incidence and risk factors for multiple antibiotic-resistant Pseudomonas aeruginosa in cystic fibrosis. Chest 2007; 132(2):562–568.
31. St Denis M, Ramotar K, Vandemheen K, et al. Infection with Burkholderia cepacia complex bacteria and pulmonary exacerbations of cystic fibrosis. Chest 2007; 131(4):1188–1196.
32. Burns JL, Gibson RL, McNamara S, et al. Longitudinal assessment of *Pseudomonas aeruginosa* in young children with cystic fibrosis. J Infect Dis 2001; 183:444–452.
33. Gibson RL, Emerson J, McNamara S, et al. Significant microbiological effect of inhaled tobramycin in young children with cystic fibrosis. Am J Respir Crit Care Med 2003; 167:841–849.
34. Ratjen F, Doring G, Nikolaizik H. Effect of inhaled tobramycin on early *Pseudomonas aeruginosa* colonisation in patients with cystic fibrosis. Lancet 2001; 358:983–984.
35. Singh PK, Schaefer AL, Parsek MR, et al. Quorum-sensing signals indicate that cystic fibrosis lungs are infected with bacterial biofilms. Nature 2000; 407:762–764.
36. Aaron SD, Ferris W, Ramotar K, et al. Single and combination antibiotic susceptibilities of planktonic, adherent, and biofilm-grown *Pseudomonas aeruginosa* isolates cultured from sputa of adults with cystic fibrosis. J Clin Microbiol 2002; 40:4172–4179.
37. Sadikot RT, Blackwell TS, Christman JW, et al. Pathogen-host interactions in Pseudomonas aeruginosa pneumonia. Am J Respir Crit Care Med. 2005; 171(11):1209–1223.
38. Donaldson SH, Boucher RC. Update on pathogenesis of cystic fibrosis lung disease. Curr Opin Pulm Med 2003; 9:486–491.
39. Schroeder TH, Lee MM, Yacono PW, et al. CFTR is a pattern recognition molecule that extracts Pseudomonas aeruginosa LPS from the outer membrane into epithelial cells and activates NF-kappa B translocation. Proc Natl Acad Sci U S A. 2002; 99(10):6907–6912.
40. Pier GB, Grout M, Zaidi TS. Role of mutant CFTR in hypersusceptibility of cystic fibrosis patients to lung infections. Science 1996; 271:64–67.
41. Prince AS. Biofilms, antimicrobial resistance, and airway infection. N Engl J Med 2002; 347:1110–1111.
42. Costerton JW, Stewart PS, Greenberg EP. Bacterial biofilms: a common cause of persistent infection. Science 1999; 284:1318–1322.
43. Grassme H, Jendrossek V, Riehle A, et al. Host defense against Pseudomonas aeruginosa requires ceramide-rich membrane rafts. Nat Med 2003; 9:322–330.
44. Cannon CL, Kowalski MP, Stopak KS, et al. Pseudomonas aeruginosa-induced apoptosis is defective in respiratory epithelial cells expressing mutant cystic fibrosis transmembrane conductance regulator. Am J Respir Cell Mol Biol 2003; 29(2):188–197.
45. Block JK, Vandemheen KL, Tullis E, et al. Predictors of pulmonary exacerbations in patients with cystic fibrosis infected with multi-resistant bacteria. Thorax 2006; 61(11):969–974.
46. Jarad NA, Giles K. Risk factors for increased need for intravenous antibiotics for pulmonary exacerbations in adult patients with cystic fibrosis. Chron Respir Dis 2008; 5(1):29–33.
47. Smith JJ, Travis SM, Greenberg EP, et al. Cystic fibrosis airway epithelia fail to kill bacteria because of abnormal airway surface fluid. Cell 1996; 85:229–236.
48. Saiman L, Prince A. *Pseudomonas aeruginosa* pili bind to asialo GM1 which is increased on the surface of cystic fibrosis epithelial cells. J Clin Invest 1993; 92:1875–1880.

49. Worlitzsch D, Tarran R, Ulrich M. Effects of reduced mucus oxygen concentration in airway *Pseudomonas* infections of cystic fibrosis patients. J Clin Invest 2002; 109:317–325.
50. Yarden J, Radojkovic D, De Boeck K, et al. Association of tumour necrosis factor alpha variants with the CF pulmonary phenotype. Thorax 2005; 60(4):320–325.
51. Shah RM, Sexauer W, Ostrum BJ, et al. High-resolution CT in the acute exacerbation of cystic fibrosis: evaluation of acute findings, reversibility of those findings, and clinical correlation. AJR Am J Roentgenol 1997; 169(2):375–380.
52. Thomas SR. The pulmonary physician in critical care. Illustrative case 1: cystic fibrosis. Thorax 2003; 58(4):357–360.
53. Harris JK, De Groote MA, Sagel SD, et al. Molecular identification of bacteria in bronchoalveolar lavage fluid from children with cystic fibrosis. Proc Natl Acad Sci U S A 2007; 104(51):20529–20533.
54. Ratjen F. Diagnosing and managing infection in CF. Paediatr Respir Rev 2006; 7:S151–S153.
55. Master V, Roberts GW, Coulthard KP, et al. Efficacy of once-daily tobramycin monotherapy for acute pulmonary exacerbations of cystic fibrosis: a preliminary study. Pediatr Pulmonol 2001; 31(5):367–376.
56. Kalish LA, Waltz DA, Dovey M, et al. Impact of Burkholderia dolosa on lung function and survival in cystic fibrosis. Am J Respir Crit Care Med 2006; 173(4):421–425.
57. Golini G, Cazzola G, Fontana R. Molecular epidemiology and antibiotic susceptibility of Burkholderia cepacia-complex isolates from an Italian cystic fibrosis centre. Eur J Clin Microbiol Infect Dis 2006; 25(3):175–180.
58. Fernandes B, Plummer A, Wildman M. Duration of intravenous antibiotic therapy in people with cystic fibrosis. Cochrane Database Syst Rev. 2008; (2):CD006682.
59. Randell SH, Boucher RC. Effective mucus clearance is essential for respiratory health. Am J Respir Cell Mol Biol 2006; 35:20–28.
60. Henke MO, Ratjen F. Mucolytics in cystic fibrosis. Paediatr Respir Rev 2007; 8(1):24–29.
61. Dovey M, Aitken ML, Emerson J, et al. Oral corticosteroid therapy in cystic fibrosis patients hospitalized for pulmonary exacerbation: a pilot study. Chest 2007; 132(4):1212–1218.
62. Moran F, Bradley JM, Jones AP, Piper AJ. Non-invasive ventilation for cystic fibrosis. Cochrane Database Syst Rev 2007; (4):CD002769.
63. Flume PA. Airway clearance techniques. Semin Respir Crit Care Med 2003; 24(6):727–736.
64. Schneiderman-Walker J, Pollock SL, Corey M, et al. A randomized controlled trial of a 3-year home exercise program in cystic fibrosis. J Pediatr 2000; 136(3):304–310.
65. Klijn PH, Oudshoorn A, van der Ent CK, et al. Effects of anaerobic training in children with cystic fibrosis: a randomized controlled study. Chest 2004; 125(4):1299–1305.
66. Bell SC, Robinson PJ. Exacerbations in cystic fibrosis: 2. Prevention. Thorax 2007; 62(8):723–732.
67. Elkins MR, Robinson M, Rose BR, et al. A controlled trial of long-term inhaled hypertonic saline in patients with cystic fibrosis. N Engl J Med 2006; 354:229–240.
68. Donaldson SH, Bennett WD, Zeman KL, et al. Mucus clearance and lung function in cystic fibrosis with hypertonic saline. N Engl J Med 2006; 354:241–250.
69. McArdle JR, Talwalkar JS. Macrolides in cystic fibrosis. Clin Chest Med 2007; 28(2):347–360.
70. Southern KW, Barker PM. Azithromycin for cystic fibrosis. Eur Respir J 2004; 24(5):834–838.
71. Lands LC, Dezateux C, Crighton C. Oral non-steroidal anti-inflammatory drug therapy for cystic fibrosis. Cochrane Database Sys Rev 1999; (2):CD001505.
72. Konstan MW, Byard PJ, Hoppel CL, et al. Effect of high-dose ibuprofen in patients with cystic fibrosis. N Engl J Med. 1995; 332(13):848–854.
73. Fennell PB, Quante J, Wilson K, et al. Use of high-dose ibuprofen in a pediatric cystic fibrosis center. J Cyst Fibros 2007; 6(2):153–158.
74. Eigen H, Rosenstein BJ, FitzSimmons S, et al. A multicenter study of alternate-day prednisone therapy in patients with cystic fibrosis. Cystic Fibrosis Foundation Prednisone Trial Group. J Pediat 1995; 126(4):515–523.

8

Community-Acquired Pneumonia

ELBIO MARIANO ESPERATTI and ANTONI TORRES MARTI
Universitat de Barcelona, CIBER de Enfermedades Respiratorias (CIBERES) and
Insitut d'Investigacions Biomèdiques August Pi i Sunyer (IDIBAPS), Barcelona, Spain

I. Introduction

The lungs are constantly exposed to microorganisms. A complex system of host defences is required to prevent these organisms from gaining access to and for removing them from the lungs. This process, however, may be breached and pathogenic microorganisms may reach the alveoli. The combined effects of microorganism multiplication and host response determine the clinical condition known as pneumonia.

Acute lower respiratory tract infections (primarily pneumonia) are a major public health problem. They cause more disease and death than any other infection, and the mortality rate in the last decades has been relatively unchanged.

II. Definition

Community-acquired pneumonia (CAP) is defined as an acute infection of the lung parenchyma accompanied by symptoms of acute illness (1). The gold standard for diagnosis should be the identification of a microbiological pathogen isolated from lung tissue, an impractical test in clinical practice. An alternative gold standard could be based on a combination of clinical symptoms and radiographic, laboratory, and microbiological findings. In the clinical and research setting, isolated findings on chest radiography are often interpreted as the gold standard for the initial diagnosis of pneumonia even though chest radiography is neither 100% sensitive nor 100% specific for this condition. Compared with high-resolution computed tomography, 31% of cases of possible pneumonia may be missed with chest X ray (2); however, strategies involving alternative radiographic techniques are not supported by current evidence (3). The most useful classification of pneumonia is based on the site of origin of the infection as this factor implies a different etiology, prognosis and treatment. The term "community-acquired pneumonia" refers to the appearance of infection in a nonhospitalized population with no risk factors for multidrug resistant pathogens while the term "hospital-acquired pneumonia" (HAP) or "nosocomial pneumonia" is used when there is no evidence that the infection was present or incubating at the time of hospital admission. This latter type of pneumonia is most frequently found in patients receiving mechanical ventilation, hence the term "ventilator-associated pneumonia."

III. Epidemiology

More than 55 million people die each year worldwide, and pneumonia is among the leading causes of death. As a group, respiratory diseases are the foremost cause of death. As a specific disease, lower respiratory tract infections (primarily pneumonia) are the third leading cause of death after ischemic heart and cerebrovascular disease, accounting for 6.6% of all deaths (4). In terms of DALYs (the disability adjusted life years, a measure to quantify the burden of disease), pneumonia is the second major cause of burden of disease accounting for 5.8% of deaths, at the same level as human immunodeficiency virus (HIV)/acquired immunodeficiency syndrome (AIDS).

Pneumonia is the leading cause of death in children, with more than 2 million children under five years of age dying from pneumonia each year, accounting for almost one in five under-five deaths worldwide; that is, pneumonia kills more children than any other illness, even more than AIDS, malaria and measles combined (5).

There are an estimated 4 million cases of CAP per year in the United States, resulting in approximately 10 million visits to the physician, 1 million hospitalizations, and 45,000 deaths (6,7). Although the precise incidence of CAP is not known in several European countries, pneumonia is the fourth cause of death in both Western and Eastern Europe. The incidence of CAP in primary care is reported to be 5 to 10 cases per 1000 patients per year, but this is highly dependent on age (8). In the adult population, the incidence starts to rise from about the age of 50, up to 15 to 30 per 1000 in the 75- to 79-year age group and 40 to 60 per 1000 in people over 85 years of age. Additionally, age is an independent risk factor for hospitalization in elderly patients (9,10). Studies indicate a male preponderance of between 60% and 64% of cases.

CAP occurs predominantly in patients with other comorbid diseases and less than 50% of cases have no comorbidity. Chronic lung disease is the most common comorbidity associated with CAP, followed by heart disease. Other comorbidities associated with increased rates of CAP and subsequent mortality include alcoholism, diabetes, chronic kidney or liver disease, cancer, dementia, cerebrovascular diseases, and immunodeficiency states (10–12). Smoking is probably the most important risk factor for pneumonia in immunocompetent nonelderly adults, particularly for invasive pneumococcal disease (13).

According to different studies, between one in 30 and one in 6 patients are admitted to the intensive care unit (ICU). This may be due, in part to the different spectrum of illness severity seen in different hospitals, but may also reflect different ICU admission criteria and facilities. There is much smaller variation in the proportion of patients receiving mechanical ventilation that represents 4% to 11% of all hospital admissions for CAP (14). The overall mortality by CAP in ambulatory patients is between 3% and 5% while that in hospitalized patients is 14%, increasing to 20% to 50% in patients requiring ICU care (12,15,16).

IV. Etiology

CAPs are predominantly of bacterial or viral origin and much less frequently parasitic or fungal. The search for microbial agents responsible for CAP is usually not carried out in the community. Therefore, data on microbial etiology are derived from either studies performed specifically for studying microbial epidemiology of CAP, or as satellite results of clinical trials testing antimicrobials or therapeutic strategies. In contrast, in the hospital evidence for microbial agents is extensively sought in patients with severe, nonresponding pneumonia or at risk of severe pneumonia. In these circumstances, as well as in clinical studies, in spite of this extensive search, the yield is quite disappointing, as no pathogen is identified in at least 50% of cases. With more invasive and complex testing such as polymerase chain reaction (PCR) to detect respiratory pathogens in lung aspirate specimens obtained by transthoracic needle aspiration, the proportion of cases of CAP in which the etiology is established increases up 83% (17). By contrast, in observational studies assessing the "real world," the proportion with defined cause can be as little as 25% among inpatients and 6% among outpatients (18).

Although many pathogens have been associated with pneumonia, a small number of key pathogens cause most cases. The predominant causative pathogen observed is *Streptococcus pneumoniae* (pneumococcus), from less than 5% to 35% among different studies (19). It is important to note that *S. pneumoniae* can represent a significant proportion of cases where the etiology is not documented by conventional testing (17). The likelihood of pneumococcal pneumonia is increased by alcoholism, chronic obstructive pulmonary disease (COPD), immunoglobulin deficiency, and HIV infection.

The incidence of other microorganisms varies according to the severity of the disease (Table 1). CAP due to *Haemophilus influenzae* usually occurs after upper respiratory tract infection. Infection by *Legionella pneumophila* may cause asymptomatic seroconversion, a lone episode of pyrexia, or pneumonia. *Legionella* spp. is a common cause of severe CAP and in several studies is the second most common identified pathogen following *S. pneumoniae*.

Gram-negative bacilli (GNB), *Enterobacteriaceae* and *Pseudomonas* spp., are common causes of HAP, but selective antimicrobial pressure and changes in the health care environment have increased the frequency of GNB CAP. Risk factors for GNB pneumonia have been established: probable aspiration, previous hospital admission, previous antimicrobial treatment, and the presence of pulmonary comorbidity. Pulmonary comorbidity and previous hospital admission are also risk factors for infection by *Pseudomonas aeruginosa* (20).

Mycoplasma pneumoniae and *Chlamydia* spp. are common causes of CAP in immunocompetent ambulatory patients. They are often refered to as "atypical" pathogens and rarely occur in the elderly (1% in patients over 80 years of age) (21). *M. pneumoniae* is exclusive to humans and can be transmitted through aerosols from

Table 1 Most Common Causative Factor in Community-Acquired Pneumonia by Patient Care Setting (in Order of Frequency)

Outpatients	Inpatients (non-ICU)	Inpatient (ICU)
S. pneumoniae	*S. pneumoniae*	*S. pneumoniae*
M. pneumoniae	*M. pneumoniae*	*Legionella* spp.
H. influenzae	*C. pneumoniae*	*H. influenzae*
C. pneumoniae	*H. influenzae*	Gram-negative bacilli
Respiratory viruses[a]	*Legionella* spp.	*Staphylococcus aureus*
	Respiratory viruses[a]	

[a]Influenza A and B, adenovirus, RSV, parainfluenza.
Abbreviation: ICU, intensive care unit.
Source: From Ref. 3.

person to person and transmission is therefore enhanced by close personal contact. Prior upper respiratory tract infection is found in about 50% of patients.

Respiratory viruses, including *influenza* A and B, *adenovirus, respiratory syncytial virus, and parainfluenza*, are important causes of CAP. In hospitalized nonimmunocompromised patients, the frequency of respiratory viral infection can be as high as 23% (22,23). Influenza is responsible for at least half of the viral pneumonias in immunocompetent adults. Pneumonia may occur immediately after the acute illness caused by the virus itself (primary pneumonia) or may result from bacterial superinfection, usually by *S. pneumoniae, H. influenzae*, or *Staphylococcus aureus*, following a period of clinical improvement (secondary pneumonia). Primary pneumonia occurs more often in association with heart failure while secondary pneumonia is seen more often in elderly patients and in those with comorbidities, such as chronic cardiovascular or respiratory disease, diabetes mellitus, or chronic hepatic or renal failure.

A substantial number of CAP may be attributed to more than one microbe. Polymicrobial pneumonia in nonimmunocompromised patients has been reported at all ages, as well as in inpatients and outpatients, with rates from 5% to 25% (24,25). The most frequent combinations of pathogens are bacteria with an atypical organism (e.g., *S. pneumoniae* and *Chlamydophila pneumoniae*) and bacteria and viruses (e.g., *S. Pneumoniae* and influenza). It is important to note that no clinical marker is useful to differentiate poly from monomicrobial pneumonia (22).

In the evaluation of an individual, physicians should consider specific risk factors for the probable etiology, especially when less frequent microorganisms should be taken into account (3) (Table 2). On the basis of the mainly on retrospective studies, a diverse

Table 2   Risk Factors Related to Specific Pathogens in CAP

Alcoholism	*S. pneumoniae, oral anaerobes, K. pneumoniae, Acinetobacter* spp. *Mycobacterium tuberculosis*
COPD and/or smoking	*H. influenzae, P. aeruginosa, Legionella* spp, *S. pneumoniae, M. cararrhalis, C. pneumoniae*
Aspiration	Enteric gram-negative, anaerobes
Lung abscess	CA-MRSA[a], oral anaerobes, *Mycobacterium tuberculosis*, atypical mycobacteria
Exposure to bat or bird droppings	*Histoplasma capsulatum*
Exposure to birds	*Chlamydophila psittaci* (if poultry: avian influenza)
Hotel or cruise ship stay in previous 2 wk	*Legionella* spp
Travel to or residence in Southeast or Eastern Asia	*Burkholderia pseudomallei*, avian influenza, SARS
Active influenza in the community	*Influenza, S. pneumoniae, S. aureus, H. influenzae*
Structural lung disease (bronchiectasis)	*P. aeuruginosa, S. aureus*
Intravenous drug use	*S. aureus, anaerobes, S. pneumoniae, Mycobacterium tuberculosis*
Endobronchial obstruction	*Anaerobes, S. pneumoniae, H. influenzae, S. aureus*
HIV infection (early)	*S. pneumoniae, H. influenzae, Mycobacterium tuberculosis*

[a]CA-MRSA, community-acquired methicillin-resistant *Staphylococcus aureus*.
Source: Modified from Ref. 3.

population of nonhospitalized patients with CAP have been found to be infected with a spectrum of pathogens that most closely resembles HAP, including multidrug-resistant pathogens, such as *Enterobacteriaceae, Pseudomonas* spp and methicillin-resistant *S. aureus.* For this heterogeneous group, the disease has been denominated health care–associated pneumonia (HCAP) and includes patients with antimicrobial therapy in the previous 90 days, hospitalization more than or equal to two days in the preceding 90 days, residence in a nursing home or extended care facility, home infusion therapy, chronic dialysis, or a family member with multidrug-resistant pathogen (26). According to the guidelines, the diagnostic and therapeutic considerations for HCAP should be the same as HAP. However, recent prospective studies in Europe have found a spectrum of etiology in these patients that resembles CAP (27). This issue, therefore, deserves more study before a definitive recommendation can be made.

An increased incidence of pneumonia due to community-acquired methicillin-resistant *S. aureus* (CA-MRSA) has recently been observed. Though resistant to fewer antibiotics than hospital-acquired MRSA, these strains often contain the Panton–Valentine leukocidine gene, a toxin associated with clinical features of shock, respiratory failure, and necrotizing pneumonia with formation of abscess and empyemas (28).

V. Pathogenesis

The mechanisms most frequently responsible for the development of pneumonia are inhalation of microorganisms into the lower airways and aspiration of oropharyngeal contents. Direct extension from contiguous spaces or hematogenous seeding from an extrapulmonary focus is less frequent.

Most microorganisms in room air reside on the surface of aerosolized particles. Only material with a diameter of less than 5 μm reaches the alveoli. Therefore inhalation is relevant for small microorganisms such as *Mycoplasma, Chlamydophila, Coxiella,* and viruses. In contrast, aspiration of oropharyngeal secretions is the main mechanism of contamination of the lower airways by large bacteria, for example, *S. pneumoniae, S. aureus, P. aeruginosa, and Klebsiella pneumoniae.* While awake the normal glottal reflex prevents aspiration. However, during sleep 50% of normal persons aspirate small volumes of pharyngeal secretions (29). Healthy adults have 10 to 100 million bacteria per milliliter of oropharyngeal secretions. This may increase in patients with periodontal disease. The ability of virulent microorganisms to colonize the oropharynx is determined by the interaction of specific microbial adhesins with cellular receptors. For example, colonization by GNB is increased in persons with lower levels of salivary fibronectin, which occurs because of alcoholism, diabetes, malnutrition, and other severe comorbidities. Despite the frequency of microaspiration, microbiological proliferation in the lower airways is normally prevented by (*i*) mechanical defenses (including cough, entrapment of microorganisms by bronchial mucus and physical carriage of mucus to the pharynx by the ciliary epithelium), (*ii*) humoral immune factors in respiratory secretions (lysozyme, lactoferrin, immunoglobulins, and complement) that kill microorganisms or inhibit their adherence to bronchial epithelium, and (*iii*) cellular components of immunity including alveolar macrophages.

Once in the alveoli, numerous or more virulent microbes elicit an inflammatory response that, despite serving to reinforce innate immunity and being essential to rid the lungs of microorganisms, contributes directly to lung injury and abnormal pulmonary function.

Microbes initiate inflammation when detected by a host cell population specialized to be sentinels: alveolar macrophages and dendritic cells, which are particularly important for sensing microbes and passing this information to other cells such as epithelial cells and lymphocytes. Additionally, epithelial cells can be directly activated by microorganisms. The identification of microbial invaders relies on host receptors called "pattern-recognition receptors" (PRR) that bind molecular moieties common to microbes (30). The diverse activation pathway converges on epithelial cells and activates the transcription of nuclear factor kappa B (NF-κB), a central molecule that induces and regulates the expression of proinflammatory mediators, including neutrophil chemokines, colony-stimulating factors, and adhesion molecules (31).

Neutrophils are the effectors of innate immunity. During infection they migrate out of the pulmonary capillaries and into the air spaces. After phagocytosis, neutrophils kill ingested microorganisms by several mechanisms, including reactive oxygen species, antimicrobial proteins, and degradative enzymes. These cells are not a dead end in these communication pathways but convey important information that direct the immune response. They generate proinflammatory signals including tumor necrosis factor alpha (TNF-α), chemokines, and chemerin, which recruit and activate dendritic cells and B-lymphocyte stimulators. Neutrophils activate T-cells through interleukin-12 (IL-12). Thus, acquired and innate immune responses against microorganisms in the lungs are shaped by signals derived from neutrophils.

Inflammation is critical for innate immunity and host defense, but it can injure the lungs. The neutrophil products generated to kill microorganisms also kill host cells and damage host tissues. Hence, lung infection is a common cause of the acute respiratory distress syndrome (ARDS) (32).

VI. Clinical Evaluation

The diagnosis of CAP is based on the presence of specific clinical features (e.g., cough, fever, sputum production, and pleuritic chest pain) (3). Unfortunately, symptoms at presentation or isolated physical signs distinguish poorly between CAP and other causes of respiratory illness and only a few combinations of findings are useful: normal heart rate ($\leq$100 beats/min), temperature ($\leq$37.8°C) and respiratory rate ($\leq$20 breaths/min) reduce the probability of CAP (negative likelihood ratio 0.18) (33). On the other hand the combination of patient history and physical examination may be relevant: the combination of acute cough, fever, tachycardia, and crackles on chest examination increase the probability of pneumonia between 18% and 42% (1). Both clinical features and respiratory findings on physical examination may be lacking or altered in elderly patients in whom nonrespiratory symptoms such as mental status change or falls may predominate (34). Neither do routine laboratory tests add much information with the exception of C reactive protein (CRP) that in some but not all studies has shown a sensitivity for CAP detection of up to 100% when the value is between 50 and 100 mg/L (35,36).

There is currently no strong evidence on which to base the decision as to when to perform a chest X ray. There are limited data on its diagnostic performance (1), although the sensitivity appears to be decreased in patients with emphysema, bullae, or other structural abnormalities of the lung; obese patients, in whom it may be difficult to discern the existence of infiltrates; and patients with very early infection, severe dehydration, or profound granulocytopenia. The consensus guidelines endorse the need for chest X ray to confirm all diagnoses of CAP (3). Although several radiological patterns have been associated with pneumonia caused by specific microorganisms, this is not reliable for diagnosing a specific pathogen (37–39).

A. Risk Stratification
The most important issue in the management of a patient with CAP is the decision as to the most appropriate care setting: outpatient, hospitalization on a medical ward, or admission to an ICU. Almost all the major decisions regarding the management of CAP, including diagnostic testing and treatment, revolve around the initial assessment of severity.

Between 30% and 50% of patients who are hospitalized are at low risk of death and may potentially be managed at home (11,40). The decision regarding hospitalization should be based on the stability of the clinical condition, the risk of death and complications, the presence or absence of other medical problems, and social characteristics. Severity or prognostic scores should be used to identify patients who may be candidates for outpatient treatment (3). The most widely used prediction score is the "pneumonia severity index" (PSI) that stratifies the patients to five risk categories (Fig. 1 and Table 3) (11); the higher the score, the higher the risk of death. Patients in classes I and II have a 30-day mortality risk of lower than 1% and can be safely treated as outpatients, while patients in class III have a risk of death of 0.9% to 2.9%. As the risk of clinical worsening—although very low—is highest during the first 24 hours after presentation and decreases thereafter (41), it is therefore prudent to observe these patients in the emergency department for a short period of time. Lastly, patients in classes IV and V have a risk of mortality of between 8.9% and 29.2 % and should be hospitalized. An easy to use version of the PSI is available at http://pda.ahrq.gov/clinic/psi/psicalc.asp.

An alternative and simpler score that may be used at bedside is the "CURB 65" score which assesses five variables, each of which is assigned one point: confusion,

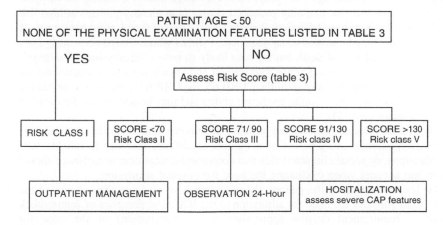

Figure 1   Risk stratification according to the Pneumonia Severity Index.

Table 3 Pneumonia Severity Index

Patient characteristics	Score assigned
Demographic factors	
Age (in yr)	
Males	Age
Females	Age −10
Nursing home resident	Age +10
Coexisting conditions	
Neoplastic disease	+30
Liver disease	+20
Congestive heart failure	+10
Cerebrovascular disease	+10
Kidney disease	+10
Initial physical examination	
Altered Mental status	+20
Respiratory rate ≥30/min	+20
Systolic Blood Pressure ≤90	+20
Temperature <35 or ≥40	+15
Heart rate ≥125/min	+10
Initial laboratory findings	
pH <7.35	+30
BUN >30 mg/dL	+20
Sodium <130	+20
Glucose ≥250 mg/dL	+10
Hematocrit <30	+10
PaO_2 < 60 or oxygen saturation < 90%	+10
Pleural effusion	+10

Source: From Ref. 11.

urea >7 mmol/L, respiratory rate >30/min, low blood pressure (systolic <90 mm Hg or diastolic ≤60 mm Hg) and age >65 years (42). This score aids in avoiding the inappropriate admission of low-risk mortality patients and may help identify patients at high risk who would benefit from hospitalization. Patients with a score of 0 or 1 point have a risk of death of 1.5% and may be treated as an outpatient. Patients with a CURB 65 score ≥2 are not only at increased risk of death but are also likely to have clinically important physiological derangements requiring active intervention and should usually be considered for hospitalization. A simplified version of the CURB 65, the CRB 65, which does not require urea levels, has demonstrated similar predictive ability and may be appropriate for decision making in primary care (43).

    Other considerations such as the presence of hypotension (systolic blood pressure lower 90), hypoxemia, exacerbation of comorbid conditions, inability to reliably take oral medications, or social characteristics that compromise treatment compliance should be taken into account when evaluating the need for hospital admission.

    On hospitalization of the patient, the next step is to evaluate the severity of the disease and to consider the need for admission to the ICU. The presence of septic shock (vasopressor requirement despite appropriate fluid resuscitation) or the need for mechanical ventilation defines severe CAP and these patients should be directly admitted to an ICU (3). However, not all patients eventually admitted to an ICU present such findings at presentation and delay in ICU transfer because of delayed respiratory failure or delayed onset of septic shock is associated with increased mortality (44). Although a high CURB 65 score or a PSI category IV or V can be used to identify candidates for ICU admission, none of these has been prospectively evaluated and all have shown a low specificity in retrospective analysis. Thus, other criteria have recently been established to predict a worse prognosis to determine intensive care requirement (3). The presence of three or more these criteria has been suggested as criteria for ICU admission: respiratory rate $\geq$30/min, arterial oxygen pressure to oxygen inspired fraction rate (PaO$_2$/FiO2) $\leq$250, multilobar infiltrates, confusion, uremia (BUN $\geq$ 20 mg/dL), leukopenia (<4000 white blood cells/mm^3), thrombocytopenia (<100,000 platelets/mm^3), hypothermia, and hypotension requiring aggressive fluid resuscitation. Prospective validation of these criteria is needed.

B. Diagnostic Testing

The length of diagnostic testing for specific pathogens should be based on the following factors: the probability that such a finding would significantly alter standard empirical management decisions, the severity and therefore care setting of the patient and suspicion of a specific pathogen on an epidemiological basis. Diagnostic tests for outpatients with suspected bacterial CAP is optional because of the low probability of treatment failure and good prognosis with recommended empirical antibiotic treatment (3). Several reasons justify such a recommendation: low diagnostic performance of routine tests, costs, potential delays in starting antibiotic therapy from the need to obtain specimens, complications of invasive tests, and additional testing for false positives. The presence of epidemiological variables that point to a specific pathogen requiring nonstandard treatment clearly justifies appropriate diagnostic tests (Table 2). Similarly diagnostic testing is recommended in the following clinical situations: severe CAP, failure of outpatient antibiotic therapy, leukopenia, structural lung disease, chronic liver disease or alcoholism, asplenia, pleural effusion, and the presence of cavitary infiltrates with the suspicion of MRSA.

Blood cultures have a poor sensitivity (5–14%), with the most common microorganism isolated being *S. pneumoniae*. Bacteremia in pneumococcal CAP does not appear to modify the prognosis in terms of time to clinical stability or mortality when compared with nonbacteremic pneumonia (45). Additionally, false positives by blood culture have been associated with more prolonged hospital stay and vancomycin use. Thus blood cultures are optional for hospitalized patients with CAP but should be performed in the groups of patients with clinical indications for more extensive testing as discussed above. The strongest indication for blood cultures is severe CAP, since these patients are more likely to be infected with pathogens other than *S pneumoniae*, such as *S. aureus*, *P. aeruginosa*, and other GNB (46), and have a higher yield of blood cultures.

A valid expectorated sputum sample for microbiological processing requires more than 25 polymorphonuclear cells and less than 10 squamous epithelial cells per low power field and should be obtained whenever possible, especially in patients with clinical indications for diagnostic testing. The same considerations for blood cultures in severe CAP are applicable to sputum samples. When valid sputum is obtained, the specificity of the Gram stain for pneumococcal pneumonia is estimated to be greater than 80% (47,48). Because of the fastidious nature of *S. pneumoniae* and *H. influenzae*, the sensitivity of sputum culture (50–60%) for these pathogens is less than that of Gram stain examination. The reverse is true *for S. aureus* and GNB as these bacteria are much hardier and may proliferate during sputum transport and processing. However, if the Gram stain of a valid sputum specimen does not corroborate the presence of these bacteria, then contamination by oral flora should be considered. Although specimens obtained after initiation of antibiotic therapy are unreliable and must be interpreted with caution, the collection of pretreatment expectorated sputum should not delay the initiation of antibiotic administration. Unfortunately, 40% or more patients with CAP are unable to produce any sputum at all or cannot produce it in a timely manner (49). An endotracheal aspirate or bronchoscopically obtained respiratory sample is always recommended for patients intubated for severe CAP.

Urinary antigen tests for *S. pneumoniae* and *L. pneumophila* are rapid and very useful tools whose main advantages are speed, simplicity and ability to detect a specific pathogen with reasonable accuracy, even after antibiotic therapy has been started. For *S. pneumoniae*, studies in adults show a sensitivity of 50% to 80% and a specificity of over 90% for the urinary antigen test. Concentrating the urine sample before antigen testing increases sensitivity and is recommended (50,51). It is a useful test when culture samples cannot be obtained or when antibiotic therapy has already been started. For *Legionella* all available assays detect only *L. pneumophila* serogroup 1, which accounts for 80% to 95% of community-acquired cases of Legionnaires disease with a sensitivity ranging from 70% to 90% and a specificity of nearly 99%. Rapid antigen detection tests for influenza can lead to consideration of antiviral therapy. Most tests available show a sensitivity of 50% to 70% and a specificity of nearly 100% (52).

VII. Management

A. Antimicrobial Treatment

Until more accurate and rapid diagnostic methods are available, the initial treatment for most patients remains empirical (Table 4) (3). Selection of antimicrobial regimens should be based on the prediction of the most likely pathogen and knowledge of local antimicrobial susceptibility patterns for these pathogens. In individual patients, physician should consider specific epidemiological risk factors as discussed above (Table 2).

In previously healthy outpatients with no risk factors for drug-resistant *S. pneumoniae* (DRSP), a macrolide (azitromycin, clarithromycin, or erythromycin) is recommended (3). The rates of *S. pneumoniae* macrolide resistance have risen to 25% in several parts of the world, and some data have suggested that resistance to macrolides results in clinical failure (53). It is, therefore, prudent to treat patients with a respiratory fluoroquinolone or β-lactam plus a macrolide in regions with recognized high resistance rates.

The prevalence of DRSP has increased worldwide, and risk factors for β-lactam resistance in *S. pneumoniae* that have been described include age >65 or <5, β-lactam treatment within the previous three months, alcoholism, medical comorbidities, and immunosuppressive disease or treatment (54,55). Despite such findings, the clinical relevance of β-lactam resistance in *S. pneumoniae* remains controversial because it does not appear to alter the clinical outcome and usually does not result in treatment failures.

In the presence of comorbidities, immunosuppression, the use of antibiotics in the last three months or other risk factors for DRSP, a respiratory fluoroquinolone, or a

Table 4 Recommended empirical antibiotics for community-acquired pneumonia

---

Outpatient treatment

1. Previously healthy and no use of antimicrobials within previous three months:
   Macrolide: azithromycin, clarithromicyn, or erythromycin
   Doxycycline
2. In regions with a high rate ($\geq$25%) of infection with high-level macrolide-resistant *S. pneumoniae*:
   A respiratory fluoroquinolone [moxifloxacin, gemifloxacin. or levofloxacin (750 mg)] *or*
   a β-lactam (amoxicillin high doses or amoxicillin clavulanate is preferred, *or* ceftriaxone,
   ceforoxime, or cefpodoxime) *plus* a macrolide.
3. Presence of comorbities (chronic lung, heart or liver disease; diabetes, alcoholism, malignancies,
   asplenia, immunosuppression) or antimicrobial use within the previous three months: the same
   agents listed in 2.

Inpatient non-ICU treatment

A respiratory fluoroquinolone [moxifloxacin, gemifloxacin, or levofloxacin (750 mg)] *or* a
β-lactam *plus* a macrolide

Inpatient ICU treatment

A β-lactam (cefotaxime, ceftriaxone, or ampicillin-sulbactam) plus *either* a respiratory fluoroquinolone *or* azithromycin (for patients allergic to penicillin, fluoroquinolone, and aztreonam).

Special concerns

If *Pseudomona* is a consideration:
   An antipneumococcal, antipseudomonal β lactam (piperacillin-tazobactam, cefepime, impipenem,
   or meropenem) **plus** *either* ciprofloxacin *or* levofloxacin
If CA-MRSA is a consideration: add vancomycin *or* linezolid.

Abbreviations: CA-MRSA, community-acquired methicillin-resistant *S. aureus*; ICU, intensive care unit.

β-lactam plus a macrolide is recommended. Anaerobic coverage is clearly indicated only
in patients with a clear risk for aspiration, for example, a history of loss of consciousness.
   CA-MRSA should be suspected in patients presenting with cavitary infiltrates
without risk factors for anaerobic aspiration. In these patients, vancomycin or linezolid
should be added, though the outcome in these patients is still very poor and optimal
management of this infection is yet to be defined (28). If the etiology of CAP has been
reliably identified, antimicrobial therapy should be directed at that pathogen (3). An
exception to this rule could be the ICU patient with pneumococcal bacteremia. In this
group, combined treatment with a β-lactam and a macrolide has been associated with a
lower mortality in observational studies (56). Early treatment, within 48 hours of
symptoms, with oseltamivir or zanamivir is recommended for patients with influenza.
Additionally, these drugs can be used to reduce viral shedding in hospitalized patients
with influenza with or without concomitant pneumonia (3).
   Antibiotic treatment should be administered as soon as possible after considering
the most likely pathogen. This recommendation is based on retrospective studies with
some methodological limitations that show lower mortality among patients who have
received early antibiotic therapy (57). A specific time window in which treatment should
be started is difficult to establish because of lack of prospective data.
   Patients should be switched from intravenous to oral therapy when they are
hemodynamically stable, clinically improved and are able to ingest medications.

Although many variables should be considered in individual patients, discharge is recommended if there is safe environment for continued care, there have been no other medical problems and the patients are clinically stable. The established criteria to define clinical stability (58) are temperature $\leq 37.8°C$, heart rate ≤ 100 beats/min, respiratory rate ≤ 24 breaths/min, systolic blood pressure ≥ 90 mm hg, arterial oxygen saturation $\geq 90\%$ or $PO_2 \geq 60$ mmHg on room air, and normal mental status.

B. Nonantimicrobial Treatment

In patients with respiratory failure and hypoxemia who are unable to achieve acceptable levels of arterial oxygenation using conventional oxygen therapy at maximal concentration, noninvasive ventilation with bi-level positive airway pressure (BiPAP) is justified. This intervention reduces the incidence of tracheal intubation, septic shock, and 90-day mortality (59). Patients with COPD or who are hypercapnic are most likely to benefit but the indication is not limited to this group. In patients complicated with ARDS who need invasive mechanical ventilation, low tidal-volume ventilation (6 mL/kg ideal body weight) should be used (60). Other aspects of the management of sepsis and septic shock in patients with CAP do not differ significantly from those implemented in patients with other sources of infection.

C. Nonresponding Pneumonia

The term "nonresponding pneumonia" is used to define a clinical situation in patients with inadequate clinical response despite antibiotic treatment. Two different patterns of nonresponding pneumonia have been described in hospitalized non-ICU patients (3). Progressive pneumonia is considered in cases with clinical deterioration with acute respiratory failure requiring ventilatory support and/or the appearance of septic shock, usually occurring within the first 72 hours of hospital admission. Persistent pneumonia is defined as the absence of or delay in achieving clinical stability. Up to 15% of the patients may to have a lack of response to empirical antibiotic treatment, with 8% experiencing early (within 24 to 48 hours) and 7% late (72 hours or more) failure (61). Mortality with nonresponding CAP is several fold higher than among responding patients (62).

The causes of nonresponding pneumonia are classified according to the etiology as infectious, noninfectious and of unknown origin. Infections account for 40% of nonresponding CAP. The most frequent microorganisms found are *S. pneumoniae, Legionella, S. aureus, and Pseudomonas* (62,63). There have been isolated cases of treatment failure related to resistance to the new fluoroquinolones, specifically levofloxacin (64), and to the macrolides (53). Rarer or unusual microorganisms may also cause nonresponding pneumonia (65), as they may not be adequately covered by the initial empirical therapy.

Several diseases can mimic CAP and behave as nonresponding pneumonia, including pulmonary hemorrhage, inflammatory diseases such as bronchiolitis obliterans with organizing pneumonia (BOOP), thromboembolic diseases, pulmonary eosinophilia, hypersensitivity pneumonitis, and others (66).

Nonresponding CAP is more frequent in severe pneumonia, in patients admitted to the ICU and in patients with liver disease (61,63). Local spread of infection such as to the pleural space is independently associated with nonresponding CAP, as is CAP due to *Legionella* pneumonia or gram-negative microorganisms. Interestingly, treatment failure is lower in influenza-vaccinated patients.

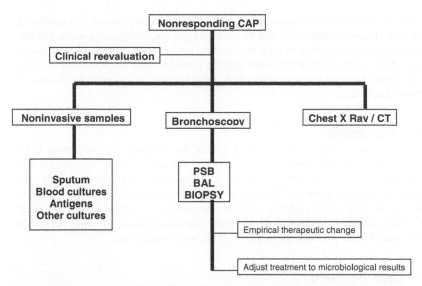

PSB, Protected Specimen Brush. BAL, bronchoalveaolar lavage. CT, computed tomography.

Figure 2 Approach to the patient with treatment failure. *Abbreviations*: PSB, protected specimen brush; BAL, bronchoalveaolar lavage; CT, computed tomography.

Figure 2 presents an approach to patients with nonresponding pneumonia. The initial evaluation of clinical response should take place within the first three days if there is no amelioration of symptoms or even before in cases with clinical progression. A careful review of the clinical history and the initial microbiological results should be undertaken to confirm the diagnosis of CAP. Important epidemiological clues for unusual microorganisms should be reviewed. On confirmation of CAP without unusual microorganisms, host factors may explain the slower resolution of infectious parameters, such as elderly patients with comorbid conditions or immunosuppression. Chest X rays may show pleural effusion, lung abscess and/or new infiltrates. Pleural effusion is a frequent cause of treatment failure and requires thoracocentesis.

In addition to further radiological studies and noninvasive samples, endoscopic methods should be considered to evaluate the airways and to obtain samples for microbiological tests and other studies. Bronchoscopy allows direct observation of the airways and the recovery of samples directly in the infected lobe. In fact, the diagnostic yield of protected specimen brush (PSB) and bronchoalveolar lavage (BAL) is 41% in treatment failures with CAP (62,63,67). BAL evaluation and cell counts are very useful in the orientation of diagnosis towards noninfectious causes (68). Thus, in the presence of >20% eosinophils, it is mandatory to rule out causes such as pulmonary eosinophilia, fungal infection, drug-induced pneumonitis, or others. Pulmonary hemorrhage is suggested by the presence of blood or hemosiderin-loaded macrophages (>20%), and an increase in lymphocyte count suggests hypersensitivity pneumonitis, sarcoidosis, or pulmonary fibrosis.

In early treatment failure, broad-spectrum antibiotic therapy should be considered. If possible new invasive samples should be obtained for microbiological studies before adjusting antibiotic therapy even though results may not be available for up to 48 hours. In nonresponding CAP, the new antibiotic regime must broaden the spectrum to cover not only the usual bacteria but also resistant *S. pneumoniae, P. aeruginosa, S. aureus,* and anaerobic bacteria.

VIII. Prevention

Vaccines against pneumococci and influenza remain the mainstay for preventing CAP. All persons ≥50 years and those in contact with high-risk persons and health care workers should receive the influenza vaccine. The pneumococcal polysaccharide vaccine is recommended for people ≥65 years, immunocompromised individuals, patients with anatomic or functional asplenia, and chronic diseases such as congestive heart failure, COPD, diabetes mellitus, liver disease, and alcoholism. Smoking cessation should be a goal for all patients, particularly those with pneumonia.

IX. Case Scenario

A 32-year-old woman presented to the emergency department because of fever and shortness of breath. She had been well until two days before, when she developed chills, myalgia, and frontal headache. There no was chest pain, hemoptysis, or cough. On initial examination, her temperature was 38.7°C, the pulse was 130, and the respiratory rate was 29. Blood pressure was 92/62 mm Hg and oxygen saturation was 93% while breathing room air. Chest X ray showed alveolar infiltrates in the upper right and lower left lobes. The white blood cell count was 18,000/mm^3 with band forms 23%, neutrophils 58%, and lymphocytes 9%; platelets were 93,000/mm^3; hematocrit was 37%. ABG breathing room air was pH 7.46/PCO$_2$ 30/PO$_2$ 64/HCO$_3$ 20.5/SO$_2$ 92%. The CRP was 23 mg/dL, and procalcitonin (PCT) was 1.6 ng/mL.

The patient was hospitalized in a general ward and levofloxacin 500 mg twice daily was started. Blood cultures and urinary antigen tests for *S. pneumoniae* and *L. pneumophila* serogroup 1 were obtained.

On the second day, respiratory distress worsened and oxygen saturation decreased to 85%, despite supplementary oxygen with a nonrebreathing mask. The patient was transferred to the ICU. Tracheal intubation was done and mechanical ventilation was started. Chest X ray showed progression of previous infiltrates with a pulmonary edema pattern. Blood cultures were negative but the urinary antigen test for *S. pneumoniae* was positive. Ceftriaxone was added to levofloxacin. The diagnosis was severe pneumococcal CAP complicated with ARDS. Progressive improvement was observed in clinical, laboratory and gas exchange variables over the following days. On the sixth day, the patient was extubated and discharged from the hospital five days later.

A. Discussion

The most important issues in this case are the prognosis and site-of-care issues. At admission, the PSI score was 32 or risk class II, representing a 30-day mortality risk of 1.5%. Theoretically, this patient could have been treated in the ambulatory setting but other considerations determined the site of care. Several of her values were just above the threshold for a more severe score: PaO_2 64, respiratory rate 29, and systolic blood pressure 92, with threshold values in the PSI score of 60, 30, and 90, respectively. Several variables at or near cut-off values justify hospitalization in patients at low risk (3). The score measured by CURB 65 for this case was I (urea > 20). Again, the respiratory rate and blood pressure were close to threshold values, which could imply clinically important physiological derangements. Additionally, although not considered in PSI and CURB 65, the patient actually met three minor criteria for severe pneumonia, thrombocytopenia, multilobar infiltrates, and an increased blood urea nitrogen (BUN) (3).

In cases in which the accuracy of risk scores is doubtful, additional tools such as inflammatory biomarkers may be useful. CRP is an early nonspecific but sensitive marker of inflammation. High-serum CRP level ($\geq$10 mg/dL) are a marker independently associated with a high risk of death in patients with lower respiratory tract infection (69). Other clinically important adverse outcomes associated with high CRP levels include longer hospital stay and a lower clinical recovery rate at eight weeks (70). In addition, among patients with PSI risk I to III, high-serum CRP levels are related to the need for hospitalization (71). Thus, the serum CRP values of 23 mg/dL support the need for hospitalization.

PCT is a prohormone that has emerged as a promising biomarker in different clinical settings. Its level increases rapidly in bacterial infections but remains low in viral diseases. PCT also seems to be a prognostic factor in sepsis and pneumonia (72,73). In community-based studies of CAP, serum procalcitonin levels correlate with severity measured by PSI. Additionally levels $\geq$0.5 ng/mL may predict death and complications (74). Likewise, when compared with CRB 65, PCT has at least comparable predictive potential for death from pneumonia because PCT of $\leq$ 0.228 ng/mL can predict survival in all risk groups with a very high negative predictive value of 98% (75). Thus, PCT may be used to identify patients who might be safely treated as an outpatient despite an increased predictive clinical score. The serum PCT level of this patient (1.6 ng/mL) was high enough to consider hospitalization and a high risk of complications.

References

1. Metlay J, Fine M. Testing strategies in the initial management of patients with community acquired pneumonia. Ann Intern Med 2003; 138(2):109–118.
2. Syrjälä H, Broas M, Suramo I, et al. High-resolution computed tomography for the diagnosis of community-acquired pneumonia. Clin Infect Dis 1998; 27:358–363.
3. Mandel LA, Wundernik RG, Anzueto A, et al. Infectious Diseases Society of America/ American Thoracic Society consensus guidelines on the management of community-acquired pneumonia in adults. Clin Infect Dis 2007; 44:S27–S72.
4. Mathers C, Bernard C, Moesgaard Iburg K, et al. WHO Global Burden of Disease in 2002: data sources, methods and results. Available at: http://www.who.int/healthinfo/paper54.pdf. Accessed April 2008.
5. WHO/UNICEF. Pneumonia: The forgotten killer of children. Available at: http://www.unicef. org/publications/index_35626.html. Accessed March 10, 2008.
6. Marston BJ, Plouffe JF, File TMJ, et al. Incidence of community-acquired pneumonia requiring hospitalization: results of a population-based active surveillance study in Ohio; The Community-Based Pneumonia Incidence Study Group. Arch Intern Med 1997; 157:1709–1718.
7. Halm EA, Teirstein AS. Management of community acquired-pneumonia. N Eng J Med 2002; 347:2039–2045.

8. Bauer TT, Ewig S, Marre R, et al. CRB-65 predicts death from community-acquired pneumonia. J Intern Med 2006; 260(1):93–101.
9. LaCroix AZ, Lipson S, Miles TP, et al. Prospective study of pneumonia hospitalizations and mortality of U.S. older people: the role of chronic conditions, health behaviors, and nutritional status. Public Health Rep 1989; 104(4):350–360.
10. Koivula I, Sten M, Makela PH. Risk factors for pneumonia in the elderly. Am J Med 1994; 96 (4):313–320.
11. Fine MJ, Auble TE, Yealy DM, et al. A prediction rule to identify low-risk patients with community-acquired pneumonia. N Engl J Med 1997; 336(4):243–250.
12. Fine MJ, Smith MA, Carson CA, et al. Prognosis and outcomes of patients with community-acquired pneumonia. A meta-analysis. JAMA 1996; 275(2):134–141.
13. Nuorti JP, Butler JC, Farley MM, et al. Cigarette smoking and invasive pneumococcal disease. Active Bacterial Core Surveillance Team. N Engl J Med 2000; 342:681–689.
14. Ruiz M, Ewig S, Marcos MA, et al. Etiology of community-acquired pneumonia: impact of age, comorbidity, and severity. Am J Respir Crit Care Med 1999; 160(2):397–405.
15. Bont J, Hak E, Hoes AW, et al. A prediction rule for elderly primary-care patients with lower respiratory tract infections. Eur Respir J 2007; 29(5):969–975.
16. Torres A, Serra-Batlles J, Ferrer A, et al. Severe community-acquired pneumonia: epidemiology and prognostic factors. Am Rev Respir Dis 1991; 144:312–318.
17. Ruiz Gonzalez A, Falguera M, Nogues A, et al. Is the Streptococcus pneumoniae the leading cause of pneumonia of unknown aetiology? A microbiologic study of lung aspirates in consecutive patients with community-acquired pneumonia. Am J Med 1999; 106:385–390.
18. Fine MJ, Stone RA, Singer DE, et al. Processes and outcome of care for patients with community acquired pneumonia: results from the Pneumonia Patient Outcome Research Team (PORT) cohort study. Arch Intern Med 1999; 159:970–980.
19. Woodhead M, Blasi F, Ewing S, et al. Guidelines for the management of adult lower respiratory tract infections. Eur Respir J 2005; 26:1138–1180.
20. Arancibia F, Bauer TT, Ewig S, et al. Community-acquired pneumonia due to gram-negative bacteria and pseudomonas aeruginosa: incidence, risk, and prognosis. Arch Intern Med 2002; 162:1849–1858.
21. Fernandez-Sabe N, Carratala J, Roson B, et al. Community-acquired pneumonia in very elderly patients: causative organisms, clinical characteristics, and outcomes. Medicine (Baltimore) 2003; 82:159–169.
22. Marcos MA, Camps M, Pumarola T, et al. The role of viruses in the aetiology of community-acquired pneumonia in adults. Antivir Ther 2006; 11:351–359.
23. de Roux A, Marcos MA, Garcia E, et al. Viral community-acquired pneumonia in non-immunocompromised adults. Chest 2004; 125:1343–1351.
24. Gutierrez F, Masia M, Rodriguez JC, et al. Community-acquired pneumonia of mixed etiology: prevalence, clinical characteristics, and outcome. Eur J Clin Microbiol Infect Dis 2005; 24:377–383.
25. Saito A, Kohno S, Matsushima T, et al. Prospective multicenter study of the causative organisms of community-acquired pneumonia in adults in Japan. J Infect Chemother 2006; 12:63–69.
26. Bonten MC, Chastre J, Craig WA, et al. Guidelines for the management of adults with hospital-acquired, ventilator-associated, and healthcare-associated pneumonia. Am J Respir Crit Care Med 2005; 171:388–416.
27. Carratalà J, Mykietiuk A, Fernández-Sabé N, et al. Health care-associated pneumonia requiring hospital admission: epidemiology, antibiotic therapy, and clinical outcomes. Arch Intern Med 2007; 167:1393–1399.
28. Rubinstein E, Kollef MH, Nathwani D. Pneumonia caused by methicillin-resistant Staphylococcus aureus. Clin Infect Dis 2008; 46:S378–S385.

29. Gleeson K, Eggli DF, Maxwell SL. Quantitative aspiration during sleep in normal subjects. Chest 1997; 111:1266–1272.
30. Akira S, Uematsu S, Takeuchi O. Pathogen recognition and innate immunity. Cell 2006; 124:783–801.
31. Mizgerd JP. Acute lower respiratory tract infection. N Engl J Med 2008; 358:716–727.
32. Bauer TT, Ewig S, Rodloff AC, et al. Acute respiratory distress syndrome and pneumonia: a comprehensive review of clinical data. Clin Infect Dis 2006; 43:748–756.
33. Gennis P, Gallagher J, Falvo C, et al. Clinical criteria for the detection of pneumonia in adults: guidelines for ordering chest roentgenograms in the emergency department. J Emerg Med 1989; 7:263–268.
34. Metlay JP, Schulz R, Li YH, et al. Influence of age on symptoms at presentation in patients with community-acquired pneumonia. Arch Intern Med 1997; 157:1453–1459.
35. Smith RP, Lipworth BJ. C-reactive protein in simple community-acquired pneumonia. Chest 1995; 107:1028–1031.
36. Albazzaz MK, Pal C, Berman P, et al. Inflammatory markers of lower respiratory tract infection in elderly people. Age Ageing 1994; 23:299–302.
37. Mac Farlane JT, Miller AC, Smith WHO, et al. Comparative radiographic features of community-acquired legionnaires' disease, pneumococcal pneumonia, Mycoplasma pneumoniae, and psittacosis. Thorax 1984; 39:28–33.
38. Sopena N, Sabria-Leal M, Pedro-Botet ML, et al. Comparative study of the clinical presentation of Legionella pneumonia and other community-acquired pneumonias. Chest 1998; 113:1195–1200.
39. Tan MJ, Tan JS, Hamor RH, et al. The radiologic manifestations of legionnaire's disease: the Ohio community-based pneumonia incidence study group. Chest 2000; 117:398–403.
40. Marrie TJ, Lau CY, Wheeler SL. A controlled trial of a critical pathway for treatment of community acquired pneumonia. JAMA 2000; 283:749–755.
41. Halm EA, Fine MJ, Marrie TJ, et al. Time to clinical stability in patients hospitalized with community-acquired pneumonia: implications for practice guidelines. JAMA 1998; 279:1452–1457.
42. Lim WS, van der Eerden MM, Laing R, et al. Defining community acquired pneumonia severity on presentation to hospital: an international derivation and validation study. Thorax 2003; 58:377–382.
43. Capelastegui A, Espana PP, Quintana JM, et al. Validation of a predictive rule for the management of community-acquired pneumonia. Eur Respir J 2006; 27:151–157.
44. Ewig S, de Roux A, Bauer T, et al. Validation of predictive rules and indices of severity for community acquired pneumonia. Thorax 2004; 59:421–427.
45. Bordo J, Peyrani P, Brock GN. The presence of pneumococcal bacteremia does not influence clinical outcomes in patients with community-acquired pneumonia. Chest 2008; 133: 618–624.
46. Ruiz M, Ewig S, Torres A, et al. Severe community-acquired pneumonia. Am J Respir Crit Care Med 1999; 160:923–929.
47. Roson B, Carratala J, Verdaguer R, et al. Prospective study of the usefulness of sputum gram stain in the initial approach to community-acquired pneumonia requiring hospitalization. Clin Infect Dis 2000; 31:869–874.
48. Reed WW, Byrd GS, Gates RH Jr., et al. Sputum gram's stain in community-acquired pneumococcal pneumonia: A meta-analysis. West J Med 1996; 165:197–204.
49. van der Eerden MM, Vlaspolder F, de Graaff CS, et al. Comparison between pathogen directed antibiotic treatment and empirical broad spectrum antibiotic treatment in patients with community acquired pneumonia: a prospective randomised study. Thorax 2005; 60:672–678.
50. Dominguez J, Gali N, Blanco S, et al. Detection of Streptococcus pneumoniae antigen by a rapid immunochromatographic assay in urine samples. Chest 2001; 119:243–249.

51. Gutierrez F, Masia M, Rodriguez JC, et al. Evaluation of the immunochromatographic Binax NOW assay for detection of Streptococcus pneumoniae urinary antigen in a prospective study of community- acquired pneumonia in Spain. Clin Infect Dis 2003; 36:286–292.

52. Landry ML, Cohen S, Ferguson D. Comparison of Binax NOW and Directigen for rapid detection of influenza A and B. J Clin Virol 2004; 31:113–115.

53. Daneman N, McGeer A, Green K, et al. Macrolide resistance in bacteremic pneumococcal disease: implications for patient management. Clin Infect Dis 2006; 43:432–438.

54. Yu VL, Chiou CC, Feldman C, et al. An international prospective study of pneumococcal bacteremia: correlation with in vitro resistance, antibiotics administered, and clinical outcome. Clin Infect Dis 2003; 37:230–237.

55. Vanderkooi OG, Low DE, Green K, et al. Predicting antimicrobial resistance in invasive pneumococcal infections. Clin Infect Dis 2005; 40:1288–1297.

56. Baddour LM, Yu VL, Klugman KP, et al. Combination antibiotic therapy lowers mortality among severely ill patients with with pneumococcal bacteremia. Am J Respir Crit Care Med 2004; 170:440–444.

57. Houck PM, Bratzler DW, Nsa W, et al. Timing of antibiotic administration and outcomes for Medicare patients hospitalized with community-acquired pneumonia. Arch Intern Med 2004; 164:637–644.

58. Menéndez R, Torres A, Rodriguez de Castro F, et al. Reaching stability in community-acquired pneumonia: the effects of the severity of disease, treatment, and the characteristics of patients. Clin Infect Dis 2004; 39:1783–1790.

59. Ferrer M, Esquinas A, Leon M, et al. Non-invasive ventilation in severe hypoxemic respiratory failure. A randomized clinical trial. Am J Respir Crit Care Med 2003; 168:1438–1444.

60. The Acute Respiratory Distress Syndrome Network. Ventilation with lower tidal volumes as compared with traditional tidal volumes for acute lung injury and the acute respiratory distress syndrome. The Acute Respiratory Distress Syndrome Network. N Engl J Med 2000; 342:1301–1308.

61. Menéndez R, Torres A, Zalacaín R, et al. Risk factors of treatment failure in community acquired pneumonia: implications for disease outcome. Thorax 2004; 59:960–965.

62. Arancibia F, Ewig S, Martinez JA, et al. Antimicrobial treatment failures in patients with community-acquired pneumonia: causes and prognostic implications. Am J Respir Crit Care Med 2000; 162:154–160.

63. Rosón B, Carratalà J, Fernández-Sabé N, et al. Causes and factors associated with early failure in hospitalized patients with community-acquired pneumonia Arch Intern Med 2004; 164:502–508.

64. Chen DK, McGeer A, de Azavedo JC, et al. Decreased susceptibility of Streptococcus pneumoniae to fluoroquinolones in Canada. Canadian Bacterial Surveillance Network. N Engl J Med 1999; 341:233–239.

65. Menéndez R, Cordero PJ, Santos M, et al. Pulmonary infection with Nocardia species: a report of 10 cases and review. Eur Respir J 1997; 10:1542–1546.

66. Kuru T, Lynch JP. Nonresolving or slowly resolving pneumonia. Clin Chest Med 1999; 20:623–651.

67. Ortqvist A, Kalin M, Lejdeborn L. Diagnostic fiberoptic bronchoscopy and protected brush culture in patients with community-acquired pneumonia Chest 1990; 97:576–582.

68. Jacobs JA, De Brauwer EI, Ramsay G, et al. Detection of non-infectious conditions mimicking pneumonia in the intensive care setting: usefulness of bronchoalveolar fluid cytology. Respir Med 1999; 93:571–578.

69. Seppa Y, Bloigu A, Honkanen PO, et al. Severity assessment of lower respiratory tract infection in elderly patients in primary care. Arch Intern Med 2001; 161:2709–2713.

70. Hedlund J. Community-acquired pneumonia requiring hospitalisation: factors of importance for the short-and long term prognosis. Scand J Infect Dis Suppl 1995; 97:1–60.

71. Stauble SP, Reichlin S, Dieterle T, et al. Community acquired pneumonia: which patients are hospitalised? Swiss Med Wkly 2001; 13:188–192.
72. Christ-Crain M, Jaccard-Stolz D, Bingisser R, et al. Effect of procalcitonin-guided treatment on antibiotic use and outcome in lower respiratory tract infections: cluster-randomised, single-blinded intervention trial. Lancet 2004; 363:600–607.
73. Christ-Crain M, Müller B. Procalcitonin in bacterial infections –hype, hope, more or less? Swiss Med Wkly 2005; 135:451–460.
74. Masiá M, Gutiérrez F, Shum C, et al. Usefulness of procalcitonin levels in community-acquired pneumonia according to the patients outcome research team pneumonia severity index. Chest 2005; 128:2223–2229.
75. Krüger S, Ewig S, Marre R, et al. Procalcitonin predicts patients at low risk of death from community-acquired pneumonia across all CRB-65 classes. Eur Respir J 2008; 31:349–355.

9
Health Care–Associated Pneumonia

ALI A. EL SOLH
State University of New York at Buffalo School of Medicine and Biomedical Sciences, and School of Public Health and Health Professions, Buffalo, New York, U.S.A.

I. Introduction

The last two decades have witnessed a major evolution in the classification of pneumonia. Traditionally, clinicians have classified pneumonia by clinical characteristics, dividing them into "acute" and "chronic" pneumonias. The term acute was linked to the presence of symptoms of less than three weeks' duration and was indicative customarily of an infectious etiology. Chronic pneumonias tended to be either noninfectious, mycobacterial, fungal, or related to opportunistic infections. With the creation of sub-specialty services and introduction of life-saving technologies (i.e., mechanical venti-lation), the classification of pneumonia has shifted to a new scheme that revolves around the patient's underlying risk factors. The advantage of this classification scheme over previous systems is that it can help guide the selection of appropriate initial treatments even before the microbiologic cause of the pneumonia is known.

Not until few years ago, there were two broad categories of pneumonia in this scheme: community-acquired pneumonia (CAP) and hospital-acquired pneumonia (HAP). The first entity referred to patients who sought medical attention for lower respiratory tract infection while residing in the community. HAP was reserved for those who developed pneumonia 48 hours after hospitalization. Over the last several years, a number of investigators (1,2) have documented that individuals who acquire infections while receiving out-of-hospital health care differ from those with community-acquired infections. In fact, because of their frequent contact with the health care environment, these patients become colonized with multidrug-resistant (MDR) pathogens that would carry over to the time of hospital admission. Hence, the term "health care–associated pneumonia" was introduced in the literature to account for this new entity.

By definition, HCAP refers to patients with pneumonia who have a history of recent hospitalization in the past 90 days, residence in a nursing home or extended care facility, treatment with chronic hemodialysis, receipt of home wound care, or exposure to a family member with drug-resistant pathogen infection (3). Semantically, HCAP may encompass not only those patients who meet the above criteria but also those who acquire pneumonia during hospitalization (HAP) or following endotracheal intubation [ventilator-associated pneumonia (VAP)] (4). While recognizing the continuum spectrum of causative agents between these entities, a recent proceeding on HCAP (5) has elected to separate these entities into four categories on the basis of their most likely organisms in attempt to maximize the likelihood of achieving a favorable patient outcome (Fig. 1).

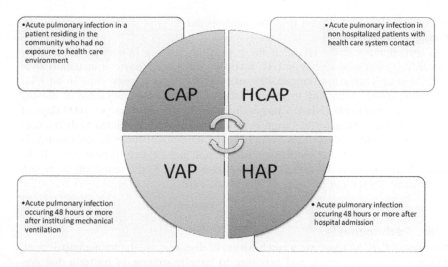

Figure 1 Alphabet soup of pneumonia.

II. Epidemiology

Health care–associated pneumonia accounts for approximately 15% of all health care–acquired infections and is the second most common health care–related infection after that of the urinary tract. The incidence of HCAP is actually unknown due to the paucity of study, but it is estimated to range between 17.3% and 67.4% depending on the population analyzed and the diagnostic techniques utilized (6). Using a large database, Kollef and colleagues (7) analyzed retrospectively the records of 4543 patients hospitalized with culture-positive pneumonia during a two-year period. Of these, 48.9% had CAP, 21.7% had HCAP, 18.4% had HAP, and 11% had VAP. The median age of patients with HCAP was 77 years. Nearly half of these patients were residing in skilled nursing facilities prior to presentation. The burden of comorbidities was higher in this population compared with those with CAP in addition to cardiovascular diseases, diabetes mellitus, and medical immunosuppression accounting for the bulk of underlying illnesses. These findings were later duplicated by Carratalà and coworkers (8) in a prospective study of 727 nonseverely immunosuppresed adults presenting to the emergency with pneumonia. HCAP accounted for 17% of hospital admissions. Forty-three percent had been hospitalized in the 90 days period prior to developing pneumonia, 31.7% received chemotherapy or visited a hospital clinic or a dialysis center in the 30 days before pneumonia, 25.4% resided in long-term care (LTC) facilities, and 14.3% were the recipient of home health care.

The incidence of HCAP is expected to increase in the coming decades and may even surpass the rate of CAP. One retrospective study from a single center reported a higher incidence of HCAP (67.4%) admitted to a single center compared with CAP (32.6%) (9). Of those, 68.9% were recently hospitalized, 39.2% were immunosuppressed, 28.1% presented from a nursing home, and 10% were on hemodialysis. The study inclusion criteria however were limited to culture-positive pneumonia, and it is likely that patients with CAP were excluded from the analysis due to prior antibiotic use or inadequate respiratory specimens.

A special entity of the HCAP is the population residing in nursing homes. The number of frail older adults living in LTC facilities is expected to rise dramatically over the next 30 years (10). An estimated 40% of adults will spend some time in an LTC facility before dying. According to several surveys, the estimated incidence of nursing home–acquired pneumonia (NHAP) ranges from 0.3 to 2.5 episodes per 1000 days of resident care (11,12). Despite the variation in incidence, which is related to differences in study design, number of facilities evaluated, and intensity of surveillance, this rate is 10 times the incidence of pneumonia in noninstitutionalized elderly persons (13). If the incidence of pneumonia in this population remains the same, by the year 2030, there will be an estimated 1.9 million episodes of NHAP annually.

III. Pathogenesis

Most episodes of HCAP represent a combination of disease-related immune impairment, acquisition of a virulent strain, and exposure to large inoculums of bacteria that predispose to pneumonia. Although there are several avenues by which potential pathogens may gain access to the lung, the most likely route in HCAP is presumed to be colonization of the upper respiratory tract followed by aspiration of bacteria laden oropharyngeal secretions into the lower respiratory tract. The presence of several factors such as bed confinement, urinary incontinence, and prior antibiotic usage, has been linked to oropharyngeal colonization by gram-negative bacteria (14,15). With increasing severity of illness, changes in epithelial glycoprotein-binding characteristics develop along with alterations in the enzymatic content of salivary and tracheal secretions (16). When coupled with decreased salivation from drug-induced antidepressants, antiparkinsonian medications, diuretics, antihypertensives, or antihistamines, the process of oropharyngeal colonization is amplified. Bacterial pneumonia follows the clinically silent aspiration of microorganisms that have been harbored in the nasopharynx. In a study assessing pulmonary aspiration in a long-term care setting, 56% of aspiration events progressed to pneumonia (17). In these patients, the susceptibility to lower respiratory tract infection is enhanced by the proportional decrease in immune response associated with the number of comorbidities (18). Following PHA stimulation, institutionalized elderly show a decrease in T-cell proliferation and interleukin (IL)-12 production while IL-10 production is increased independent of age compared to young healthy males.

IV. Clinical Presentation

Excluding institutionalized patients, available reports indicate only few variations in the clinical presentation of HCAP compared with CAP (8). Yet, investigations involving patients residing in LTC facilities showed that the classic signs of infections might be lacking. Compared with patients with CAP, patients with NHAP were less likely to have a productive cough (61% vs. 35%), chills (58% vs. 24%), myalgia (33% vs. 7%), or arthralgia (10% vs. 0%) (19). A retrospective cohort analysis comparing the clinical presentations of NHAP and CAP found similarly that patients with NHAP were more likely to have altered mental status (55.9% vs. 11.3%), tachypnea (40.9% vs. 22.8%), and hypotension (7.0% vs. 1.1%) (20). These atypical findings could be responsible for a delay in diagnosis and treatment, contributing to increased morbidity and mortality in this group of patients.

V. Etiologic Agents

To date, no multicenter studies have used comprehensive testing to establish the etiology of HCAP. While the bacteriologic yield of respiratory samples in HCAP is generally higher than those reported in patients with CAP (8), the preponderant microbial pathogens responsible for HCAP may remain undetermined due to the variations in epidemiologic studies vis-à-vis the demographics of the HCAP population under investigation, the type of techniques used to collect respiratory specimens, and the yield of diagnostic tests chosen. Carratalà and colleagues (6) reviewed the etiology of HCAP using three contemporary trials and reported a broad spectrum of causative pathogens. *Streptococcus pneumoniae* and *Staphylococcus aureus* were the most frequent gram-positive organisms accounting for 5.5% to 27.8% and 2.4% to 46.7% of cases, respectively. A significant proportion of patients in this category were infected with methicillin-resistant *Staph. aureus* (MRSA) (0.8–30.6%). Penicillin- and erythromycin-resistant pneumococcal strains were also more prevalent in HCAP with estimated frequency of 33.3% and 41.7%, respectively. Among the gram-negative bacteria, *Pseudomonas aeruginosa* was by far the most frequently reported organisms and was isolated in 1.6% to 25.5%. *Escherichia coli*, *Klebsiella pneumoniae*, and other nonfermenting gram-negative rods occurred in 2.4% to 5.2%, 0% to 7.6%, and 0% to 19%. Of interest, atypical pathogens like *Mycoplasma*, *Chlamydia*, and *Legionella* represented a small fraction (<2%) of the total pathogens isolated. Whether the prevalence of these organisms is truly underestimated or simply represents a rare occurrence in HCAP, antimicrobial coverage against these agents has been recommended until further studies are available.

Only one study of patients with pneumonia undergoing long-term hemodialysis was reported (21). The rate of microbial identification was limited to 18.2%. In patients with microbiologically confirmed pneumonia, the most common pathogens were *S. pneumoniae* (18.7%), *P. aeruginosa* (15.4%), *Klebsiella* spp. (8.8%), and *Haemophilus influenzae* (8.2%). Despite high rates of colonization with MRSA in the dialysis population, *Staphylococcus* spp. were infrequently the causative pathogen (2.2%). As for patients receiving home care, a single prospective case-control study of 175 patients with MRSA infection (22) identified a highly significant association between MRSA infection and prior receipt of home nursing care such as a nursing home infusion therapy, prior hospitalization, and transfer from another institution.

More substantial literature exists on the microbial etiology responsible for pneumonia in LTC facilities. Agents causing NHAP share some similarities with those responsible for CAP and HAP. Muder (23) reviewed 18 studies of NHAP published between 1978 and 1994 in which the infection was sought using sputum cultures. Only 5 of the 18 studies used strict criteria for sputum quality established by Murray and Washington (24) requiring the presence of >25 polymorphonuclear leucocytes and <10 epithelial cells per 100 power microscopic field on Gram stain. On the basis of a yield of 22% to 42%, *S. pneumoniae* (4–16%), *H. influenzae* (0–10%), *Moraxella catarrhalis* (0–5%), gram-negative bacilli (0–12%), and *Staph. aureus* (1–4%) were the predominant isolates (25–29). The remaining studies that used modified criteria or no criteria for determining sputum validity reported *S. pneumoniae* in 0% to 30%, *Staph. aureus* in 0% to 27%, *H. influenzae* in 0% to 19%, and gram-negative bacilli in 3% to 55% of all cultures. In a more comprehensive diagnostic work up that included standard bacteriologic cultures, serology, and culture for respiratory viruses, Loeb and coworkers (12) were able to obtain adequate sputum specimens for culture in only 9% of the 272 episodes of lower respiratory tract infection. Although the etiology was indeterminate in 42%, respiratory viruses accounted for 22% of all episodes, suggesting that viruses may have a greater role in causing NHAP than previously thought.

Residents of LTC facilities are at particularly high risk for developing MDR pneumonia. Kupronis and colleagues (30) performed an analysis of 2402 cases of invasive pneumococcal disease among hospitalized residents of LTC facilities and community-dwelling older adults. The risk of invasive pneumococcal disease was reported to be more than fourfold higher in older adults residing in LTC facilities compared with older adults from the community (risk ratio 4.4, 95% CI, 4.2–4.5). In severe cases of NHAP requiring intubation and mechanical ventilation, the prevalence of MDR pathogens is more pronounced. In a prospective study of 47 patients with severe NHAP, *Staph. aureus* (29%), including methicillin-resistant isolates, surpassed *S. pneumoniae* (9%) as the most common organisms isolated by quantitative cultures (31). Those who failed to respond to an initial course of antibiotic therapy at the nursing home, the most frequent pathogens recovered by bronchoscopy were MRSA (33%), enteric gram-negative rods (24%), and *Pseudomonas* spp. (14%) (32).

VI.   Diagnostic Strategies

There is no gold standard that is established for the diagnosis of HCAP. The combination of fever, purulent cough with a new infiltrate on chest X ray remains the norm in establishing the diagnosis of pneumonia. The role of ancillary testing in making the diagnosis of HCAP has not been thoroughly investigated. Some of the recommendations are rather an extrapolation of the data that have emerged over the years with our experience in the treatment of CAP/HAP/VAP.

A.   Sputum Gram stain

The potential value of sputum Gram stain in nonintubated HCAP remains to be determined. Although the presence of a predominant bacterial phenotype on a Gram stain has been consistently taunted as highly valuable in directing initial therapy, there are several limitations to the diagnostic utility of Gram stain that raise a number of questions about its routine use in clinical settings of HCAP. The central problem with sputum Gram stain relates of how accurately expectorated sputum represents lower respiratory tract infection secretions without contamination from the oropharynx (Table 1). Colonization of the upper respiratory tract by both gram-negative bacteria and gram-positive bacteria is more prevalent in recently hospitalized or institutionalized patients and is related more to the burden of systemic illness and degree of care than to age itself (33,34). In one particular population, oropharyngeal colonization by gram-negative bacteria has been documented in 22% to 37% of older patients residing in LTC facilities (35). Previous antibiotic therapy, smoking, malnutrition, decrease in functional status, and urinary tract

Table 1 Colonization Rates of the Upper Respiratory Tract Flora by Suspected Pathogens

Pathogen	Colonization rate (%)	Risk groups
Streptococcus pneumoniae	35–69	Carrier rates increased in children, day care workers, and during winter months
Staphylococcus aureus	5–50	Carrier rates increased in hospitalized patients, institutionalized elderly, and with prior antibiotic use
Enteric gram-negative bacilli	3–65	Carrier rates increased in institutionalized elderly, in patients with comorbid diseases, and in alcoholics

incontinence have all been identified as factors to colonization of the upper respiratory tract by these pathogens (33).

In addition, patients with HCAP may not raise a diagnostic specimen for Gram stain that meets strict quality standards for interpretation. Gram stains can be subject to misinterpretation and the final report may vary depending of the skills and experience of the operator (36). Furthermore, the likelihood of obtaining a positive specimen is reduced further in those who have received prior antibiotics (37). The greatest concern lies in the failure of Gram stain to detect atypical pathogens that may cause HCAP. In the absence of adequate data on the prevalence of atypical pathogens in HCAP, there are concerns about not providing adequate coverage for these infections. Published data from trials in CAP have indicated that mortality and morbidity may be higher when antibiotic regimens do not include these pathogens in their spectrum (38). Until the sensitivity and specificity of Gram stain are better delineated in nonintubated HCAP, sputum Gram stain should be considered complementary to the clinical evaluation when determining antimicrobial therapy.

B. Blood Culture

Blood cultures are positive in 8.7% to 30.9% (8,9) in patients with HCAP. *Pneumococcus* remains the most commonly isolated organisms followed by MRSA and *P. aeruginosa*. The yield is strongly influenced by prior antibiotic therapy, which raises the question of its utility and cost effectiveness in a population that are frequently exposed to antimicrobial therapy. However, the unequivocally convincing nature of isolating a respiratory pathogen from blood, the opportunity to test the antimicrobial sensitivity of the isolate, and the relative simplicity of blood for culture argue to continue the current practice until the question is tested more rigorously.

C. Urinary Antigen Detection

A variety of urinary antigen tests are commercially available that can be used for the diagnosis of HCAP. Compared with blood or sputum cultures, antigen studies have the advantage of being less affected by prior antibiotic usage and also by remaining positive longer after treatment has been initiated. Although not tested specifically in HCAP, testing for pneumococcal antigens can improve the diagnostic yields of lung aspirates (39). Overall the specificity is high (>90%) but the sensitivity is low to moderate and ranging between 0% and 58%. An exception is the urinary antigen for *Legionella pneumophila* type 1 that has a sensitivity of 70% and specificity approaching 100% (40). This test does not reliably detect any of the other 14 serogroups of *L. pneumophila* or the more than 40 other species of *Legionella*.

D. Serologic Studies
Serology can be useful in epidemiologic studies but has limited application in the determining the etiologic diagnosis of HCAP.

E. Invasive Procedures
Transtracheal aspiration and bronchial washings are a more accurate means of obtaining specimens for Gram stain and culture, although this procedure is rarely practical in the outpatient setting. The use of fiberoptic bronchoscopy in HCAP is most appropriate in patients who are severely ill, most notably if endotracheal intubation and mechanical ventilation are necessary. Gram stain of BAL specimens can provide early clues to a diagnosis of pneumonia. The identification of intracellular bacteria in more than 2% to 4% of cells has accurately predicted positive quantitative culture in ventilated patients (41). To be of greatest value however, bronchoscopic specimens for culture and Gram stain should be collected before antibiotic therapy. This would be practical if carrying out the procedure would not significantly delay initiation of treatment. Alternatively, obtaining endotracheal aspirates for quantitative cultures might be considered a reasonable compromise. Unlike in patients with VAP where colonization of the endotracheal tube reduces the diagnostic accuracy of endotracheal aspirates, contamination of tracheal aspirates is less likely to occur in newly intubated patients with HCAP. In a study of 75 patients with NHAP requiring artificial ventilation, diagnostic accuracy of quantitative endotracheal aspirates (QEA) was most favorable at 10^4 cfu/mL. QEA findings correlated significantly with both PSB and BAL quantitative cultures ($r = 0.71$ and $r = 0.77$, respectively) (42).

VII. Approach to Antimicrobial Therapy
Current treatment of pneumonia is largely based on timely prescription of adequate antibiotic therapy. However, antimicrobial treatments are hampered by the ever-increasing problem of resistant strains, and the prospects for introduction of novel antibiotics in the near future are limited.

Most epidemiologic investigations have clearly demonstrated that the indiscriminate administration of antimicrobial agents has serious consequences which contribute to the emergence of multiresistant pathogens and increase the risk of superinfections with potentially increased morbidity and mortality in addition to antibiotic-related toxicity and higher cost (3). Conversely, it has been demonstrated that inappropriate empiric antimicrobial therapy was strongly associated with poor outcome (31). Two factors seem to render the choice of antibiotics particularly difficult in patients with HCAP. First, the sampling techniques, particularly in nonintubated HCAP, are not specific enough to differentiate colonizing bacteria from infecting pathogens. Second, the spectrum of bacterial pathogens is too broad to have one or two agents to cover all the microorganisms potentially responsible for HCAP.

Data emerging from recent investigations have indicated that patients with HCAP were at higher risk of receiving inadequate antimicrobial therapy compared to CAP and were also more likely to have a worse outcome (7,8). Among the reasons for this discrepancy between HCAP and CAP is the lack of adequate coverage for MDR pathogens. Micek and colleagues (9) identified MRSA, *P. aeruginosa*, and other non-fermenting gram-negative rods as the common pathogens responsible for inadequacy of the initial antimicrobial regimen. Those patients were more likely to die than did patients treated with appropriate initial regimen (32.2% vs. 15.7%). Alternatively, numerous trials have documented the safety and efficacy of antibiotic regimens in patients with HCAP who received therapy not directed at MDR pathogens. HCAP arising in nursing homes have been treated successfully with oral quinolones (26) with fewer hospital transfer and lower costs (43).

Three factors have been shown to predict the presence of MDR pathogens in HCAP. These pathogens were recovered from severely ill patients requiring admission to an intensive care unit, with low functional status (ADL > 12), who had prior exposure to antibiotics for more than three days in the preceding six months (44). Accordingly, the treatment of HCAP may be divided into two categories: those who require limited spectrum coverage (CAP-like) and those who need broad-spectrum antibiotics (HAP-like) (Fig. 2). Limited-spectrum therapy may include a quinolone or a combination of β-lactam (ceftriaxone, ertapenem) plus a macrolide. Patients in this category can be treated in the nursing home or in the community with oral quinolone. Broad-spectrum therapy should be given to those who exhibit at least two out of the three factors indicative of the presence of MDR pathogens. The proposed regimens would include a combination of anti-pseudomonal β-lactam (piperacillin/tazobactam, cefipime, imipenem, or meropenem) plus an antipseudomonal quinolone (ciprofloxacin or high-dose levofloxacin). In cases where there is a recent history of prior treatment with a fluoroquinolone (within the prior

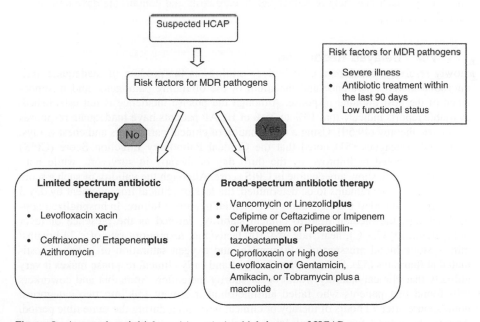

Figure 2 Approach to initial empiric antimicrobial therapy of HCAP.

3 months), an aminoglycoside (gentamicin, tobramycin, or amikacin) should be substituted along with the addition of a macrolide to cover for possible legionellosis and fluoroquinolone-resistant pneumococcus (45). Similarly, prior treatment with co-trimoxazole or clarithromycin or azithromycin is predictive of pneumococcal infections resistant to these agents. Hence, health care providers need to determine if any of these agents has been used recently so that an alternative is considered to avoid treatment failure.

Adding an agent against MRSA should be evaluated in the context of patient's recent contact with health care systems. Among the risk factors associated with MRSA infection include diabetes, renal failure, recent influenza, home nursing care, prior hospitalization, transfer from another hospital or nursing home, and previous use of antibiotics (22,44). Unfortunately, there is a significant heterogeneity in the prevalence of MRSA among the HCAP population and in the impact of omitting such coverage on outcome (46,47). Until prospective controlled trials are made available, the opinion is to provide initial coverage with either vancomycin or linezolid for those HCAP patients who require broad-spectrum therapy. Once the results of respiratory cultures and the in vitro susceptibility of the isolated pathogens are made available, de-escalation therapy should be considered. In the event that an offending agent could not be identified, antibiotic therapy should not be modified if clinical criteria are showing evidence of clinical stability or radiographic clearance.

In the absence of strong evidence to guide the optimal duration of therapy, treatment for seven days is recommended except when *P. aeruginosa* or *Acinetobacter* spp. are isolated. Longer duration (>8 days) of therapy is suggested for *P. aeruginosa* or *Acinetobacter* spp. infection as relapse may occur in up to 25% of patients. These recommendations are based on data derived from hospitalized patients with VAP (48). Such an approach may help to reduce health care costs and contain the development of bacteria resistance.

VIII. Delayed Resolution

Slowly resolving pneumonia of infectious etiology is the product of inadequate antimicrobial therapy, virulence and inoculum of the offending pathogens, and incompetence of the host immune response. Although the precise incidence is not established, available reports indicate that 10% to 25% of HCAP patients have inadequate responses to empiric therapy (49,50). Using a combination of clinical parameters and chest X rays, Luna and colleagues (51) noted that the Clinical Pulmonary Infection Score (CPIS) scores were noted to improve by the third day of therapy in survivors, while nonsurvivors failed to show any decline in CPIS score. Although the validity of such a score in intubated HCAP remains to be determined, the lack of clinical improvement by day 3 of therapy should alert the physicians for potential treatment failure. In hospitalized non-ICU settings, the median time to clinical stability, defined as the presence of fever (temperature, $\leq 37.2°C$), heart rate of ≤ 100 beats/min, respiratory rate of ≤ 24 breaths/min, systolic blood pressure of >90 mmHg, and oxygen saturation of $\geq 90\%$, is estimated at four days (52). Failure to have a rapid and early clinical response makes it very unlikely that clinical stability would occur shortly thereafter. Arancibia and coworkers (50) found that patients who failed antimicrobial treatment fell into two categories: nonresponse after 72 hours of therapy or clinical worsening during the same time period. Among the causes for treatment failure included an unsuspected primary infecting pathogen, a persistent (often drug-resistant) pathogen, acquisition of nosocomial infection, or a noninfectious process. Tuberculin skin testing and sputum smears and cultures for acid-fact bacteria may be indicated in the patient with risk factors or clinical features suggestive of *Mycobacterium tuberculosis*. Past travel history or exposures may suggest exposure to endemic fungi (*Histoplasma capsulatum* or *Coccidioides immitis*). Fiberoptic bronchoscopy with BAL and transbronchial biopsy is the preferred initial invasive procedure in evaluating treatment failure. The yield would depend on the demographics, radiographic features, and pretest likelihood. In rare instances, surgical biopsy may be necessary to diagnose refractory, nonresolving pneumonia.

IX. Summary

HCAP is a recently recognized entity of respiratory infections with important clinical ramifications for patients in and out of the hospital. Those afflicted are at high risk for being colonized with MDR pathogens because of their frequent contact with health care environment. On the basis of available data, patients with HCAP are more likely to have higher burden of comorbidities, receive inadequate antimicrobial coverage, and have worse outcome than patients with community acquired pneumonia. The approach to therapy is not standardized because there are limited studies conducted in this population. Future investigations are needed to determine duration of antibiotic usage, course of illness, and mortality specific factors in HCAP.

References

1. Naimi TS, LeDell KH, Como-Sabetti K, et al. Comparison of community- and health care-associated methicillin-resistant *Staphylococcus aureus* infection. JAMA 2003; 290:2976–2984.
2. Tambyah PA, Habib AG, Ng TM, et al. Community-acquired methicillin-resistant *Staphylococcus aureus* infection in Singapore is usually "healthcare associated." Infect Control Hosp Epidemiol 2003; 24:436–438.
3. Niederman MS, Craven DE, Bonten MJ, et al. Guidelines for the management of adults with hospital-acquired, ventilator-associated, and healthcare-associated pneumonia. Am J Respir Crit Care Med 2005; 171:388–416.
4. Craven D, Palladino R, McQuillen D. Health-care associated pneumonia in adults: management principles to improve outcome. Infect Dis Clin North Am 2004; 18:939–962.
5. Kollef M, Morrow L, Baughman R, et al. Health care-associated pneumonia: a critical appraisal to improve identification, management, and outcomes-proceedings of the HCAP summit. Clin Infect Dis 2008; 46:S296–S334.
6. Carratalà J, Garcia-Vidal C. What is health care–associated pneumonia and how is it managed? Curr Opin Infect Dis 2008; 21:168–173.
7. Kollef MH, Shorr A, Tabak YP, et al. Epidemiology and outcomes of health-care–associated pneumonia: results from a large US database of culture-positive pneumonia. Chest 2005; 128:3854–3862.
8. Carratalà J, Mykietiuk A, Fernández-Sabé N, et al. Healthcare-associated pneumonia requiring hospital admission: epidemiology, antibiotic therapy, and clinical outcomes. Arch Intern Med 2007; 167:1393–1399.
9. Micek ST, Kollef K, Reichley R, et al. Health care-associated pneumonia and community-acquired pneumonia: a single center experience. Antimicrob Agents Chemother 2007; 51:3568–3573.
10. Richards C. Infections in residents of long-term care facilities: an agenda for research. Report of an expert panel. J Am Geriatr Soc 2002; 50:570–576.

11. Muder RR. Pneumonia in residents of long-term care facilities: epidemiology, etiology, management, and prevention. Am J Med 1998; 105:319–330.
12. Loeb M, McGeer A, McArthur M, et al. Risk factors for pneumonia and other lower respiratory tract infections in elderly residents of long-term care facilities. Arch Intern Med 1999; 159:2058–2064.
13. Muder RR. Approach to the problem of pneumonia in long-term care facilities. Compr Ther 2000; 26:255–262.
14. Verghese A, Berk SL. Bacterial pneumonia in the elderly. Medicine 1983; 62:271–285.
15. Cunha BA. Pneumonia in the elderly. Clin Microbiol Infect 2001; 7:581–588.
16. Quinn M, Miller V, Dal Nogare A. Increased salivary exoglycosidase activity during critical illness. Am J Respir Crit Care Med 1994; 150:179–183.
17. Pick N, McDonald A, Bennett NN, et al. Pulmonary aspiration in a long-term care setting: clinical and laboratory observations and an analysis of risk factors. J Am Geriatr Soc 1996; 44:763–768.
18. Castle S, Uyemura K, Rafi A, et al. Comorbidity is a better predictor of impaired immunity than chronological age in older adults. J Am Geriatr Soc 2005; 53:1565–1569.
19. Marrie TJ, Blanchard W. A comparison of nursing home-acquired pneumonia patients with patients with community-acquired pneumonia and nursing home patients without pneumonia. J Am Geriatr Soc 1997; 45:50–55.
20. Meehan TP, Chua-Reyes JM, Tate J, et al. Process of care performance, patient characteristics, and outcomes in elderly patients hospitalized with community-acquired or nursing home-acquired pneumonia. Chest 2000; 117:1378–1385.
21. Slinin Y, Foley RN, Collins AJ. Clinical epidemiology of pneumonia in hemodialysis patients: the USRDS waves 1, 3, and 4 study. Kidney Int 2006; 70:1135–1141.
22. Lescure FX, Locher G, Eveillard M, et al. Community-acquired infection with healthcare-associated methicillin-resistant *Staphylococcus aureus*: the role of home nursing care. Infect Control Hosp Epidemiol 2006; 27:1213–1218.
23. Muder R. Pneumonia in residents of long-term care facilities: epidemiology, etiology, management, and prevention. Am J Med 1998; 105:319–330.
24. Murray P, Washington J. Microscopic and bacteriologic analysis of expectorated sputum. Mayo Clinic Proc 1975; 50:339–344.
25. Marrie T, Durant H, Kwan C. Nursing home acquired pneumonia: a case-control study. J AM Geriatr Soc 1986; 34:697–702.
26. Peterson P, Stein D, Guay DR, et al. prospective study of lower respiratory tract infections in an extended care nursing home program: potential role of oral ciprofloxacin. Am J Med 1988; 85:164–171.
27. Hirata-Dulas CAI, Stein D, Guay DR, et al. A randomized study of ciprofloxacin versus ceftriaxone in the treatment of nursing home acquired lower respiratory tract infections. J Am Geriatr Soc 1991; 39:979–985.
28. Marrie T, Durant H, Yates L. Community-acquired pneumonia requiring hospitalization: 5-year prospective study. Rev Infect Dis 1989; 11:586–599.
29. Drinka P, Gauerke C, Voeks S, et al. Pneumonia in a nursing home. J Gen Intern Med 1994; 9:650–652.
30. Kupronis BA, Richards CL, Whitney CG. Invasive pneumococcal disease in older adults residing in long-term care facilities and in the community. J Geriatr Soc 2003; 51:1520–1525.
31. El Solh A, Sikka P, Ramadan F, et al. Etiology of severe pneumonia in the very elderly. Am J Respir Crit Care Med 2001; 163:645–651.
32. El Solh A, Aquilina A, Dhillon R, et al. Impact of invasive strategy on management of antimicrobial treatment failure in institutionalized older people with severe pneumonia. Am J Respir Crit Care Med 2002; 166:1038–1043.

33. Valenti WM, Trudell RG, Bentley DW. Factors predisposing to oropharyngeal colonization with gram-negative bacilli in the aged. N Engl J Med 1978; 298:1108–1111.

34. Johanson WG, Pierce AK, Sanford JP. Changing pharyngeal bacterial flora of hospitalized patients. Emergence of gram-negative bacilli. N Engl J Med 1969; 281:1137–1140.

35. Palmer LB, Albulak K, Fields S, et al. Oral clearance and pathogenic oropharyngeal colonization in the elderly. Am J Respir Crit Care Med 2001; 164:464–468.

36. Fine M, Orloff J, Rihs J, et al. Evaluation of housestaff physicians' preparation and interpretation of sputum gram stains for community-acquired pneumonia. J Gen Intern Med 1991; 6:189–191.

37. Kalin M, Lindberg A. Diagnosis of pneumococcal pneumonia: a comparison between microscopic examination of expectorate, antigen detection, and cultural procedures. Scand J Infect Dis 1983; 15:153–160.

38. Houck P, MacLehose R, Niederman M, et al. Empiric antibiotic therapy and mortality among Medicare pneumonia inpatients in 10 Western States: 1993, 1995, and 1997. Chest 2001; 119:1420–1426.

39. Ruiz-Gonzalez A, Nogues A, Falguera M, et al. Rapid detection of pneumococcal antigen in lung aspirates: comparison with culture and PCR technique. Respir Med 1997; 91:201–206.

40. Plouffe J, File T, Breiman R, et al. Reevaluation of the definition of Legionnaires' disease: use of the urinary antigen assay. Clin Infect Dis 1995; 20:1286.

41. Dupont H, Chalhoub V, Plantefeve G, et al. Variation of infected cell count in bronchoalveolar lavage and timing of ventilator-associated pneumonia. Intensive Care Med 2004; 30:1557–1563.

42. El Solh AA, Akinnusi M, Pineda L, et al. Diagnostic yield of quantitative endotracheal aspirates in patients with severe nursing home-acquired pneumonia. Crit Care 2007; 11:R57.

43. Loeb M, Carusone SC, Goeree R, et al. Effect of a clinical pathway to reduce hospitalizations in nursing home residents with pneumonia: a randomized controlled trial. JAMA 2006; 295:2503–2510.

44. El Solh AA, Pietrantoni C, Bhat A, et al. Indicators of potentially drug-resistant bacteria in severe nursing home-acquired pneumonia. Clin Infect Dis 2004; 39:474–480.

45. Vanderkooi O, Low D, Green K, et al. Predicting antimicrobial resistance in invasive pneumococcal disease. Clin Infect Dis 2005; 40:1288–1297.

46. Wenisch C, Krause R, Szell M, et al. Moxifloxacin versus standard therapy in patients with pneumonia hospitalized after failure of preclinical anti-infective treatment. Infection 2006; 34:190–195.

47. Yakovlev SV, Stratchounski LS, Woods GL, et al. Ertapenem versus cefepime for initial empirical treatment of pneumonia acquired in skilled-care facilities or in hospitals outside the intensive care unit. Eur J Clin Microbiol Infect Dis 2006; 25:633–641.

48. Chastre J, Wolff M, Fagon JY, et al. Comparison of 8 vs 15 days of antibiotic therapy for ventilator-associated pneumonia in adults: a randomized trial. JAMA 2003; 290:2588–2598.

49. Menendez R, Perpina M, Torres A. Evaluation of non resolving and progressive pneumonia. Semin Respir Infect 2003; 18:103–111.

50. Arancibia F, Ewig S, Martinez J, et al. Antimicrobial treatment failures in patients with community-acquired pneumonia: causes and prognostic implications. Am J Respir Crit Care Med 2000; 162:154–160.

51. Luna CM, Blanzaco D, Niederman MS, et al. Resolution of ventilator-associated pneumonia: prospective evaluation of the clinical pulmonary infection score as an early clinical predictor of outcome. Crit Care Med 2003; 31:676–682.

52. Menéndez R, Torres A, Rodriguez de Castro F, et al. Reaching stability in community-acquired pneumonia: the effects of the severity of disease, treatment, and the characteristics of patients. Clin Infect Dis 2004; 39:1783–1790.

10
Managing Ventilator-Associated Pneumonia: Antibiotic Therapy and Targeted Prevention

ALEXANDRA CHRONEOU and NIKOLAOS ZIAS
Lahey Clinic Medical Center, Burlington, Massachusetts, U.S.A.

DONALD E. CRAVEN
Lahey Clinic Medical Center, Burlington, and Tufts University School of Medicine, Boston, Massachusetts, U.S.A.

I. Introduction

Ventilator-associated pneumonia (VAP), defined as pneumonia developing ≥48 hours after intubation, is the most common serious infection in intensive care unit (ICU) patients leading to increased mortality, morbidity, and health care costs (1–3). Bacterial pathogens causing VAP vary by patient population and type of ICU. Leakage of bacteria around the endotracheal tube (ETT) cuff is a major route of access to the lower respiratory tract and a vital target for VAP prevention efforts (1–4).

Over the past decade, initial antibiotic therapy for VAP has been modified because of dramatic increases in infections caused by multidrug-resistant (MDR) pathogens, such as *Pseudomonas aeruginosa* and methicillin-resistant *Staphylococcus aureus* (MRSA) (1–3). Risk factors for colonization and infection with MDR pathogens include prior antibiotic treatment, contact with the health care system, poor hand hygiene, environmental sources, and the duration of mechanical ventilation (1–3).

This chapter focuses on antibiotic therapy for VAP in immunocompetent adults and effective, evidence-based prevention strategies to improve patient outcomes. It highlights recent advances, current guidelines, and selected primary references.

II. Definition and Pathogens

VAP is defined as pneumonia that occurs in a patient receiving mechanical ventilation for ≥48 hours (1,2). Early-onset VAP (<5 days) includes patients without risk factors for MDR pathogens who are more likely to be infected with pathogens seen in community-acquired pneumonia, such as *Streptococcus pneumoniae* (pneumococcus), *Haemophilus influenzae*, methicillin-sensitive *S. aureus* and enteric gram-negative bacilli, such as *Klebsiella pneumonia* (1,3). Pathogens causing MDR or late-onset VAP (≥5 days) include MRSA and *P. aeruginosa* (1,3) (Table 1).

III. Epidemiology

Rates of VAP vary by type of ICU with a pooled mean of 7.3/1000 ventilator days for medical versus 13.2 for surgical ICUs (1). The 50th percentile (median) was 6.0/1000 ventilator days for medical and 11.6/1000 ventilator days for surgical ICUs (1).

Table 1 Summary of Common MDR Pathogens Causing VAP, Initial Therapy, and Evolving Issues

MDR pathogen	Antibiotic therapy (2)	Clinical comments (selected references)
MRSA	Vancomycin 15 mg/kg every 12 hr. Adjust dose for renal function. (Target vancomycin blood trough level = 15–20 µg/mL) *or* Linezolid 600 mg IV/PO every 12 hr	Hospital-acquired MRSA and community-acquired MRSA clones (United States 300/400) are emerging in hospitals (5). High doses of vancomycin are recommended due to treatment failures possibly related to inadequate dosing (1,6). High doses of vancomycin may cause greater renal toxicity in the severely ill, those with renal failure, or on therapy with other nephrotoxic medications (6,7). Linezolid achieves high concentrations in the lung fluid (7) and inhibits toxin production and may be useful in patients with renal failure or nonresponse to vancomycin (6,8,9). Increasing resistance to vancomycin (sensitive = MICs ≤2 µg/mL) or vancomycin intermediate-resistant *S. aureus* (VISA) are associated with poorer outcomes and may be missed with current microbiological methods (6,10).
P. aeruginosa	Cephalosporins third generation (e.g., cefepime or ceftazidime) *or* fourth generation (cefepime) *or* Carbapenem (imipenem, meropenem, doripenem) *or* Piperacillin-tazobactam *plus* Aminoglycoside (amikacin, gentamicin, or tobramycin) *or* Antipseudomonal fluoroquinolone (ciprofloxacin or levofloxacin)	Has the capacity to develop resistance to all antibiotics except polymyxin (11). Automated in vitro susceptibility testing for β-lactam antibiotic may have a high rate of false susceptibility and resistance when compared to disk diffusion and E-tests (12). Extended infusion of piperacillin-tazobactam improves time above the MIC and may reduce mortality (13). The use of combination therapy (β-lactam *plus* an aminoglycoside) vs. monotherapy does not reduce resistance emergence or improve patient outcomes (14,15). If *P. aeruginosa* is suspected combination therapy should be used until antibiotic sensitivity is available (1). Caution is advised for empiric use of fluoroquinolones due to excessive prescribing, greater resistance, and risk for MRSA (1).
Acinetobacter spp.	Carbapenem (imipenem, meropenem) *plus* Aminoglycoside (amikacin, gentamicin, or tobramycin) *or* Polymyxin B (Colistin®)	Treatment of *Acinetobacter* VAP is limited due to widespread antibiotic resistance (16). There are reports of discordance between in vitro susceptibility testing and clinical responses to carbapenems and other antibiotics (17). Initial antibiotic therapy for highly resistant isolates may be limited to polymyxin B (Colistin) *plus* aminoglycosides *or* rifampin. Also, aerosolized polymyxin may be useful (18).

(Continued)

Table 1 Summary of Common MDR Pathogens Causing VAP, Initial Therapy, and Evolving Issues (*Continued*)

MDR pathogen	Antibiotic therapy (2)	Clinical comments (selected references)
ESBL *plus* *Klebsiella* *pneumoniae* *plus* *Escherichia* *coli*	Carbapenem (imipenem, meropenem, doripenem ± aminoglycoside (amikacin, gentamicin, or tobramycin)	ESBL *plus* strains are rapidly evolving and carbapenems are the surest agents for therapy (for ESBL *plus* organisms), although carbapenem resistance is beginning to increase (19). Concerns have been raised on the accuracy of in vitro antibiotic sensitivity testing for detecting ESBL *plus* isolates (11,20). The hallmark of ESBL *plus* *Klebsiella* *pneumoniae* or *Escherichia coli* is a variable response to cephalosporins and thus third- and fourth-generation agents should be avoided as monotherapy (11,20). The most reliable empiric choice is a carbapenem ±an aminoglycoside (1,11,20).
Enterobacter spp.		Third- and fourth-generation cephalosporins should not be used for treatment of *Enterobacter* spp. VAP because of the high frequency of resistance of this pathogen to this therapy (19).

Abbreviations: VAP, ventilator-associated pneumonia; MDR, multidrug resistant; MRSA, methicillin-resistant *Staphylococcus aureus*; MIC, minimum inhibitory concentration; ESBL, extended-spectrum β-lactamase.

Rates of VAP increase with the duration of mechanical ventilation, with attack rates previously estimated to be approximately 3% per day (1–3). Crude mortality rates for VAP ranging from 20% to 60%, largely reflect the impact of age, severity of underlying disease, presence of organ failure, infection by specific MDR pathogen(s), and type of ICU patient population (1–3).

Prevention strategies are critically important to improve clinical outcomes such as mortality, morbidity, and reduced health care costs (1,2,4). An average episode of VAP has been estimated to increase hospitalization by 12 days, ventilator days by 6 days, ICU stay by 6 days, and hospital costs from $12,000 to $40,000 (1–3).

IV. Etiology

The wide spectrum of MDR pathogens causing VAP are dynamic and vary over time by ICU type and patient population, underscoring the importance of timely, ICU-specific surveillance data (1–3). Bacteria causing VAP may originate from many sources, including the patient's endogenous flora or cross-contamination from other patients, staff, contaminated devices, or the environment (1–3). Prior hospitalization, care in chronic care facilities and especially precedent antibiotic therapy are important predisposing factors for colonization and infection with MDR versus other pathogens (1–3). VAP is often caused by more than one type of bacteria, because of aspiration or leakage of mixed bacterial flora colonizing the oropharynx, that enter the lower respiratory tract (1–3).

Candida albicans is a common fungal colonizer of the lower airway secretions, but rarely causes VAP (1,3). By comparison, in patients with chronic underlying diseases, *Aspergillus fumigatus* is an emerging pathogen and can be difficult to diagnose using conventional VAP diagnostic methods (21). The incidence of VAP caused by viruses is low, but includes seasonal viruses, such as influenza A and B, parainfluenza, adenovirus, and respiratory syncytial virus (1). Interest has also increased in purulent tracheobronchitis or VAP due to herpes simplex virus (HSV) (22).

V. Pathogenesis

VAP pathogenesis invariably begins with bacterial colonization that may progress to ventilator-associated tracheobronchitis (VAT) and in some patients to VAP. Most patients will have low numbers of bacteria colonizing the trachea that are held in check by the host's mechanical, humoral, and cellular defenses (1–3,23).

In contrast to healthy people, critically ill patients and those with VAP have high rates of oropharyngeal colonization with bacterial pathogens (1–3,23). Host factors, types of bacteria colonizing the pharynx, and the use of antibiotics may alter colonization and adherence of MDR pathogens resulting in progression to VAT or VAP (24,25). Oral epithelial cells rich in fibronectin bind gram-positive organisms such as *Streptococci* and *S. aureus*, conversely those poor in fibronectin preferentially bind gram-negative bacilli such as *P. aeruginosa* (23). Retrograde colonization of the oropharynx from the stomach may contribute to increased levels of oropharyngeal colonization and subsequent lower respiratory tract infection (1–3).

Mucociliary and mechanical clearance in the trachea are important factors in the defense against infection (23,24). Cell-mediated immune response by polymorphonuclear leukocytes (PMNs) and macrophages is controlled by a complex array of lipids, peptides, and cytokines, including interleukins, interferons, growth factors, and chemotactic factors.

The ETT can also be a nidus for colonization and biofilm formation (1,3,23,24) (Fig. 1). Bacterial biofilm formation on the ETT provides a shelter from host defenses and antibiotics. Biofilm emboli to the distal alveoli during routine nasotracheal suctioning or bronchoscopy are also a concern. The result of this war between the bacteria and host defenses will determine if the patient has only colonization, VAT, or VAP (1,3,23–25).

VI. Diagnosis

Intubated patients have excellent access to lower respiratory tract bacteria, as there is primarily one way to enter and exit the lung. The diagnosis of VAT and VAP overlap in terms of clinical signs, symptoms, and microbiological examination of endotracheal sputum (cultures and Gram stains) (Table 2) (1–3,23–25). A diagnosis of VAP requires the presence of a new or progressive radiographic infiltrate.

The clinical diagnosis of bacterial VAP needs confirmation by smears of sputum and a culture with significant concentrations of a bacterial pathogen using semiquantitative (SQ) or quantitative (Q) endotracheal aspirates (ETA) (1). The presence of

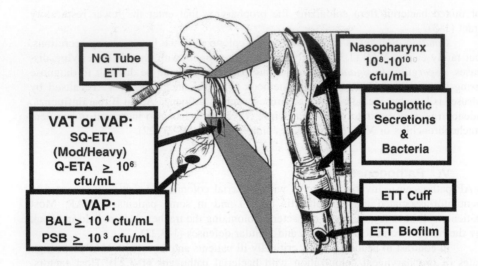

Figure 1 An intubated patient with oropharyngeal bacterial colonization. Note subglottic secretions with high concentrations of bacteria (millions per milliliter) pooled above the ETT cuff may leak around the cuff. The ETT and its cuff also prevent mechanical clearance of bacteria and secretions from the trachea. Bacteria encased in biofilm may form in the lumen of an ETT. Aspiration of subglottic secretions reduces bacterial entry into the trachea. Note the number of bacteria needed for the diagnosis of VAT or VAP using ETA or more distal sampling by bronchoscopic or nonbronchosopic BAL or PSB. Taken with permission from Craven (24). *Abbreviations*: ETT, endotracheal tube; NG, nasogastric tube; SQ, semiquantitative; Q, quantitative; ETA, endotracheal aspirates; VAT, ventilator-associated tracheobronchitis; VAP, ventilator-associated pneumonia; BAL, bronchoalveolar lavage; PSB, protected specimen brush.

bacteria on Gram stain (smear) correlates with approximately $>10^5$ bacteria per milliliter of sputum. SQ-ETA with moderate (+++) or heavy (++++) growth of a pathogen suggests the diagnosis of VAT or VAP. ETA growth reported as rare (+) or few (++) growth probably represents tracheal colonization. Some microbiology labs report Q-ETA in there is a pathogen $\geq 10^6$ colony-forming units/mL (CFU/mL), indicating a diagnosis of VAT or VAP.

SQ-ETAs and Q-ETAs can be obtained quickly and are most commonly used to diagnose VAP. Both have high sensitivity for detecting VAP, but a lower specificity (accuracy of VAP diagnosis) than specimens obtained by quantitative bronchoscopic bronchoalveolar lavage (B-BAL) or nonbronchoscopic (NB-BAL) methods used to sample the distal airway in the lung.

B-BAL or NB-BAL $\geq 10^4$ CFU/mL or protective specimen brush (B-PSB $\geq 10^3$ CFU/mL) have good diagnostic sensitivity and higher diagnostic specificity than ETA samples but are not widely available on demand in most hospitals and are more expensive (1,3,26). All cultures and smears should be obtained before starting or changing antibiotics. This is critical for later de-escalation of empiric antibiotics (1,3).

Table 2 Comparison of Diagnostic Criteria for VAP or VAT

	VAP	VAT
Clinical signs and symptoms	Temperature (>38°C *or* 100.4°F) *or* leukocyte count >12,000/mm³ *or* leukopenia <4,000/mm³ (at least one of these) *plus* New onset of purulent endotracheal secretions or change in sputum [VAP may have new rales, bronchial breath sounds, and worsening oxygen requirements (increasing FiO₂)][a]	
Radiology: Chest X ray, CT scan	New and persistent infiltrate *or* Consolidation *or* Cavitation	Transient infiltrate *or* No new infiltrate *or* Nondiagnostic (e.g., atelectasis, ARDS, or CHF)
Microbiology	ETA: Gram stain with PMNs ± bacteria (note morphology and color) SQ-ETA (moderate to heavy growth) or Q-ETA >10⁵⁻⁶ CFU/mL Bronchoscopic or nonbronchoscopic samples Cytospin: PMN ± bacteria BAL ≥10⁴CFU/mL *or* PSB ≥10³ CFU/mL	Bronchoscopic or nonbronchoscopic samples not done *or* Cytospin smear negative BAL: <10⁴ CFU/mL *or* PSB <10³ CFU/mL

[a]FiO₂, fraction of inspired oxygen.
Note that diagnosis of each requires specific clinical, radiological, and microbiological criteria that may overlap, making the specificity of the diagnosis difficult for clinicians.
Abbreviations: VAP, ventilator-associated pneumonia; VAT, ventilator-associated tracheobronchitis; ARDS, acute respiratory distress syndrome; CHF, congestive heart failure; ETA, endotracheal aspirate; PMNs, polymorphonuclear leukocytes; SQ, semiquantitative; Q, quantitative, BAL, bronchoalveolar lavage; PSB, protective specimen brush.
Source: From Ref. 24.

The advantages of ETA over distal sampling by BAL/PSB remain controversial (27,28). In one large, prospective, randomized trial of VAP diagnosis, patients having B-BAL/B-PSB had a significantly lower 14-day mortality rate, reduced mean sepsis-related organ failure ($p = 0.04$), and more antibiotic-free days ($p < 0.001$) than patients having a clinical diagnosis and sputum SQ-ETA (27), but more patients in the bronchoscopic group received "adequate" therapy than those in the ETA group. On the contrary, no differences in outcomes were observed between the two groups in length of stay in the hospital, ICU, or 28-day mortality in a recent randomized study by a Canadian Critical Care Trials group, in which patients were randomly assigned to undergo B-BAL versus SQ-ETA (28). Both groups were also randomized to receive empirical combination antibiotic therapy or monotherapy.

The clinical pulmonary infection score (CPIS), used in some ICUs, gives points for clinical, radiographical, physiological (PaO₂/FiO₂) and microbiological data for a single numerical result. CPIS scores of >6, correlate well with the presence of clinical pneumonia (1–3). Biological markers, such as procalcitonin (PCT), C-reactive protein (CRP), and soluble triggering receptor expressed on myeloid calls (sTREM-1), may be helpful adjuncts for the diagnosis and management of VAP (29). PCT is secreted as part of the systemic inflammatory response to infection. Ramirez et al. established the cutoff point of

2.9 mg/mL for PCT in combination with the simplified CPIS that had specificity for VAP diagnosis (30). PCT may also be helpful as a guide to shorten antibiotic treatment (31).

VII. Antibiotic Management

A. Step 1: Initial, Empiric Antibiotic Choices

The first principle of therapy is that the initial antibiotic regimen be started early and be appropriate (pathogen sensitive in vitro) and adequate (proper dosing, route, and lung penetration) (1). The selection of antibiotics should be based on the presence or absence of risk factors for MDR pathogens, the severity of infection, and be broad enough to cover all of the likely pathogens, until further microbiological culture and sensitivity are available. The management issues and appropriate therapy for common MDR pathogens are summarized in the 2005 American Thoracic Society/Infectious Diseases Society of America (ATS/IDSA) guidelines (Table 1) (1).

Risk factors for MDR pathogens include prior antibiotic therapy, prior hospitalization, late-onset VAP, chronic dialysis, residence in chronic health care facilities, immunocompromisation, and the presence of endemic ICU pathogens. Initiation of early, appropriate, and adequate therapy for VAP is particularly important for elderly, debilitated patients who are in shock or have multiple organ failure. Blood cultures and respiratory sputum samples should be collected before antibiotics are initiated to assure proper therapy and optimal de-escalation of antibiotics (1).

Adequate doses of antibiotics are needed to obtain maximum penetration and concentration in the lung parenchyma to obtain better control of the infection, minimize tissue damage, and reduce morbidity and mortality (1). For example, if there are from 100,000 to 10 million MDR organisms per milliliter of fluid in the BAL sample, the total concentration of bacteria in the lung is enormous. This underscores the importance of administering early, appropriate concentrations of antibiotic to the lung parenchyma, which is above the minimum inhibitory concentration (MIC) of the pathogen and sufficient to reduce the bacterial burden. Keep in mind, MICs performed in vitro on agar are crude surrogates and may not reflect concentrations of lung bacteria in vivo and, therefore, have limitations for extrapolation in vivo (11,20). There can also be other variables in vivo such as necrotic tissue, abscess formation, inflammation, poor blood supply, and presence of a foreign body (e.g., ETT with biofilm-encased bacteria) that can affect bacterial killing (26).

Finally, the timing of administration and initial dose of the antibiotic (e.g., a β-lactam) needed to achieve maximal time above the MIC of the specific pathogen(s) also appear important to achieve better clinical outcomes. Lodise and coworkers using a nonrandomized trial design reported that mortality rates in patients who had 3.375 g of piperacillin-tazobactam given by a four-hour infusion every eight hours were significantly lower than rates in patients given the same dose by a 30-minute infusion every four to six hours (13). Similar concepts for dosing also apply to carbapenems.

B. Step 2: Assessing Clinical Response and Antibiotic
De-escalation

Initial antibiotic coverage should be liberal and sufficiently broad enough to cover all suspected pathogens, but de-escalation or streamlining antibiotic therapy, based on the patient's clinical response and microbiological data, is of critical importance.

De-escalation improves patient outcomes and minimizes antibiotic use (1). Patients without evidence of VAP should have their antibiotics stopped and a search initiated for other diagnoses.

C. Step 3: Limiting Duration of Therapy

In a large trial, patients with VAP randomized to seven to eight days of antibiotic therapy had significantly fewer recurrences and less resistance than patients treated for 14 to 15 days. There was a trend toward higher rates of recurrence in patients with VAP due to *P. aeruginosa* in the seven- to eight-day group, but no significant differences were noted in mortality or other important clinical response parameters (32). The ATS/IDSA guideline recommends seven days of therapy for uncomplicated hospital-acquired pneumonia or VAP with close follow-up for any signs of relapse, especially in patients with VAP due to *P. aeruginosa* (1). The use of PCT levels and oxygenation parameters may provide clues to patients who are more likely to relapse or need a longer duration of antibiotic therapy (31).

In most patients, clinical improvement takes 24 to 48 hours; therefore, the selected antimicrobial regimen should not be changed during this time unless there is evidence of progressive deterioration (1). Possible causes for clinical deterioration or failure to improve include *wrong diagnosis* [pulmonary embolism with infarction, atelectasis, pulmonary hemorrhage, neoplastic or connective tissue disease, or acute respiratory distress syndrome (ARDS) with diffuse alveolar damage, other source of infection]; *wrong therapy* (drug resistant pathogen, inadequate dosing, or wrong antimicrobial agent); *wrong pathogen* (tuberculosis, fungal, parasitic, or viral infection, *Legionella* spp. infection); or *complication* (empyema or lung abscess, *Clostridium difficile* colitis, bacterial or *A. fumigatus* superinfection, or drug fever) (1).

VIII. Targeted Prevention

Tremendous progress has been made in reducing health care–associated infections in the past five years (1–4,23,33–36) Prevention in the ICU is a team sport that requires leadership, organization, goals, clearly defined roles, "checklists," quality improvement targets, and multidisciplinary staff meetings with data feedback (2,4,23,34). An overview of selected prevention strategies taken from detailed, evidence-based national guidelines and review articles are discussed and summarized in Table 3 (1–4,33–36).

Effective prophylaxis of VAP should begin with a team armed with evidence-based goals and targeted interventions, adequate staffing ratios, and involvement of nurses and respiratory therapists along with effective staff education (Table 3) (1–4,34). In one study, use of a self-study module, with in-service teaching programs, fact sheets, and posters resulted in a 58% reduction in VAP and cost savings between $425,000 and >$4,000,000 following 12 months period after intubation (36).

Proper isolation and effective infection control practices with adequate environmental cleaning are cornerstones for VAP prevention (1,2,4,35). Unfortunately, staff compliance with proven infection control measures, such as hand hygiene, remains inconsistent in many hospitals. Antibiotic stewardship programs play an important role in reducing the risk for all health care–associated infections and reduces the risk of colonization with MDR pathogens and complications such as *C. difficile* infections (1,2,4).

Table 3 Summary of Prevention Strategies for VAP

Strategy	Comments
Model: multidisciplinary team, with a "champion" to lead, goals, "bundles," checklists, monitoring, and data feedback	Multidisciplinary team with a "champion" to set goals. Use of evidence-based data, goals, checklists, and feedback of data suggested. Benchmarks should be discussed and re-evaluated regularly
Staff education and proper ICU staffing for nurses and respiratory therapists	Staff education programs for physicians, nurses, and respiratory therapists to improve awareness; provide current data. Proper staffing and patient nurse ratios critical for patient safety. Adherence to guidelines, protocols, and infection control standards.
Infection control	Data support effective hand hygiene to reduce spread of MDR pathogens Environmental cleaning needed. Surveillance of MDR pathogens, outbreaks, data feedback changes. Screening for MRSA suggested and debated.
Antibiotic control	Antibiotic stewardship reduces inappropriate antibiotic use, costs, and risk of infection with MDR pathogens. Designated pharmacist of infectious disease physician review or computer programs are beneficial
Use of ICU bundles	Use of IHI and other team bundles to reduce risk of VAP (semi-upright patient positioning, stress bleeding prophylaxis, deep venous thrombosis prophylaxis, and sedation vacation)
Semi-upright position (avoiding supine positioning)	Maintain patient semi-upright ($>30°$, if possible). Do no keep patient supine, especially when receiving enteral nutrition
Oral care (37,38)	Oral care is widely used to prevent VAP. Doesn't reach subglottic area. Effective in comparative, nonrandomized trials.
Stress bleeding prophylaxis	Data suggest that histamine type 2 receptor blockers or PPIs are more effective than sucralfate in preventing serious gastrointestinal bleeding, may have trend toward increased VAP (2). PPIs may increase the risk of *C. difficile* infection.
Enteral feedings	Enteral feeding preferred to parenteral nutrition. Protocols help standardize implementation and monitoring.
Targeting colonization CHX ±other antibiotics (2,39,40) SDD (41)	Randomized controlled trials demonstrate efficacy. Greatest effect in cardiac patients. Combinations of antibiotics given orally (down the NG tube) ±systemically in randomized clinical trials demonstrate reduced rates of lower respiratory tract infections compared to controls; decreased mortality noted in SDD patients receiving systemic antibiotics. SDD should be used selectively in the United States due to widespread presence of MDR pathogens; more widely used in Europe (1,2,42). A randomized study of SOD vs. SDD is currently underway in the Netherlands.

(Continued)

Table 3 Summary of Prevention Strategies for VAP (*Continued*)

Strategy	Comments
Targeting the ETT:	
Sedation vacation with awakening and breathing trials (42–45)	Implement standard protocols to limit sedation, assess use of continuous sedation enhance awakening to reduce duration of intubation.
	Use of spontaneous awakening and breathing trials that increase earlier extubation, reduce length of stay, and mortality (10).
NIPPV (46)	NIPPV to prevent intubation is supported by several clinical trials to reduce pneumonia and improves patient outcomes (35).
	NIPPV especially useful in patients with COPD and CHF (35)
CASS (47)	VAP significantly decreases VAP in several randomized clinical trials (19,36).
	Requires more staff time and cost.
s-ETT (48)	In a randomized VAP trial, colloidal s-ETT reduced microbiologically confirmed VAP by 36% overall ($p < 0.002$) and 48% ($p < 0.005$) in first 10 days (49).
	No difference was noted in secondary outcomes: mortality, length of stay, antibiotic use.
Early tracheostomy (50)	Three randomized trials suggest possible benefit from early tracheostomy; some methodological concerns, but may be helpful in critically ill patients who will probably need long term intubation and later tracheostomy.
Vaccination	Pneumococcal and influenza vaccination are recommended (1,2).
Smoking cessation	Smoking cessation programs strongly recommended (1,2).
Nutritional counseling and physical therapy	Counsel for malnutrition, obesity, and early physical therapy effective (1).
Prevention of aspiration	Check sedation, head of the bed after extubation, avoid reintubation; check speech and swallow studies to prevent recurrent aspiration (1).

Abbreviations: VAP, ventilator-associated pneumonia; ICU, intensive care unit; PPI, proton pump inhibitors; MDR, multidrug resistant; MRSA, methicillin-resistant *Staphylococcus aureus*; CHX, chlorhexidine; SDD, selective decontamination; NG, nasogastric tube; SOD, selective oral decontamination; ETT, endotracheal tube; NIPPV, noninvasive positive pressure ventilation; CASS, continuous aspiration of subglottic secretions.
Source: Taken in part from Refs. 1, 2, 4, 19, and 34.

The use of the Institute for Healthcare Improvement (IHI) "bundles" have been credited with increased awareness and marked reductions in VAP rates nationwide. The IHI bundle recommendations for VAP include maintaining patients in a semi-upright position (avoiding supine patient positioning) and implementing sedation vacations than facilitating earlier extubation (33,42–45).

A. Targeting VAT to Prevent VAP

In recent years, there has been an increased interest in treating VAT as a strategy to prevent VAP. VAT is thought to be an intermediary step between colonization and VAP that occurs in approximately 10% of patients ventilated for more than 48 hours and is associated with longer duration of mechanical ventilation (24,25). In a recent, randomized controlled trial, serial Q-ETA were used to diagnose VAT (defined as the presence of a pathogen $>10^6$ CFU/mL of sputum and no infiltrate on chest X ray). Patients diagnosed with VAT were randomized to receive targeted, appropriate parenteral antibiotics or no therapy (24). The study was stopped early because of a significant increase in mortality ($p < 0.05$) for patients who had therapy delayed (18% vs. 47%, $p < 0.001$). In addition, patients treated with antibiotics had a significant decrease in subsequent VAP episodes (14% vs. 47% $p < 0.01$). The data are compelling and suggest that VAT may be a better target that VAP to initiate "targeted" antibiotic therapy rather that the current model of "empiric" therapy followed by de-escalation (1,23,24). Clearly, further research is needed in this area.

B. Targeting the ETT and Biofilm

The ETT facilitates bacterial entry into the lower respiratory tract by leakage around the cuff and limiting effective removal of secretions from the lower respiratory tract that need removal by endotracheal suctioning (1–4). In addition, the ETT becomes colonized and is a nidus for biofilm growth (24). Bacteria encased in biofilms are sheltered from killing by antibiotics, host cellular defenses in the lung (macrophages and PMNs), and lysis by antibody and complement (1–4). Efforts to reduce entry of oropharyngeal bacteria around the cuff into the lower respiratory tract and limiting the use of sedative and paralytic agents that depress cough and maintaining endotracheal cuff pressure at >20 cmH$_2$O are important VAP prevention strategies (42–45).

Sedation and Weaning Protocols

Standardized weaning protocols reduce days of mechanical ventilation, facilitate ETT removal, and lower rates of VAP. In a more recent study, patients were randomized to a spontaneous awakening trial (SAT) or the intervention SAT plus a spontaneous breathing trial (SBT), and the combined group had significantly reduced mechanical ventilator and ICU days and lower mortality ($p < 0.01$) (43).

Noninvasive Positive Pressure Ventilation

Noninvasive positive pressure ventilation (NIPPV) provides ventilatory support without the need for intubation and is an effective alternative for patients with acute exacerbations of chronic obstructive pulmonary disease (COPD) or acute hypoxemic respiratory failure. NIPPV is associated with decreased rates of pneumonia, antibiotic use, and reduced patient mortality (1,2,46).

Continuous Subglottic Secretion Drainage

Continuous aspiration of subglottic secretions (CASS) through use of specially designed ETTs with a wider, elliptical hole helps facilitate drainage of subglottic secretions and reduces bacteria entering the trachea. A recent Cochrane review reported that CASS decreased mortality [risk ratio (RR) 0.41, 95% CI, 0.22–0.76], lowered rates of VAP (RR 0.57, 95% CI 0.33–0.97); decreased length of ICU and hospital stays (47). A recent meta-analysis demonstrated that CASS reduced the risk of VAP by half

(RR = 0.51, 95% CI = 0.37–0.71), shortened ICU stay by three days (95% CI, 2.1–3.9), and delayed the onset of VAP by six days. CASS also was cost effective, saving $4992 per episode of VAP prevented or $1872 per patient; mortality was not affected (47). Limitations have been tube cost, identifying patients that would be intubated >48 hours, and need for increased staff time for monitoring.

Silver-Coated ETT
The North American Silver-Coated Endotracheal Tube (NASCENT) study was a randomized one that compared a colloidal silver-coated-endotracheal tube (s-ETT) with a control ETT (c-ETT) (48). An overall 36% reduction in microbiologically confirmed VAP ($p < 0.03$) in patients randomized to the s-ETT versus the c-ETT and a 48% reduction in VAP during the first 10 days of intubation ($p < 0.005$) was seen. No significant differences were noted between patients in terms of length of stay, antibiotic use, and mortality. Although the s-ETT is more expensive, it does not require additional nursing time but would require a strategy to identify persons who would be intubated >48 hours.

C. Targeting Airway Colonization
Oral Care and Oral Antiseptics
The oral antiseptic chlorhexidine has demonstrated efficacy in reducing VAP, especially in cardiac surgery patients (38,39). In a recent multicenter, double-blind, randomized clinical trial of VAP outcomes, subjects treated with 2% chlorhexidine (CHX) paste were compared with patients randomized to 2% CHX plus 2% colistin (paste) or placebo (40). Although the risk of VAP was reduced by 65% in the CHX group ($p = 0.01$), no difference was noted in ventilator days, length of stay, or mortality.

Antibiotic Prophylaxis
Modulation of oropharyngeal colonization, by combinations of oral antibiotics, with or without systemic therapy or selective decontamination of the digestive tract (SDD) is effective in preventing VAP, but data are difficult to assess because of differences in methodological study quality, spectrum of regimens used, study populations, and clinical impact (1,2,41). The clinical evidence for the efficacy of SDD was recently reviewed in a Cochrane review reporting a reduction in respiratory tract infections and overall mortality, without an increase in antibiotic resistance in adult patients receiving intensive care (41). Because of increased concerns over rapid increases in MDR pathogens and *C. difficile* in hospitals in the United States, recent guidelines have suggested that SDD should be limited to selected ICU patient populations and "not used routinely" for widespread VAP prevention.

IX. Case Scenarios
A. Case 1
A 76-year-old man with an acute stroke and probable aspiration pneumonia was intubated in the emergency room and admitted to the ICU and treated with IV meropenem for seven days.

Three days later, his temperature spiked to 103°F, with hypotension, increased white blood cell (WBC) count of 16,000/mm^3 with 20% bands and 62% neutrophils, increased oxygen demand (FiO$_2$), and a new left upper lobe consolidation. He had purulent sputum. Gram stain showed many PMNs and numerous gram-positive cocci in clusters. He was started in vancomycin 1 g intravenously every 12 hours (weight is 65 kg) without clinical improvement at 48 hours. His cultures were positive for MRSA, MIC to vancomycin was reported as ≤2 µg/mL, but by E-test the MIC was high (2 µg). A repeat sputum Gram stain on therapy showed many bacteria and his PCT level was elevated. He was switched to IV linezolid and improved clinically over the next 48 hours with decreased temperature, WBC, and improved oxygenation. The computerized tomography (CT) lung scan indicated several lung abscesses.

Four days later, he again developed a temperature to 101°F, his WBC count was 9200/mm^3 with no left shift, and his sputum Gram stain had many PMNs but no bacteria. A "cold sore" was noted on his lip. The ETA smear had multinucleated giant cells (Fig. 2A); culture was positive for HSV, and he was started on acyclovir.

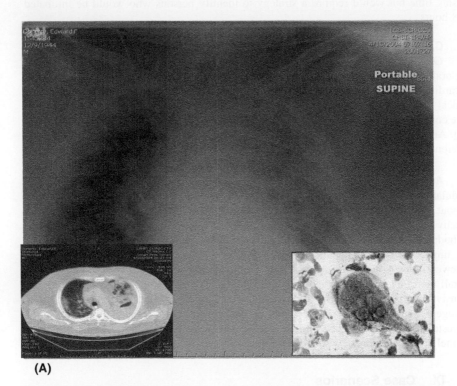

(A)

Figure 2 (*See color insert*) (**A**) Case 1: CT scan shows lung abscess not seen on chest X ray secondary to MRSA pneumonia. Sputum smear taken on day 9 of intubation demonstrated multinucleated giant cells. Culture and PCR were positive for herpes simplex virus. (**B**) Case 2: Initial chest X ray and lung biopsy taken on day 12 of intubation demonstrating narrow-branching, fungal septate hyphae, later identified as *Aspergillus fumigatus*. *Abbreviations:* MRSA, methicillin-resistant *Staphylococcus aureus*; PCR, polymerase chain reaction.

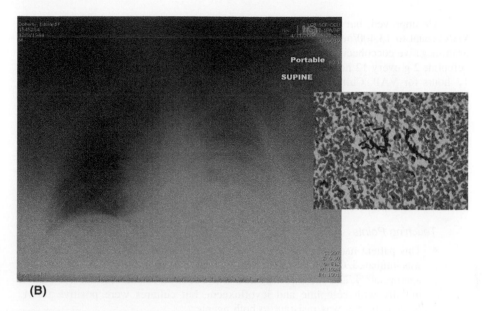

Figure 2 *(See color insert)* *(Continued)*

Teaching Points

- He did not respond clinically to vancomycin therapy perhaps because the initial dose was inadequate (not initially dosed by weight), concentrations in the lung may have been too low, and the MRSA isolate had a high MIC, which is not routinely detected by microbiology laboratories and is associated with a poorer clinical response than strains with a low MIC of 0.5 µg/mL (6,10).
- Lack of clinical response, presence of bacteria on Gram stain, and the elevated PCT level are further confirmation of inadequate therapy. The CT scan suggested lung abscesses that were not clearly seen on chest X ray, which would require that linezolid therapy be extended beyond seven days.
- Later-onset fever, purulent tracheobronchitis/VAP due to HSV was diagnosed by the presence of multinucleated giant cells on smear and the growth of HSV on culture. HSV tracheobronchitis or VAP has been associated with late clinical deterioration and poorer outcomes; macroscopic oral-labial and bronchial lesions that are smear or culture positive are helpful for diagnosis (22).

B. Case 2

A 62-year-old man was admitted with multiple trauma and a history of diabetes mellitus and chronic lung disease with many exacerbations that were treated with steroids and antibiotics. He was intubated, had a temperature of 100°F and changes on chest X ray in the lower lobe that were felt to be due to trauma or aspiration. He was started on ceftriaxone 2 g daily and clindamycin 600 mg every eight hours. His blood cultures on admission were positive for pneumococcus.

He improved, but two days later spiked a temperature to 102°F with increased WBC count to 13,400/mm^3 and increased oxygen demand. His ETA had pleomorphic, gram-negative coccobacilli and many PMNs. He was empirically started on intravenous cefepime 2 g every 12 hours, levofloxacin 750 mg daily, and vancomycin 1.25 g every 12 hours for VAP. Cultures were positive for *Acinetobacter baumannii*, resistant to cefepime and levofloxacin, but sensitive to meropenem and aminoglycosides. He was switched to meropenem and given aerosolized gentamicin therapy.

Five days later his fever persisted, and his chest CT scan suggested a possible cavity. Bronchoscopy specimens had many PMNs, no organisms, and both smears and cultures were negative for bacteria, fungi, viruses, *Legionella* and mycobacteria. Because of clinical deterioration, an open lung biopsy was performed that demonstrated many narrow-branching septate hyphae (Fig. 2B). He was started on IV voriconazole; biopsy cultures contained *A. fumigatus*.

Teaching Points

- This patient had several chronic underlying diseases, acute chest trauma, and was intubated. On admission he had pneumococcal bacteremia that was treated appropriately, and subsequently had VAP due to *A. baumannii* that was treated initially with cefepime and levofloxacin, but cultures were positive for *A. baumannii* that was resistant to both agents.
- Many *Acinetobacter* spp. are resistant to cefepime and levofloxacin, and this patient had received levofloxacin many times before. Initial coverage with a carbapenem plus an aminoglycoside would have been effective; most strains are sensitive to polymyxin with or without rifampin.
- Invasive aspergillosis may be a cause of VAP in ICU patients who have cirrhosis, COPD, or diabetes mellitus, neutropenia, steroid therapy, or an underlying hematological disorder or malignancy.
- This patient underscores the fact that clinical manifestations in invasive aspergillosis may be subtle and difficult to diagnose in critically ill, mechanically ventilated patients (21). Positive cultures for Aspergillus are present in <50% of patients. Thus, *Aspergillus galactomannan* (GM) in the BAL and serum appear to be helpful for this diagnosis (21). Voriconazole provides effective antifungal therapy for invasive aspergillosis.

X. Summary

There has been great progress in our understanding of VAP management that includes three simple and effective steps. Step 1: Initiate early, appropriate, and adequate antibiotic therapy, until definitive cultures and clinical response can be assessed. Step 2: De-escalate initial antibiotics on the basis of clinical response, culture, and antibiotic sensitivity data, as available. Step 3: Stop antibiotic treatment at seven days to reduce the risk of superinfection, unless there is a complication. An alternative strategy may be to target VAT.

Prevention of VAP and other health care–associated infections has moved from the back to the front seat. IHI has been a force for "sowing seeds of change." However, more may be needed to prevent VAP in some institutions than just "implementing the IHI bundle." Clearly, prevention should be the primary focus and the key to reducing

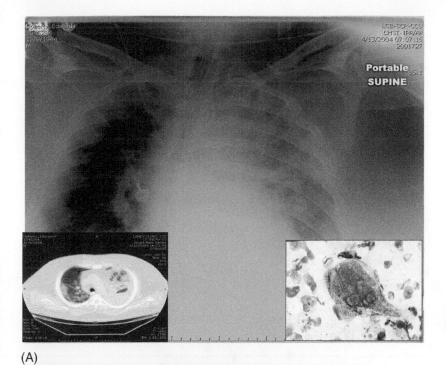

(A)

(B)

Figure 10.2 (**A**) Case 1: CT scan shows lung abscess not seen on chest X ray secondary to MRSA pneumonia. Sputum smear taken on day 9 of intubation demonstrated multinucleated giant cells. Culture and PCR were positive for herpes simplex virus. (**B**) Case 2: Initial chest X ray and lung biopsy taken on day 12 of intubation demonstrating narrow-branching, fungal septate hyphae, later identified as *Aspergillus fumigatus*. *Abbreviations:* MRSA, methicillin-resistant *Staphylococcus aureus*; PCR, polymerase chain reaction.

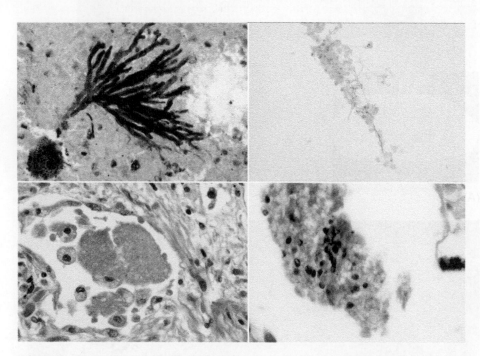

Figure 12.1 Pathology of opportunistic infections. (*Top left*) Hyphae of *Aspergillus* spp. are seen with GMS stain and are septate, with dichotomous branching at 45° angles. (*Top right*) *Nocardia* spp. is seen as long, delicate filaments that can easily be overlooked. (*Bottom left*) *P. jiroveci* infection typically has a frothy eosinophilic intra-alveolar exudate filling acini. (*Bottom right*) Cysts of *Pneumocystis* are seen with GMS and have a delicate capsular wall with variable shapes, including collapsed forms. *Abbreviation*: GMS, Gomori methenamine silver.

mortality, morbidity, and health care costs. Hospital administrators need to realize that "investing in an ounce of prevention is definitely worth more than a pound of cure," particular if payments to hospitals are reduced for patients who develop health care–associated infections. Proper implementation of effective VAP prevention measures will take teamwork, thought, investment, and a change in culture, and spreading the seeds of prevention will be needed in chronic care hospitals, rehabilitation facilities, and nursing homes that are an integral part of our changing health care system. In the future, health care facilities will need to reevaluate their strategies and priorities, perhaps adapting the following old philosophy:

"Don't wait for the ship to come in, row out to meet it."

References

1. Niederman MS, Craven DE, Bonten M. et al. American Thoracic Society and the Infectious Diseases Society of America Guideline Committee guidelines for the management of adults with hospital-acquired, ventilator-associated, and health care-associated pneumonia. Am J Respir Crit Care Med 2005; 171:388–416.
2. Tablan OC, Anderson LJ, Besser R, et al. Guidelines for preventing health-care–associated pneumonia, 2003: recommendations of CDC and the Healthcare Infection Control Practices Advisory Committee. MMWR Recomm Rep 2004; 53:1–36.
3. Chastre J, Fagon JY. Ventilator-associated pneumonia. Am J Respir Crit Care Med 2002; 165:867–903.
4. Kollef MH. Prevention of hospital-associated pneumonia and ventilator-associated pneumonia. Crit Care Med 2004; 32:1396–405.
5. Popovich KJ, Weinstein RA, Hota B. Are community-associated methicillin-resistant Staphylococcus aureus (MRSA) strains replacing traditional nosocomial MRSA strains? Clin Infect Dis 2008; 46:787–794.
6. Deresinski S. Counterpoint: Vancomycin and Staphylococcus aureus–an antibiotic enters obsolescence. Clin Infect Dis 2007; 44:1543–1548.
7. Hidayat LK, Hsu DI, Quist R, et al. High-dose vancomycin therapy for methicillin-resistant Staphylococcus aureus infections: efficacy and toxicity. Arch Intern Med 2006; 166: 2138–2144.
8. Stevens DL, Ma Y, Salmi DB, et al. Impact of antibiotics on expression of virulence-associated exotoxin genes in methicillin-sensitive and methicillin-resistant Staphylococcus aureus. J Infect Dis 2007; 195:202–211.
9. Conte JE Jr., Golden JA, Kipps J, et al. Intrapulmonary pharmacokinetics of linezolid. Antimicrob Agents Chemother 2002; 46:1475–1480.
10. Moise PA, Forrest A, Bhavnani SM, et al. Area under the inhibitory curve and a pneumonia scoring system for predicting outcomes of vancomycin therapy for respiratory infections by Staphylococcus aureus. Am J Health Syst Pharm 2000; 57(suppl 2):S4–S9.
11. Paterson DL, Ko WC, Von Gottberg A, et al. Antibiotic therapy for Klebsiella pneumoniae bacteremia: implications of production of extended-spectrum beta-lactamases. Clin Infect Dis 2004; 39:31–37.
12. Sader HS, Fritsche TR, Jones RN. Accuracy of three automated systems (MIcroScan, WalkAway, VITEK and VITEK 2) for susceptibility testing of *Pseudomonas aeruginosa* against five broad-spectrum beta-lactam agents. J Clin Microbiol 2006; 44(3):1101.
13. Lodise TP, Jr., Lomaestro B, Drusano GL. Piperacillin-tazobactam for Pseudomonas aeruginosa infection: clinical implications of an extended-infusion dosing strategy. Clin Infect Dis 2007; 44:357–363.

14. Paul M, Benuri-Silbiger I, Soares-Weiser K, et al. Beta lactam monotherapy versus beta lactam-aminoglycoside combination therapy for sepsis in immunocompetent patients: systematic review and meta-analysis of randomised trials. BMJ 2004; 328:668.

15. Bliziotis IA, Samonis G, Vardakas KZ, et al. Effect of aminoglycoside and beta-lactam combination therapy versus beta-lactam monotherapy on the emergence of antimicrobial resistance: a meta-analysis of randomized, controlled trials. Clin Infect Dis 2005; 41:149–158.

16. Munoz-Price LS, Weinstein RA. Acinetobacter infection. N Engl J Med 2008; 358:1271–1281.

17. Manikal VM, Landman D, Saurina G, et al. Endemic carbapenem-resistant Acinetobacter species in Brooklyn, New York: citywide prevalence, interinstitutional spread, and relation to antibiotic usage. Clin Infect Dis 2000; 31:101–106.

18. Linden PK, Paterson DL. Parenteral and inhaled colistin for treatment of ventilator-associated pneumonia. Clin Infect Dis 2006; 43(suppl 2):S89–S94.

19. Chow JW, Fine MJ, Shlaes DM, et al. Enterobacter bacteremia: clinical features and emergence of antibiotic resistance during therapy. Ann Intern Med 1991; 115:585–590.

20. Jacoby GA, Munoz-Price LS. The new beta-lactamases. N Engl J Med 2005; 352:380–391.

21. Meersseman W, Van Wijngaerden E. Invasive aspergillosis in the ICU: an emerging disease. Intensive Care Med 2007; 33:1679–1681.

22. Luyt CE, Combes A, Deback C, et al. Herpes simplex virus lung infection in patients undergoing prolonged mechanical ventilation. Am J Respir Crit Care Med 2007; 175:935–942.

23. Craven DE, Steger Craven K, Duncan RA. Hospital-acquired pneumonia. In: Jarvis W, ed. Hospital Infections. Boston: Little Brown, 2009.

24. Craven DE, Chroneou A, Zias N, et al. Ventilator-associated tracheobronchitis: the Impact of targeted antibiotic therapy on patient outcomes. Chest 2009; 135(2):521–528.

25. Nseir S, Favory R, Jozefowicz E, et al. Antimicrobial treatment for ventilator-associated tracheobronchitis: a randomized, controlled, multicenter study. Crit Care 2008; 12(3):R62.

26. Prince AS. Biofilms, antimicrobial resistance, and airway infection. N Engl J Med 2002; 347:1110–1111.

27. Fagon JY, Chastre J, Wolff M, et al. Invasive and noninvasive strategies for management of suspected ventilator-associated pneumonia. A randomized trial. Ann Intern Med 2000; 132:621–630.

28. Canadian Clinical Trials Group. A randomized trial of diagnostic techniques for ventilator-associated pneumonia. N Engl J Med 2006; 355:2619–2630.

29. Gibot S, Cravoisy A, Levy B, et al. Soluble triggering receptor expressed on myeloid cells and the diagnosis of pneumonia. N Engl J Med 2004; 350:451–458.

30. Ramirez P, Garcia MA, Ferrer M, et al. Sequential measurements of procalcitonin levels in diagnosing ventilator-associated pneumonia. Eur Respir J 2008; 31:356–362.

31. Christ-Crain M, Jaccard-Stolz D, Bingisser R, et al. Effect of procalcitonin-guided treatment on antibiotic use and outcome in lower respiratory tract infections: cluster-randomised, single-blinded intervention trial. Lancet 2004; 363:600–607.

32. Chastre J, Wolff M, Fagon JY, et al. Comparison of 8 vs 15 days of antibiotic therapy for ventilator-associated pneumonia in adults: a randomized trial. JAMA 2003; 290:2588–2598.

33. Resar R, Pronovost P, Haraden C, et al. Using a bundle approach to improve ventilator care processes and reduce ventilator-associated pneumonia. Jt Comm J Qual Patient Saf 2005; 31: 243–248.

34. Craven DE. Preventing ventilator-associated pneumonia in adults: sowing seeds of change. Chest 2006; 130:251–260.

35. Eggimann P, Pittet D. Infection control in the ICU. Chest 2001; 120:2059–2093.

36. Zack JE, Garrison T, Trovillion E, et al. Effect of an education program aimed at reducing the occurrence of ventilator-associated pneumonia. Crit Care Med 2002; 30:2407–2412.

37. Mori H, Hirasawa H, Oda S, et al. Oral care reduces incidence of ventilator-associated pneumonia in ICU populations. Intensive Care Med 2006; 32:230–236.

38. Chan EY, Ruest A, Meade MO, et al. Oral decontamination for prevention of pneumonia in mechanically ventilated adults: systematic review and meta-analysis. BMJ 2007; 334:889.
39. Chlebicki MP, Safdar N. Topical chlorhexidine for prevention of ventilator-associated pneumonia: a meta-analysis. Crit Care Med 2007; 35:595—602.
40. Koeman M, van der Ven AJ, Hak E, et al. Oral decontamination with chlorhexidine reduces the incidence of ventilator-associated pneumonia. Am J Respir Crit Care Med 2006; 173: 1348–1355.
41. Liberati A, D'Amico R, Pifferi, et al. Antibiotic prophylaxis to reduce respiratory tract infections and mortality in adults receiving intensive care. Cochrane Database Syst Rev 2004:CD000022.
42. Marelich GP, Murin S, Battistella F, et al. Protocol weaning of mechanical ventilation in medical and surgical patients by respiratory care practitioners and nurses: effect on weaning time and incidence of ventilator-associated pneumonia. Chest 2000; 118:459–467.
43. Girard TD, Kress JP, Fuchs BD, et al. Efficacy and safety of a paired sedation and ventilator weaning protocol for mechanically ventilated patients in intensive care (Awakening and Breathing Controlled trial): a randomised controlled trial. Lancet 2008; 371:126–134.
44. Schweickert WD, Gehlbach BK, Pohlman AS, et al. Daily interruption of sedative infusions and complications of critical illness in mechanically ventilated patients. Crit Care Med 2004; 32:1272–1276.
45. Kress JP, Pohlman AS, O'Connor MF, et al. Daily interruption of sedative infusions in critically ill patients undergoing mechanical ventilation. N Engl J Med 2000; 342:1471–1477.
46. Burns KE, Adhikari NK, Meade MO. A meta-analysis of noninvasive weaning to facilitate liberation from mechanical ventilation. Can J Anaesth 2006; 53:305–315.
47. Dezfulian C, Shojania K, Collard HR, et al. Subglottic secretion drainage for preventing ventilator-associated pneumonia: a meta-analysis. Am J Med 2005; 118:11–18.
48. Kollef MH, Afessa B, Anzueto A, et al. Silver-coated endotracheal tubes and incidence of ventilator-associated pneumonia: the NASCENT randomized trial. JAMA 2008; 300(7): 805–813.
49. Fox MY. Toward a zero VAP rate: personal and team approaches in the ICU. Crit Care Nurs Q 2006; 29:108–114; quiz 115–116.
50. Griffiths J, Barber VS, Morgan L, et al. Systematic review and meta-analysis of studies of the timing of tracheostomy in adult patients undergoing artificial ventilation. BMJ 2005; 330:1243.

11
Pneumonia in ARDS

JEAN-DAMIEN RICARD and DIDIER DREYFUSS
Institut National de la Santé et de la Recherche Médicale, INSERM U722, Paris; UFR de Médecine Paris Diderot – Paris 7, and Assistance Publique–Hôpitaux de Paris, Hôpital Louis Mourier, Service de Réanimation Médicale, Colombes, France

DAMIEN ROUX
Institut National de la Santé et de la Recherche Médicale, INSERM U722, Paris; UFR de Médecine Paris Diderot – Paris 7, France

I. Introduction

Acute lung injury (ALI) and the acute respiratory distress syndrome (ARDS) are important causes of admission to the intensive care unit (ICU) and are still associated with high mortality rates (1,2) despite recent improvement in their prognosis (3,4). The relationship between ALI/ARDS and bacterial infection is complex. Sepsis (both from pulmonary and extrapulmonary origin) is indeed a leading etiology of ALI/ARDS (1–4). In particular, lung infection may account for 50% of cases of ARDS (2,5). On the other hand, bacterial lung superinfection may be frequent during ARDS, because of impaired host defenses and prolonged mechanical ventilation (6,7). This may promote multiple organ failure and increase mortality (7,8). After a review of the epidemiology and the pathophysiology of pneumonia acquired during ARDS, this chapter focuses on its clinical management including recognition, treatment, and prevention. Viral pneumonia is not covered in this chapter, though recent observations suggest that herpesvirus pneumonia might occur during mechanical ventilation (9).

II. Definition

Pneumonia can be defined as microbial invasion of the normally sterile lower respiratory tract and lung parenchyma. During mechanical ventilation of ARDS, ventilator-associated pneumonia (VAP) will be defined as an inflammation of the lung parenchyma caused by infectious agents not present or incubating at the onset of mechanical ventilation (10).

III. Epidemiology
A. Incidence and Time of Occurrence of VAP During ARDS

VAP often complicates the course of ARDS leading to the development of sepsis, multiple organ failure, and death. Clinical studies indicate that between 34% and more than 70% of patients with ARDS are affected by pulmonary infection. Autopsy studies have found that up to 73% of patients who died of ARDS had histological evidence of pneumonia (6,7). Because some of the diagnostic criteria for VAP are key features of ARDS (radiological infiltrates, and hypoxemia), the diagnosis of pulmonary infection in patients with ARDS is often difficult. Physicians' inability to accurately diagnose nosocomial pneumonia during ARDS using clinical criteria only has been long recognized (6).

Recently, five studies have evaluated incidence and outcome of VAP during ARDS (5,11–14) (Table 1). They all used sampling techniques of distal airways, including bronchoalveolar lavage (BAL), protected specimen brushing (PSB), or plugged telescopic catheter (PTC), that avoid contamination by proximal secretions and allow quantitative culturing to distinguish between colonization and infection. Despite similar diagnostic techniques, the incidence varied markedly between studies (Table 1), ranging from 15% to 60%. This very low incidence of 15% may be explained by the fact that sampling was performed at predetermined time rather than depending on clinical suspicion of pneumonia in this study (11). Thus, false-negative results may have been frequent because of the prescription of new antibiotics before sampling was performed. All four others studies found much higher incidences, ranging from 36.5% to 60% (5,12–14). This variability may be accounted for by the fact that all studies (12–14) but one (5) were conducted in a single center, which may bias the estimate. Incidence of VAP was 36.5% in this multicenter study (5). One can reasonably conclude that the actual incidence of VAP during ARDS is higher than one third of patients, which is much more than the global incidence of VAP in the general ICU population (10). As a matter of fact, the only multicenter study compared the incidence of VAP in 134 patients with ARDS to that observed in 744 patients without ARDS on mechanical ventilation during the same period (5). Despite similar disease severity, non-ARDS patients had a much lower incidence of VAP (23%), suggesting that ARDS patients are at a higher risk for this complication. The same observations were made in a single-center study, where VAP occurred in 55% ARDS patients, whereas it affected only 28% of cases of mechanically ventilated patients without ARDS, despite similar severity of disease (13). In the vast majority of patients, VAP occurs late, i.e., after more than one week of mechanical ventilation (5,12,13) (Table 2). This may be explained by the fact that most patients were on antibiotics (broad-spectrum in most cases) before the occurrence of VAP (Table 2), which favors the occurrence of late-onset VAP (15). In addition, almost 30% of patients had more than one episode of VAP (Table 2).

IV. Etiology

A. Type of Causative Microorganisms

As could be expected from the predominance of late-onset VAP in patients receiving broad-spectrum antibiotics, difficult-to-treat organisms are predominantly involved in these patients. Methicillin-resistant staphylococci and gram-negative nonfermenting rods (*Pseudomonas aeruginosa*, *Acinetobacter baumannii*, and *Stenotrophomonas maltophilia*) accounted for 44% and 65% of causative pathogens in a single-center study and in a multicenter study, respectively (5,13) (Table 2). Enterobacteriaceae were the third most frequent group of causative pathogens (5,13).

B. Risk Factors

As mentioned above, ARDS per se seems to be an important risk factor for VAP (5,13). Only one study has prospectively assessed potential risk factors for VAP acquisition during ARDS (5). Several risk factors were identified by multivariate analysis. The

Table 1 Epidemiology of VAP During ARDS

| | Number ARDS | % VAP | Diagnosis[a] | Duration of MV | | Mortality | | | |
| | | | | | | Patients with ARDS | | Patients without ARDS | |
				VAP+	VAP−	VAP+	VAP−	VAP+	VAP−
Sutherland et al. (11)	105	15	PSB/BAL	No difference		6/16 (38%)	40/89 (45%)	NR	NR
Delclaux et al. (12)	30	60	PTC/BAL	24±13	13±13[b]	14/18 (78%)	11/12 (92%)	NR	NR
Meduri et al. (14)	94	43	BAL	NR	NR	63%	NR	NR	NR
Chastre et al. (13)[c]	56	55	PSB/BAL	34±32	17±19[d]	16/31 (52%)	18/25 (72%)	25/53 (47%)	38/134 (28%)[e]
Markowicz et al. (5)[f]	134	37	PSB/BAL/PTC	33±21	11±9[g]	28/49 (57%)	50/85 (59%)	67/162 (41%)[e]	225/582 (39%)[e]

[a]Sampling of the lung was performed because of clinical suspicion in all studies except in the one by Sutherland et al, where sampling was performed at predetermined times.

[b]$p < 0.05$.

[c]53/187 (28%) non-ARDS patients had VAP during the same period.

[d]$p < 0.005$.

[e]$p < 0.001$ vs. patients with ARDS.

[f]173/744 (23%) non-ARDS patients had VAP during the same period, in this multicenter study (8 medical and 3 medical-surgical units).

[g]$p < 0.0001$ vs. patients with VAP.

Abbreviations: ARDS, acute respiratory distress syndrome; MV, mechanical ventilation; VAP, ventilator-associated pneumonia; PSB, protected specimen brush; BAL, bronchoalveolar lavage; PTC, plugged telescopic catheter; NR, not reported.

Table 2 Clinical and Bacteriological Features of VAP During ARDS

	Delclaux et al. (12)	Chastre et al. (13)	Markowicz et al. (5)
Percentage of patients on antibiotics	43	94	90
Percentage of patients on broad-spectrum antibiotics	–	61	84
Day of first VAP	12	>7day in 90%	12
Percentage of patients with >1 VAP	28	32	31
Percentage of polymicrobial episodes	25	55	24
Percentage of gram-negative nonfermenters	29	21	47
Percentage of MRSA	–	23	18

Abbreviations: VAP, ventilator-associated pneumonia; MRSA, methicillin-resistant *Staphylococcus aureus*.

presence, but not the duration, of enteral nutrition was found to be significantly associated ($p = 0.049$) with VAP occurrence. Surprisingly, the most important risk factor for VAP was the use of sucralfate. Indeed, a highly significant association ($p < 0.0002$) was found between both its use and the duration of its use and the occurrence of VAP. Interestingly, a recent study confirmed that, at least for early-onset pneumonia, sucralfate might be a risk factor for VAP in mechanically ventilated patients (16). Finally, the use of histamine H2-blockers was not associated with VAP occurrence (5). This was also the case for the use of sedatives and muscle relaxants.

V. Pathogenesis

A. Relationship Between Lung Injury, Mechanical Ventilation, and Infection

Experimental Lung Injury and Infection

Bacterial Superinfection in Animals with Acute Lung Injury

This has been an important subject of experimental investigation since the pioneer work conducted by Johanson et al., who studied the effect of hyperoxia-induced lung injury on bacterial dissemination during lung infection in hamsters (17). Exposure to 100% oxygen for several days enhanced lung bacterial growth in animals that received an intratracheal instillation with *P. aeruginosa*. Indeed, air-breathing animals developed focal bronchopneumonia but viable organisms were not recovered from the lungs after three days. In contrast, oxygen-exposed animals had diffuse alveolar damage (a classical feature of oxygen-induced injury) and lung cultures yielded high bacterial counts. In addition, bacterial systemic dissemination, as assessed by bacterial cultures of liver tissue, was much more frequent in oxygen-exposed animals. These results suggested that bacterial superinfection of injured lungs may account for both worsening of lung function and systemic diffusion of infection. These results were confirmed by the same team in a model of ALI induced by paraquat intoxication (8). Hamsters that received paraquat only had moderate lung injury and 12% mortality, while those who were intratracheally inoculated with *P. aeruginosa* only had focal bronchopneumonia and survived. In striking contrast, animals that received both injuries, paraquat followed by bacterial challenge three days later, had severe diffuse alveolar damage and 100% mortality. Lung bacterial counts were markedly (almost 3 log) higher in animals that received both injuries than in those inoculated with *Pseudomonas* only. Systemic diffusion of infection was also more marked in animals with combined injury, as assessed by liver bacterial culture. Although these two studies indicate increased susceptibility of injured lungs to infection, the situation may be more complex. Indeed, a study by Jean and coworkers showed that previous intratracheal endotoxin (lipopolysaccharide, LPS) lung instillation might protect against a subsequent lung bacterial challenge (18). Rats received an intratracheal instillation of either endotoxin alone, or *P. aeruginosa* alone, or both. Animals that received LPS alone or combined instillation had reduced mortality and improved bacterial lung clearance. This suggested that alveolar neutrophil recruitment by LPS was able to protect against subsequent infection.

Effect of Mechanical Ventilation on Bacterial Growth

Very recently, Pugin and his team elegantly showed that cyclic cell stretch (mimicking mechanical ventilation) favoured bacterial growth (19). Human alveolar type II–like A549 cells along with human bronchial BEAS-2B cells, human MRC-5 fibroblasts, and murine RAW 264.7 macrophages were submitted in vitro to prolonged cyclic stretch. Bacteria were cultured in conditioned supernatants from cells submitted to stretch and from control static cells. *Escherichia coli* had a marked growth advantage in conditioned supernatants from the stretched cells. Interestingly, stretched cells compared with control static cells acidified the milieu by producing increased amounts of lactic acid. Alkalinization of supernatants from stretched cells blocked *E. coli* growth. In contrast, acidification of supernatants from control cells stimulated bacterial growth.

Influence of Mechanical Ventilation on Lung and Systemic Inflammation

The deleterious effects of mechanical ventilation on lung function and structure have been unambiguously demonstrated in the experimental context and termed ventilator-induced lung injury (20). Lesions are induced by lung overdistension and result in permeability-type pulmonary edema and diffuse alveolar damage. These experimental observations raised the possibility that injurious mechanical ventilation, with too high a tidal volume, may contribute to ARDS mortality in humans. Recently, this concept has been validated clinically, with low tidal volume ventilation in ARDS demonstrating increased survival. In addition, injurious mechanical ventilation may promote release from the lung into the systemic circulation of both proinflammatory and anti-inflammatory cytokines that may modify lung and systemic reaction to injury (21–23). This remains however a controversial issue, and it is, at the present time, quite difficult to draw a comprehensive theory linking mechanical ventilation and systemic inflammation and organ failure since, depending on the study, one may conclude that injurious ventilation does not affect cytokine balance (24,25), is proinflammatory (26,27), or is anti-inflammatory (28). It may be that lung priming by a previous injury is necessary for cytokine release to occur during injurious mechanical ventilation, i.e., a two-hit injury. This was demonstrated in rats subjected to injurious mechanical ventilation after either mesenteric ischemia-reperfusion injury (29), or hemorrhagic shock (30). Animals that received both injuries had a markedly greater inflammatory response than animals that were subjected to one injury only (29,30).

Influence of Mechanical Ventilation on Systemic Diffusion of Lung Infection

Several studies investigated the possibility of translocation from the lung to systemic circulation of bacteria or bacterial products such as endotoxin because of injurious mechanical ventilation. Bacteremia was more frequent in animals ventilated with an injurious high tidal volume, after intratracheal instillation of *E. coli* in dogs (31) or *Klebsiella pneumoniae* in rats (32). Even normal tidal volume ventilation may promote systemic spread of infection when compared with spontaneous breathing, as assessed by culture of contralateral lung, spleen and liver in rats with unilateral *P. aeruginosa* pneumonia (33). In these animal models, ventilation with positive end-expiratory pressure reduced bacterial dissemination (31–33). Exogenous surfactant administration also reduced bacterial dissemination from the lung during group B *Streptococcal* pneumonia in surfactant-depleted piglets (34). Interestingly, previous lung injury by mechanical ventilation may also promote the subsequent development of lung infection in spontaneously breathing rats (35). Finally, injurious ventilation may favor the translocation of endotoxin from lungs to systemic circulation (36).

B. Microbial Mechanisms
Bacterial Virulence

There is no doubt bacterial virulence plays a significant role during severe pneumonia, at least with certain pathogens. *Staphylococcus aureus* strains carrying the Panton–Valentine leukocidin (PVL) gene have been associated with highly lethal necrotizing pneumonia in young immunocompetent patients (37). PVL is a synergohymenotropic toxin that creates lytic pores in the cell membranes of neutrophils and induces release of neutrophil chemotactic factors. Intense lung inflammation in response to PVL mediates tissue necrosis accounting for the clinical and radiographic presentation in these patients. To date however, it seems that such strains are very rarely responsible for VAP (38). The other major pathogen responsible for VAP during ARDS is *P. aeruginosa,* which possesses a large arsenal of virulence factors. One of them is a type III secretion system (TTSS) (39), which upon cell contact deploys a needlelike secretion machinery to inject toxins directly into the cytoplasm of the host cell (40). Exoenzyme U (ExoU), one of the four TTSS effector molecules, is a necrotizing toxin with phospholipase activity (41) that leads to rapid lysis of mammalian cells. Recently, El-Solh et al. searched for virulent factors associated with persistent *P. aeruginosa* VAP (42). Although the study was not designed to include specifically ARDS patients, a number of them had at least ALI with PaO_2/FiO_2 ratios below 250. Of the *Pseudomonas* isolates from patients with VAP, 71% were capable of secreting type III effector proteins. There was a significant difference in BAL neutrophil apoptosis rate at VAP onset between those patients infected with strains that secreted cytotoxins and those that did not. Neutrophil elastase levels in BAL were positively correlated with the rate of neutrophil apoptosis. Despite adequate antimicrobial therapy, 13 out of 25 TTSS plus isolates were recovered at day 8 post-VAP, whereas eradication was achieved in all patients who had undetectable levels of type III secretion proteins (42). Other studies have reported that similar percentages of *Pseudomonas* VAP are caused by strains that secrete TTSS proteins (43,44). TTSS secretory isolates are predominantly either ExoU/PcrV or ExoS/PcrV phenotypes.

Role of Fungal Colonization

Recent data suggests that *Candida* spp. colonization of the airway of ventilated patients might favor the development of bacterial pneumonia, *Pseudomonas* VAP in particular. We investigated this possibility by comparing rate of *P. aeruginosa* pneumonia in rats that were or were not colonized by *Candida albicans* (45). We found that rats colonized by *C. albicans* that receive an inoculum of *P. aeruginosa* (that otherwise does not lead to pneumonia development) had a much greater incidence of *P. aeruginosa* pneumonia in comparison with rats not colonized by *C. albicans*. The underlying mechanism seems to be related, at least in part, to macrophage impairment in reactive oxygen species production (45).

C. Host Mechanisms

Altered Immunity During ALI and Mechanical Ventilation

Many experimental and clinical studies have evaluated whether acute lung injury changes lung and systemic defense against infection. In particular, alveolar macrophage and neutrophil functions were studied as well as the influence of lung injury on the inflammatory cytokines network. It is beyond the scope of this chapter to review the abundant literature on this field in detail, especially in the light of multiple uncertainties.

Experimental Studies

Despite the fact that hamsters with paraquat-induced lung injury become prone to lung superinfection and systemic bacterial dissemination, phagocytosis and intracellular killing of *S. aureus* by leucocytes recovered from the lung by lavage from these animals was normal (8). Similarly, intratracheal endotoxin instillation, which induced local recruitment of neutrophils, did not seem to affect their function in rats (18), possibly explaining why these animals were protected against the development of pneumonia after *P. aeruginosa* tracheal instillation (18). Finally, ventilator-induced lung injury is associated with neutrophil infiltration, which may participate in the generation of inflammatory lesions (20,22,46,47). Alveolar macrophages may be adversely affected during acute lung injury. For instance, alveolar macrophages retrieved by BAL in dogs with endotoxin-induced ALI exhibited reduced bacterial phagocytosis and killing (48). Inflammatory cytokine networks may also be affected by acute lung injury, resulting in an anti-inflammatory orientation and decreased systemic antibacterial defense (35,49).

Human Studies

Lungs of patients mechanically ventilated for ARDS undergo both the injury due to initial disease and possibly lesions due to mechanical ventilation (4,20). Both may affect lung and systemic antibacterial defenses. Neutrophils were implicated in the pathogenesis of ARDS more than 20 years ago (50). The functional capacity of neutrophils that infiltrate ARDS lungs was the subject of important recent investigation. Indeed, they can participate in the genesis of ARDS lesions and in the occurrence of lung superinfection if their functions are altered. For instance, neutrophils obtained from BAL fluid of patients shortly after the onset of ARDS exhibited decreased chemotactic responses and microbicidal activity (51), alterations that may favor the occurrence of lung infection. Similarly, BAL neutrophils recovered from patients with ARDS were found to be activated but hyporesponsive to ex vivo bacterial stimulation, which could partly account for increased susceptibility to infection (52). Finally, a decrease in *S. aureus* killing capabilities of blood neutrophils was evidenced in the days preceding the occurrence of a nosocomial infection in critically ill patients (53).

There are close relationships between neutrophils and the cytokine network. Indeed, the degree of activation of lung neutrophils correlated with the levels of inflammatory cytokines in ARDS patients (52). The extremely complex cytokine network is affected both by ALI and by mechanical ventilation and may influence lung and systemic antibacterial defenses. In experimental models, systemic cytokine network may be oriented toward anti-inflammation after lung injury and promote immunosuppression (49). The effects of mechanical ventilation strategy on lung cytokine balance during ARDS are under investigation. One study showed that use of low tidal volume plus high positive end-expiratory pressure (frequently used during mechanical ventilation of ARDS and considered as "protective" against further mechanical lung injury) resulted in less inflammatory cytokine production than a strategy that used a higher tidal volume and a lower end-expiratory pressure (54). However, another study showed that the protective strategy was responsible for an orientation of the cytokine network toward anti-inflammation (55). Our understanding of the physiology of lung cytokine response to mechanical ventilation is too imprecise to draw any firm conclusion on its potential role in the occurrence of organ failure (22).

In conclusion, the hypothesis that ALI and mechanical ventilation may favor lung and systemic infection and initiate a vicious circle together with infection is extremely attractive and has been the matter of extensive investigation and speculation (7,56).

VI. Diagnostic Approach

Clinical, radiological, and biological abnormalities that should lead clinicians to suspect VAP are listed in Table 3. To help clinicians decide whether or not ongoing lung infection is involved, a clinical pulmonary infection score (CPIS) score has been developed (57), based on six variables: body temperature, blood leukocytes, abundance and purulence of tracheal secretions, oxygenation, pulmonary radiography, and culture of endotracheal aspirates. Each variable is given a value ranging from 0 to 2 depending on their association with pneumonia. CPIS >6 has a good positive predictive value for pneumonia. Adjustments of this score have been made to take into account Gram stain examination of BAL or PTC samples (58).

Table 3 Clinical, Biological, and Radiological Features of Suspected VAP

Clinical findings	Biological findings	Radiological findings
Persistent fever or new febrile episode abundant and purulent respiratory secretions oxygen desaturation tachycardia hemodynamic instability or septic shock	Hypoxemia hyperleukocytosis	Persistent or new pulmonary infiltrate

Abbreviation: VAP, ventilator-associated pneumonia.

A. Microbiological Diagnosis

Because a majority of mechanically ventilated ARDS patients harbor many of the risk factors for VAP caused by multidrug resistant pathogens, efforts should be made to identify the causative pathogen. Respiratory tract cultures can be obtained from endotracheal aspirate, BAL, PSB, or PTC. Contrary to endotracheal aspirates, the invasive methods (BAL, PSB, and PTC) prevent contamination of the distal airway specimens by the proximal flora. In addition, quantitative cultures of these samples help distinguish colonization from true pulmonary infection. Local expertise and availability guide the choice of the method, however invasive bronchoscopic methods have been found to improve outcomes and reduce antibiotic use (59). Efforts should be made to obtain bacteriological samples before initiating or modifying antibiotic treatment.

VII. Management

Antimicrobial Treatment

Initial Empiric Treatment

As soon as bacterial samples are obtained, antibiotic therapy must be started or modified. Antibiotic recommendations (60) depend on the time of VAP occurrence (i.e., early-onset vs. late-onset VAP) and on the presence of risk factors for multidrug resistant pathogens.

Given the high prevalence of multidrug-resistant pathogens in VAP in ARDS patients, empiric intravenous antibiotic therapy should cover *P. aeruginosa*, Enterobacteriaceae, and *Acinetobacter* spp. (Table 4). Moreover, methicillin-resistant *S. aureus* (MRSA) should be suspected in the presence of MRSA colonization or high local incidence. The initial antibiotic (Table 4) therapy should combine (*i*) an antipseudomonal β-lactam, (*ii*) either an antipseudomonal fluoroquinolone or an aminoglycoside, and (*iii*) vancomycin or linezolid if MRSA is suspected (60).

Direct examination of the respiratory tract specimen enables to focus antibiotic therapy on suspected pathogens, for instance, to avoid empiric use of vancomycin or linezolid if only gram-negative bacilli are observed (Table 4, type C). If the patient has received antimicrobials within the past two weeks, the empiric antibiotic therapy should not include agents from the same antibiotic class. Aminoglycosides are usually injected once a day and should not be used for more than three to five days in patients who clinically respond to treatment. Vancomycin can be injected twice a day or continuously (61), with an aim to maintain a trough level of 20 to 30 μg/mL.

Treatment Adjustment According to Culture Results

The negative predictive value for VAP of properly obtained respiratory tract cultures is very high, so that a negative culture can rule out VAP. It is thus, as stated earlier, important to obtain samples before initiating antibiotic treatment. On the other hand, a nonquantitative positive culture cannot distinguish between true pneumonia and airway colonization, justifying the need for quantitative cultures. Table 5 shows the different quantitative thresholds for each sampling technique above which VAP is confirmed. Quantitative culture results below the threshold represent colonization or contamination.

After identification of the etiologic pathogen, antibiotic therapy should be deescalated or adjusted, taking into account antibiotic susceptibility of the causative pathogen. In case of negative culture and clinical improvement on day 2 or 3, antibiotic

Table 4 Initial Empiric Antibiotic Therapy for VAP

	VAP	
Type	Microorganisms	Therapy
A: Early-onset VAP and no risk factor for multidrug-resistant bacteria	*Streptococcus pneumoniae* *H. influenzae* Sensitive enteric gram-negative bacilli Methicillin-sensitive *S. aureus*	Mono-antibiotic IV therapy Ampicillin/sulbactam *or* third-generation cephalosporin (cefotaxime, ceftriaxone) *or* fluoroquinolone (levofloxacin, moxifloxacin)
B: Late-onset VAP or risk factor for multidrug-resistant bacteria	*P. aeruginosa* Methicillin-resistant *S. aureus*[a] Resistant enteric gram-negative bacilli *A. baumanii*	Combination IV therapy Selected antipseudomonal β-lactam (cefepime, ceftazidime piperacillin/tazobactam, imipenem, or meropenem) *plus* aminoglycoside (amikacin or tobramycin) *or* antipseudomonal quinolone (ciprofloxacin or levofloxacin) *plus* vancomycin[a] *or* linezolid[a]
C: Late-onset VAP and gram-negative bacilli on Gram stain of protected distal airway specimen	*P. aeruginosa* Resistant enteric gram-negative bacilli *A. baumanii*	Combination IV therapy Selected antipseudomonal β-lactam (cefepime, ceftazidime piperacilline/tazobactam, imipenem, or meropenem) *plus* aminoglycoside (amikacin or tobramycin) *or* antipseudomonal quinolone (ciprofloxacin or levofloxacin)

[a]Only if risk factor for MRSA or high local incidence
Abbreviation: VAP, ventilator-associated pneumonia.
Source: Adapted from Ref. 60.

Table 5 Microbiological Culture Thresholds for the Diagnosis of VAP

	Endotracheal aspirate	Bronchoalveolar lavage	Protected specimen brush	Plugged telescopic catheter
Quantitative culture threshold (cfu/mL)	10^6	10^4	10^3	10^3

Abbreviation: VAP, ventilator-associated pneumonia.

therapy should be stopped, as diagnosis of VAP is unlikely. In case of negative culture and absence of clinical improvement, other pathogens or diagnoses, such as extrapulmonary site of infection, empyema or noninfectious diseases must be considered.

Shorter duration of antibiotic therapy decreases colonization and superinfection with antibiotic resistant bacteria. If initial antibiotic therapy is appropriate and clinical response is satisfactory, duration of therapy should not exceed eight days (62). In case of complicated course of VAP, particularly with *P. aeruginosa*, the duration of therapy may be extended to14 days.

VIII. Prevention

VAP prevention during ARDS should not differ from general VAP prevention guidelines. Briefly, general hygiene precautions must be applied, including washing hands with alcohol-based solutions. Although sometimes difficult to obtain (63), semirecumbent patient positioning should be applied (64). Oral rinse should be regularly performed with chlorhexidine (65). Stress-ulcer prophylaxis should not be systemically used, recent data indicating that prophylaxis does not influence the clinically significant gastrointestinal bleeding rate in ICU patients (66). In addition, recent data suggest that sucralfate is an independent risk factor for VAP in ARDS patients (5), a finding confirmed in a much wider ICU population (16). The same holds true for proton-pump inhibitors whose use has been recently found to be statistically associated with the risk of acquiring HAP (67). At this stage, it is difficult to define which patients should benefit from stress-ulcer prophylaxis. Considering the latest literature, one could legitimately answer none. This attitude might be excessive, but one has to admit that the benefit of such therapy should be balanced against the risk of nosocomial pneumonia. In the authors' institution, stress ulcer prophylaxis is only given to patients with both severe respiratory failure (namely ARDS) and renal failure. Closed, rather than open, tracheal suctioning systems should be used, perhaps not for their effect on VAP (which is still debated) but certainly because they prevent desaturation and lung derecruitment during tracheal suctioning (68) and also because they reduce the risk of cross contamination with multidrug resistant microorganisms (69). Heat and moisture exchangers should be preferred overheated humidifiers, not because of their putative effect on VAP rates (70) but simply for economical reasons (70,71). However, with significant permissive hypercapnia, heated humidifiers should be used. Recent data suggest that continuous subglottic suctioning is associated with a significant reduction in early-onset VAP in postcardiac surgery patients (72). Encouraging results in terms of early-onset VAP reduction are also seen with new endotracheal tubes with polyurethane cuffs that considerably reduce leakage around the cuff (73,74). Systematic use of these new endotracheal tubes, with subglottic drainage, polyurethane cuff, or a combination, cannot however be recommended, given that VAP episodes during ARDS are mostly late-onset VAP.

In conclusion, VAP is a frequent complication in ARDS patients. Most instances are late-onset episodes, with difficult-to-treat organisms. Although VAP does not seem to influence the already high mortality of these severely ill patients, it has an important impact on morbidity as attested by a very significant attributable increase in the duration of mechanical ventilation.

References

1. Roupie E, Lepage E, Wysocki M, et al. Prevalence, etiologies and outcome of the acute respiratory distress syndrome among hypoxemic ventilated patients. SRLF Collaborative Group on Mechanical Ventilation. Societe de Reanimation de Langue Francaise [see comments]. Intensive Care Med 1999; 25:920–929.

2. Brun-Buisson C, Minelli C, Bertolini G, et al. Epidemiology and outcome of acute lung injury in European intensive care units. Results from the ALIVE study. Intensive Care Med 2004; 30:51–61.

3. Milberg JA, Davis DR, Steinberg KP, et al. Improved survival of patients with acute respiratory distress syndrome (ARDS): 1983–1993. JAMA 1995; 273:306–309.

4. The Acute Respiratory Distress Syndrome Network. Ventilation with lower tidal volumes as compared with traditional tidal volumes for acute lung injury and the acute respiratory distress syndrome. N Engl J Med 2000; 342:1301–1308.

5. Markowicz P, Wolff M, Djedaini K, et al. Multicenter prospective study of ventilator-associated pneumonia during acute respiratory distress syndrome. Incidence, prognosis, and risk factors. ARDS Study Group. Am J Respir Crit Care Med 2000; 161:1942–1948.

6. Andrews CP, Coalson JJ, Smith JD, et al. Diagnosis of nosocomial bacterial pneumonia in acute, diffuse lung injury. Chest 1981; 80:254–258.

7. Bell RC, Coalson JJ, Smith JD, et al. Multiple organ system failure and infection in adult respiratory distress syndrome. Ann Intern Med. 1983; 99:293–298.

8. Seidenfeld JJ, Mullins RC, III, Fowler SR, et al. Bacterial infection and acute lung injury in hamsters. Am Rev Respir Dis 1986; 134:22–26.

9. Luyt CE, Combes A, Deback C, et al. Herpes simplex virus lung infection in patients undergoing prolonged mechanical ventilation. Am J Respir Crit Care Med 2007; 175:935–942.

10. Chastre J, Fagon JY. Ventilator-associated pneumonia. Am J Respir Crit Care Med 2002; 165:867–903.

11. Sutherland KR, Steinberg KP, Maunder RJ, et al. Pulmonary infection during the acute respiratory distress syndrome. Am J Respir Crit Care Med 1995; 152:550–556.

12. Delclaux C, Roupie E, Blot F, et al. Lower respiratory tract colonization and infection during severe acute respiratory distress syndrome: incidence and diagnosis. Am J Respir Crit Care Med 1997; 156:1092–1098.

13. Chastre J, Trouillet JL, Vuagnat A, et al. Nosocomial pneumonia in patients with acute respiratory distress syndrome. Am J Respir Crit Care Med 1998; 157:1165–1172.

14. Meduri GU, Reddy RC, Stanley T, et al. Pneumonia in acute respiratory distress syndrome. A prospective evaluation of bilateral bronchoscopic sampling. Am J Respir Crit Care Med 1998; 158:870–875.

15. Trouillet JL, Chastre J, Vuagnat A, Joly-Guillou ML, et al. Ventilator-associated pneumonia caused by potentially drug-resistant bacteria. Am J Respir Crit Care Med 1998; 157:531–539.

16. Bornstain C, Azoulay E, De Lassence A, et al. Sedation, sucralfate, and antibiotic use are potential means for protection against early-onset ventilator-associated pneumonia. Clin Infect Dis 2004; 38:1401–1408.

17. Johanson WG Jr., Higuchi JH, Woods DE, et al. Dissemination of Pseudomonas aeruginosa during lung infection in hamsters. Role of oxygen-induced lung injury. Am Rev Respir Dis 1985; 132:358–361.

18. Jean D, Rezaiguia-Delclaux S, Delacourt C, et al. Protective effect of endotoxin instillation on subsequent bacteria-induced acute lung injury in rats. Am J Respir Crit Care Med 1998; 158:1702–1708.

19. Pugin J, Dunn-Siegrist I, Dufour J, et al. Cyclic stretch of human lung cells induces an acidification and promotes bacterial growth. Am J Respir Cell Mol Biol 2008; 38:362–370.

20. Dreyfuss D, Saumon G. Ventilator-induced lung injury: lessons from experimental studies. Am J Respir Crit Care Med 1998; 157:294–323.
21. Dreyfuss D, Saumon G. From ventilator-induced lung injury to multiple organ dysfunction? [editorial]. Intensive Care Med 1998; 24:102–104.
22. Dreyfuss D, Ricard J-D, Saumon G. On the Physiologic and Clinical Relevance of Lung-borne Cytokines during Ventilator-induced Lung Injury. Am J Respir Crit Care Med 2003; 167:1467–1471.
23. Slutsky AS, Tremblay LN. Multiple system organ failure. Is mechanical ventilation a contributing factor? Am J Respir Crit Care Med 1998; 157:1721–1725.
24. Verbrugge SJC, Uhlig S, Neggers SJCM, et al. Different ventilation strategies affect lung function but do not increase tumor necrosis factor-α and prostacyclin production in lavaged rat lungs in vivo. Anesthesiology 1999; 91:1834–1843.
25. Ricard JD, Dreyfuss D, Saumon G. Production of inflammatory cytokines in ventilator-induced lung injury: a reappraisal. Am J Respir Crit Care Med 2001; 163:1176–1180.
26. Tremblay L, Valenza F, Ribeiro SP, et al. Injurious ventilatory strategies increase cytokines and c-fos m-RNA expression in an isolated rat lung model. J Clin Invest 1997; 99:944–952.
27. Slutsky AS. Basic science in ventilator-induced lung injury: implications for the bedside. Am J Respir Crit Care Med 2001; 163:599–600.
28. Whitehead TC, Zhang H, Mullen B, et al. Effect of mechanical ventilation on cytokine response to intratracheal lipopolysaccharide. Anesthesiology 2004; 101:52–58.
29. Bouadma L, Schortgen F, Ricard JD, et al. Ventilation strategy affects cytokine release after mesenteric ischemia-reperfusion in rats. Crit Care Med 2004; 32:1563–1569.
30. Bouadma L, Dreyfuss D, Ricard JD, et al. Mechanical ventilation and hemorrhagic shock-resuscitation interact to increase inflammatory cytokine release in rats. Crit Care Med 2007; 35:2601–2606.
31. Nahum A, Hoyt J, Schmitz L, et al. Effect of mechanical ventilation strategy on dissemination of intratracheally instilled Escherichia coli in dogs. Crit Care Med 1997; 25:1733–1743.
32. Verbrugge SJ, Sorm V, van't Veen A, et al. Lung overinflation without positive end-expiratory pressure promotes bacteremia after experimental Klebsiella pneumoniae inoculation. Intensive Care Med 1998; 24:172–177.
33. Schortgen F, Bouadma L, Joly-Guillou ML, et al. Infectious and inflammatory dissemination are affected by ventilation strategy in rats with unilateral pneumonia. Intensive Care Med 2004; 30:693–701.
34. van Kaam AH, Lachmann RA, Herting E, et al. Reducing atelectasis attenuates bacterial growth and translocation in experimental pneumonia. Am J Respir Crit Care Med 2004; 169:1046–1053.
35. Lin CY, Zhang H, Cheng KC, et al. Mechanical ventilation may increase susceptibility to the development of bacteremia. Crit Care Med 2003; 31:1429–1434.
36. Murphy DB, Cregg N, Tremblay L, et al. Adverse ventilatory strategy causes pulmonary-to-systemic translocation of endotoxin. Am J Respir Crit Care Med 2000; 162:27–33.
37. Gillet Y, Issartel B, Vanhems P, et al. Association between Staphylococcus aureus strains carrying gene for Panton-Valentine leukocidin and highly lethal necrotising pneumonia in young immunocompetent patients. Lancet 2002; 359:753–759.
38. Micek ST, Dunne M, Kollef MH. Pleuropulmonary complications of Panton-Valentine leukocidin-positive community-acquired methicillin-resistant Staphylococcus aureus: importance of treatment with antimicrobials inhibiting exotoxin production. Chest 2005; 128:2732–2738.
39. Yahr TL, Goranson J, Frank DW. Exoenzyme S of Pseudomonas aeruginosa is secreted by a type III pathway. Mol Microbiol 1996; 22:991–1003.
40. Hueck CJ. Type III protein secretion systems in bacterial pathogens of animals and plants. Microbiol Mol Biol Rev 1998; 62:379–433.

41. Hauser AR, Kang PJ, Engel JN. PepA, a secreted protein of Pseudomonas aeruginosa, is necessary for cytotoxicity and virulence. Mol Microbiol 1998; 27:807–718.

42. El Solh AA, Akinnusi ME, Wiener-Kronish JP, et al. Persistent infection with Pseudomonas aeruginosa in ventilator-associated pneumonia. Am J Respir Crit Care Med 2008; 178: 513–719.

43. Hauser AR, Cobb E, Bodi M, et al. Type III protein secretion is associated with poor clinical outcomes in patients with ventilator-associated pneumonia caused by Pseudomonas aeruginosa. Crit Care Med 2002; 30:521–528.

44. Song Y, Lynch SV, Flanagan J, et al. Increased plasminogen activator inhibitor-1 concentrations in bronchoalveolar lavage fluids are associated with increased mortality in a cohort of patients with Pseudomonas aeruginosa. Anesthesiology 2007; 106:252–261.

45. Roux D, Gaudry S, Dreyfuss D, El-Benna J, et al. *Candida albicans* impairs macrophage function and facilitates *Pseudomonas aeruginosa* pneumonia in rat. Crit Care Med 2009; 37 (3):1062–1067.

46. Belperio JA, Keane MP, Burdick MD, et al. Critical role for CXCR2 and CXCR2 ligands during the pathogenesis of ventilator-induced lung injury. J Clin Invest 2002; 110:1703–1716.

47. Martin TR. Neutrophils and lung injury: getting it right. J Clin Invest 2002; 110:1603–1605.

48. Jacobs RF, Kiel DP, Balk RA. Alveolar macrophage function in a canine model of endotoxin-induced lung injury. Am Rev Respir Dis 1986; 134:745–751.

49. Munford RS, Pugin J. Normal responses to injury prevent systemic inflammation and can be immunosuppressive. Am J Respir Crit Care Med 2001; 163:316–321.

50. Tate RM, Repine JE. Neutrophils and the adult respiratory distress syndrome. Am Rev Respir Dis 1983; 128:552–559.

51. Martin TR, Pistorese BP, Hudson LD, et al. The function of lung and blood neutrophils in patients with the adult respiratory distress syndrome. Implications for the pathogenesis of lung infections. Am Rev Respir Dis 1991; 144:254–262.

52. Chollet-Martin S, Gatecel C, Kermarrec N, et al. Alveolar neutrophil functions and cytokine levels in patients with the adult respiratory distress syndrome during nitric oxide inhalation. Am J Respir Crit Care Med 1996; 153:985–990.

53. Stephan F, Yang K, Tankovic J, et al. Impairment of polymorphonuclear neutrophil functions precedes nosocomial infections in critically ill patients. Crit Care Med 2002; 30:315–322.

54. Ranieri VM, Giunta F, Suter PM, et al. Mechanical ventilation as a mediator of multisystem organ failure in acute respiratory distress syndrome. JAMA 2000; 284:43–44.

55. Stuber F, Wrigge H, Schroeder S, et al. Kinetic and reversibility of mechanical ventilation-associated pulmonary and systemic inflammatory response in patients with acute lung injury. Intensive Care Med 2002; 28:834–841.

56. Montgomery AB, Stager MA, Carrico CJ, et al. Causes of mortality in patients with the adult respiratory distress syndrome. Am Rev Respir Dis 1985; 132:485–489.

57. Pugin J, Auckenthaler R, Mili N, et al. Diagnosis of ventilator-associated pneumonia by bacteriologic analysis of bronchoscopic and nonbronchoscopic "blind" bronchoalveolar lavage fluid. Am Rev Respir Dis 1991; 143:1121–1129.

58. Fartoukh M, Maitre B, Honore S, et al. Diagnosing pneumonia during mechanical ventilation: the clinical pulmonary infection score revisited. Am J Respir Crit Care Med 2003; 168:173–179.

59. Fagon JY, Chastre J, Wolff M, et al. Invasive and noninvasive strategies for management of suspected ventilator-associated pneumonia. A randomized trial. Ann Intern Med 2000; 132:621–630.

60. Guidelines for the Management of Adults with Hospital-acquired, Ventilator-associated, and Healthcare-associated Pneumonia. Am J Respir Crit Care Med 2005; 171:388–416.

61. Wysocki M, Delatour F, Faurisson F, et al. Continuous versus intermittent infusion of vancomycin in severe Staphylococcal infections: prospective multicenter randomized study. Antimicrob Agents Chemother 2001; 45:2460–2467.

62. Chastre J, Wolff M, Fagon JY, et al. Comparison of 8 vs 15 days of antibiotic therapy for ventilator-associated pneumonia in adults: a randomized trial. JAMA 2003; 290:2588–2598.

63. van Nieuwenhoven CA, Vandenbroucke-Grauls C, van Tiel FH, et al. Feasibility and effects of the semirecumbent position to prevent ventilator-associated pneumonia: a randomized study. Crit Care Med 2006; 34:396–402.

64. Drakulovic MB, Torres A, Bauer TT, et al. Supine body position as a risk factor for nosocomial pneumonia in mechanically ventilated patients: a randomised trial. Lancet 1999; 354:1851–1858.

65. Chan EY, Ruest A, Meade MO, et al. Oral decontamination for prevention of pneumonia in mechanically ventilated adults: systematic review and meta-analysis. BMJ 2007; 334:889.

66. Faisy C, Guerot E, Diehl JL, et al. Clinically significant gastrointestinal bleeding in critically ill patients with and without stress-ulcer prophylaxis. Intensive Care Med 2003; 29:1306–1313.

67. Herzig SJ, Howell MD, Ngo LH, et al. Acid-suppressive medication use and the risk for hospital-acquired pneumonia. JAMA 2009; 301:2120–2128.

68. Maggiore SM, Lellouche F, Pigeot J, et al. Prevention of endotracheal suctioning-induced alveolar derecruitment in acute lung injury. Am J Respir Crit Care Med 2003; 167:1215–1224.

69. Ricard JD, Eveillard M, Martin Y, et al. Closed system tracheal suctioning reduces health care workers hand and equipment contamination. Intensive Care Med 2006; 32:S230 (abstr).

70. Ricard JD, Boyer A, Dreyfuss D. The effect of humidification on the incidence of ventilator-associated pneumonia. Respir Care Clin North Am 2006; 12:263–273.

71. Ricard JD. Gold standard for humidification: heat and moisture exchangers, heated humidifiers, or both? Crit Care Med 2007; 35:2875–2876.

72. Bouza E, Perez MJ, Munoz P, et al. Continuous aspiration of subglottic secretions in the prevention of ventilator-associated pneumonia in the postoperative period of major heart surgery. Chest 2008; 134:938–946.

73. Lorente L, Lecuona M, Jimenez A, et al. Influence of an endotracheal tube with polyurethane cuff and subglottic secretion drainage on pneumonia. Am J Respir Crit Care Med 2007; 176:1079–1083.

74. Poelaert J, Depuydt P, De Wolf A, et al. Polyurethane cuffed endotracheal tubes to prevent early postoperative pneumonia after cardiac surgery: a pilot study. J Thorac Cardiovasc Surg 2008; 135:771–776.

12
Pulmonary Infections in Immunosuppressed Patients

RANA KAPLAN and DOROTHY A. WHITE
Memorial Sloan-Kettering Cancer Center and Weill Medical College of Cornell University, New York, New York, U.S.A.

I. Introduction

The population of immunocompromised hosts (ICH) susceptible to pulmonary infection continues to grow. This is due to prolonged survival of patients with cancer, wider use of solid organ transplants (SOT) and hematologic stem cell transplants (HSCT), and introduction of new, targeted but powerful immunosuppressive agents for hematologic, autoimmune, dermatologic, and renal diseases (1–3). Strategies to reduce infection, including prophylactic agents and nonmyeloablative regimens for HSCT, are being employed, but pneumonia is still common (4). Some infections, such as opportunistic fungal pneumonia, are increasing in frequency, and new pathogens are emerging (5–7). When respiratory failure develops from pneumonia in the ICH, mortality is high (2,8).

Initial signs and symptoms of pneumonia in the ICH can be nonspecific and, in some cases, minimal. Radiographic evaluation with chest computerized tomography (CT) is sensitive for detecting infection at an early stage in some settings, but findings are not commonly pathognomonic of a particular infection. An understanding of the nature of host immune defects and knowledge of the usual presentation of pulmonary infections is helpful for early recognition and treatment. This chapter gives an overview of the typical clinical and radiographic features of common infections in immunosuppressed patients and discusses diagnosis, management, and prophylactic strategies.

II. Definition

Immunosuppressed patients are those with an increased propensity for opportunistic infections, which are infections of low virulence not typically seen in the normal population. Immune defects may be due to underlying disease or treatment given. The chapter emphasizes classic opportunistic infections, but mentions infections that present or are approached differently in the ICH. Discussion of noninfectious etiologies of pulmonary infiltrates is beyond the scope of this chapter and human immune deficiency (HIV)-related infections will be discussed in a separate chapter.

III. Epidemiology and Etiology

The type, severity, and duration of immunologic defects impact the likelihood of developing pneumonia. Knowledge of the immune defects that occur with different diseases and treatments, as well as the organisms associated with infections in these settings, is fundamental to developing an approach in the ICH (Table 1).

Neutropenia, usually defined as an absolute neutrophil count below 1000 cells/mm^3, is commonly encountered in cancer patients. Bacterial and fungal pneumonias are most frequent in neutropenic patients, but other infections, such as viral pneumonia, may be more severe in this setting. Treatment with growth factors can reduce the risk by shortening the period of neutropenia postchemotherapy in many cases. Neutrophil dysfunction also occurs in some congenital immune deficiency syndromes, with a resultant disposition to bacterial and fungal pneumonias.

B-cell dysfunction resulting in low total levels of immunoglobulin, subclass deficiencies or an inability to respond to antigen challenge, leads to susceptibility particularly to encapsulated bacteria that require opsonization for clearance. When immunoglobulin G levels fall below 200 mg/dL, there is a high risk of developing recurrent bacterial infections, especially sinusitis, bronchitis, and pneumonia (9). Defects in cellular immunity, characterized by T-cell dysfunction, are seen in a wide variety of diseases, as well as because of use of corticosteroids and various chemotherapeutic regimens or immunosuppressive agents (3). T cell–mediated immunity is integral to the defense against some bacterial pathogens and a variety of fungi, viruses and parasites. Patients with T-cell defects present a particular challenge when they develop pulmonary infiltrates, because of the wide variety of possible pathogens.

IV. Pathogenesis and Clinical Features
A. Fungal Infections
Aspergillus

The incidence of invasive fungal infections has increased dramatically over the past two decades (6,10). Diagnosis and treatment remain challenging. The most common opportunistic fungus to cause pneumonia remains *Aspergillus*, which is a ubiquitous filamentous fungus found in soil, water, and decaying matter. Spores are found in unfiltered air and conidia enter the lungs by inhalation. They can colonize the airways, especially in the presence of structural lung disease. Hyphae form with germination and are characteristically acutely branched and septate (Fig. 1). Host defense against aspergillosis depends on alveolar macrophages that ingest conidia and neutrophils that attack and ingest hyphae. More recently, T-lymphocytes have also been recognized as having protective immunity against the fungus (11). *Aspergillus fumigatus* spp. accounts for up to 70% of cases of infection in humans, followed by *A. flavus* and *A. terreus* (12,13).

Invasive *Aspergillus* infection in immunosuppressed patients is most commonly pulmonary, but disseminated disease also occurs. Patients at highest risk are those with hematologic malignancies, particularly during periods of neutropenia. In addition, SOT and HSCT recipients and those receiving high doses of steroids are at risk. A recent large, multicenter prospective study in the United States showed a cumulative incidence of *Aspergillus* infection of 3% after allogeneic HSCT and 2.4% after lung transplantation (14). This is lower than in prior reports, possibly reflecting changes in

Table 1 Defects in Host Defense, Associated Immunodeficiency and Pathogens

Type of immune defect	Disease or condition	Common associated organisms

Neutrophil dysfunction	Cytotoxic chemotherapy
	Leukemia
	Aplastic anemia
	Myelofibrosis
	HIV infection
	Chédiak–Higashi syndrome
	Chronic granulomatous disease
	Job's syndrome
	Malnutrition
		Bacteria
		  Staphylococcus spp.
		  Streptococcus spp.
		  Enterococci
		  Pseudomonas aeruginosa
		  Klebsiella pneumoniae
		  Haemophilus influenzae
		  Enterobacteriaceae
		
		Fungi
		  Aspergillus spp.
		  Zygomycetes
		  Candida spp.
		  Fusarium spp.
		  Trichosporon beigelii

Humoral immune dysfunction (B-cell mediated)	Splenectomy
	Chronic lymphocytic leukemia
	Non-Hodgkin's lymphoma
	Multiple myeloma
	Dysglobulinemia
	Agammaglobulinemia
		Bacteria
		  Streptococcus pneumoniae
		  Haemophilus influenzae
		  Moraxella catarrhalis
		  Neisseria meningitidis
		  Klebsiella pneumoniae
		  Escherichia coli
		  Mycoplasma pneumoniae
		Fungi
		  Pneumocystis jiroveci

Cellular immune dysfunction (T-cell mediated)	AIDS
	Hodgkin's disease
	T-cell lymphoma
	T-cell depleting drugs
	Thymic aplasia or hypoplasia
	Mucocutaneous candidiasis
	DiGeorge syndrome
	Severe combined
	  immunodeficiency
		Bacteria
		  Legionella pneumophila
		  Nocardia spp.
		  Rhodococcus equi
		  Mycobacterium spp.
		  Listeria monocytogenes
		Fungi
		  Candida spp.
		  Cryptococcus neoformans
		  Aspergillus spp.
		  Pneumocystis jiroveci
		  Coccidioides immitis
		  Histoplasma capsulatum
		Viruses
		  Cytomegalovirus
		  Herpes simplex virus
		  Influenza virus
		  Adenovirus
		  Varicella-zoster virus
		  Respiratory syncytial virus
		Parasites
		  Toxoplasma gondii
		  Strongyloides stercoralis

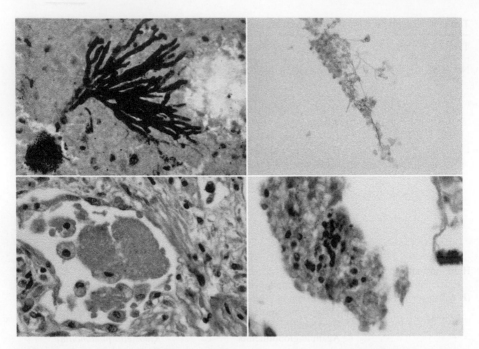

Figure 1   (*See color insert*) Pathology of opportunistic infections. (*Top left*) Hyphae of *Aspergillus* spp. are seen with GMS stain and are septate, with dichotomous branching at 45° angles. (*Top right*) *Nocardia* spp. is seen as long, delicate filaments that can easily be overlooked. (*Bottom left*) *P. jiroveci* infection typically has a frothy eosinophilic intra-alveolar exudate filling acini. (*Bottom right*) Cysts of *Pneumocystis* are seen with GMS and have a delicate capsular wall with variable shapes, including collapsed forms. *Abbreviation*: GMS, Gomori methenamine silver.

transplantation practice. It still remains a disease of high morbidity and mortality. In SOT recipients, most infections occur within the first six months after transplantation. With HSCT recipients, there is an early incidence in the preengraftment phase for both allogeneic and autologous transplants and a later occurrence as well, at approximately 100 days in allogeneic transplants. An increasing frequency of invasive pulmonary aspergillosis outside of the period of neutropenia has been noted, and risk factors are graft-versus-host disease (GVHD), cytomegalovirus (CMV) disease, or use of high doses of corticosteroids (15).

Presenting symptoms include fever, chest pain, dyspnea, cough, and/or hemoptysis. Their frequency is variable and some patients have minimal or no complaints. In one study in allogeneic HSCT, 64% of infected patients had dyspnea and 32% were febrile (16). Another study of both neutropenic and nonneutropenic patients with invasive aspergillosis found fever was present in 85% of cases, dyspnea in 65%, cough in 51%, chest pain in 24%, and hemoptysis in 7% (17). Nonneutropenic patients, compared with those with neutropenia, were less likely to have symptoms. Hemoptysis can occasionally be severe because of the angioinvasive nature of the fungus. The physical examination of the chest is frequently normal. Chest radiographs are not

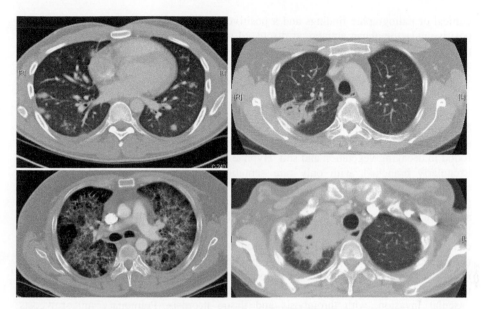

Figure 2 Radiographic manifestations of opportunistic infections. (*Top left*) Multiple nodular densities and areas of consolidation in this patient with leukemia are highly suggestive of invasive pulmonary aspergillosis. (*Top right*) Focal mass with cavitation is also a common presentation of *Aspergillus*, as occurred in a patient with a brain tumor on high doses of corticosteroids. (*Bottom left*) Interstitial infiltrates are commonly observed on chest radiograph with *P. jiroveci*, while the CT scan characteristically shows patchy areas of ground glass consolidation. (*Bottom right*) A cavitary lung mass as seen in the lung apex in this patient postallogencic stem cell transplant is a common presentation of *Nocardia*.

adequate for diagnosis of aspergillosis in ICH and chest CT should be used. Typical radiographic features are single or multiple nodular densities, wedge-shaped peripheral infiltrates (suggestive of an infarct) or a cavitary lesion(s) (Fig. 2). The "halo sign," which is an area of ground glass attenuation surrounding nodules or mass-like infiltrates reflecting bleeding, is highly suggestive of a mold infection, usually aspergillosis (18). A rounded mass within a cavity, with air around the mass ("the air crescent sign") may develop on CT chest, but is a late finding and usually occurs as neutropenia resolves (19).

Aspergillus tracheobronchitis occasionally occurs as a sole process or in association with invasive pulmonary aspergillosis. It is characterized by the presence of *Aspergillus* organisms in the airway mucosa deep to the basement membrane, with tracheobronchial ulceration, pseudomembranes, or plugs of necrotic debris and fungal elements. Radiographs may be normal, but atelectasis may occur due to proximal airway obstruction. Tracheal or bronchial wall thickening may be seen on CT chest. Although uncommon in most ICH, this phenomenon occurs in approximately 5% of lung transplant recipients with local invasion at the site of anastomosis (20).

The diagnosis of invasive pulmonary aspergillosis is frequently empiric in neutropenic patients. Criteria for definite diagnosis requires demonstration of the fungus in tissue, but a probable diagnosis is often made in a high-risk setting with characteristic clinical or radiographic findings and a positive respiratory culture for *Aspergillus* or a positive galactomannan antigen, as discussed under diagnosis (21). Mortality in HSCT patients is high, with only a 20% one-year survival rate (22). Risk factors for mortality are persistent and severe neutropenia, central nervous system involvement, uncontrolled GVHD, elevated creatinine, bilirubin, and fungal load (22,23).

Mucorales

Mucormycosis is caused by fungi of the group of Zygomycetes of the order Mucorales, and include *Mucor*, *Rhizopus*, *Cunninghamella*, and *Absidia*. Spores are ubiquitous and found in decaying vegetation and soil. Hyphae of *Mucor* are distinctive; they are broad, irregularly branched, with only rare septations, and can be morphologically distinguished from *Aspergillus* spp. Pulmonary infections are most likely to occur in patients with hematologic malignancy, particularly if neutropenic or post-HSCT, but are also seen in those with diabetes mellitus, renal failure, and in the setting of iron overload. Pulmonary infections due to Zygomycetes appear to be increasing in frequency in cancer patients, in part related to breakthrough infections in patients with hematologic malignancy while on voriconazole prophylaxis (24–26). These fungi have innate resistance to voriconazole. *Mucor* causes infection in the sinuses, central nervous system, skin, and gastrointestinal tract, as well as in the lungs, and has a propensity for vascular invasion, with thrombosis and tissue necrosis. Pulmonary mucormycosis presents as an acute rapidly progressive pneumonia, with fever, cough, and pleuritic chest pain being the most common symptoms; hemoptysis may occur. Radiographically, infiltrates or nodular mass lesions, with subsequent cavitation, and pleural effusions are seen (27). One study showed that the presence of concomitant sinusitis, more than 10 pulmonary nodules, pleural effusions, and prior use of voriconazole were independent predictors of presence of Zygomycetes rather than *Aspergillus* spp. (28). The mortality rate is high, ranging 70% to 90% in those with hematologic malignancy (24,29), and treatment involves both antifungal therapy and surgical debridement, if possible.

Other Opportunistic Fungi

Other emerging fungi include *Fusarium*, *Scedospium* spp., *and Trichosporon* (10). Mucocutaneous disease with *Candida* species is very common in ICH, but pneumonia due to *Candida* is rare, even in the setting of severe neutropenia (30). Hematogenous seeding of the lungs during fungemia can occur and can be with nonalbicans species, particularly with use of prophylactic antifungal agents.

Cryptococcus

Cryptococcus neoformans is encapsulated yeast that is found worldwide. Following inhalation, the organism grows and produces a carbohydrate capsule and a cell-mediated response, with a granulomatous reaction developing in some patients (31). Approximately 50% of cases occur in patients with defects in cell-mediated immunity, particularly those on corticosteroids or with chronic lymphocytic leukemia, chronic myelogenous leukemia, Hodgkin's disease, and post-SOT (31–33). *Cryptococcus* has a predilection for the central nervous system (CNS), with minimal fungemia potentially leading to either meningitis or disseminated disease. Most patients with cryptococcal pneumonia are asymptomatic, but fever, cough, chest pain, or malaise may develop.

Radiographic findings are usually a localized, discrete infiltrate or mass, which may enlarge, mimicking malignancy (34). Single or multiple nodules, miliary infiltrates, pleural effusions, and mediastinal lymphadenopathy may also be seen. Diagnosis can be made by finding classic encapsulated yeast forms in sputum, bronchoalveolar lavage (BAL), or lung tissue. Cryptococcal antigen is elevated in many, but not all cases of pneumonia. In the ICH, involvement of the CNS needs to be excluded.

Endemic fungi

Histoplasma capsulatum and *Coccidioides immitis* are endemic fungi with specific geographic distributions. Initial presentation may be similar to that seen in normal hosts, but ICH are at increased risk for more severe disease and dissemination of primary infection, as well as reactivation of prior disease (35–37). Patients with leukemia or lymphoma, transplant recipients, or patients receiving corticosteroids have been considered at highest risk, but recently, studies have reported the infection more commonly in those with solid tumors where lymphopenia is identified as the major risk factor (37). With histoplasmosis in the ICH, radiographic abnormalities are more commonly subcentimeter nodular opacities or linear opacities in a diffuse distribution (38). Focal airspace opacities, pleural effusions, and adenopathy are less common. With coccidioidomycosis, lobar airspace, nodular airspace, reticular interstitial, and miliary interstitial opacities can be seen (39).

Pneumocystis jiroveci

Pneumocystis jiroveci, formerly known as *Pneumocystis carinii*, is a fungal pathogen that causes pneumonia in the ICH, mainly by reactivation of infection, though aerosol transmission of infection may also occur. B- and T-cell functions are important for host defense, but intact cellular immunity is most protective. In HIV infection, circulating CD4+ T-lymphocyte counts less than $200/mm^3$ predict a risk threshold for infection. The level of T cells predisposing to infection is less well defined in non-HIV infected patients. One study showed that CD4 counts less than $300/mm^3$ were present in only 52% of cases of *Pneumocystis* in the non-HIV population (40).

Pneumocystis pneumonia is seen in patients with hematologic malignancies, transplant recipients, and in those with autoimmune and inflammatory diseases. It is less likely with solid tumors, but can occur with use of high doses of corticosteroids (41,42). Prophylaxis during high-risk periods in the six months posttransplantation has markedly reduced the incidence in these populations. Use of corticosteroids is commonly associated with development of this infection in the non-HIV population, being received by approximately 90% of patients within one month of diagnosis in one study; the median daily dose of corticosteroids was equivalent to 30 mg of prednisone (43). Another study in cancer patients with *Pneumocystis* found steroids being used in all solid tumor patients and in 45.5% of those with hematologic malignancy (41). *Pneumocystis* has been noted to occur in some patients at the time of tapering of corticosteroid therapy or immunosuppressive therapy (44). Other drugs associated with development of *Pneumocystis* are alemtuzamab, tumor necrosis factor alpha (TNFα) inhibitors (infliximab, etanercept, and adalimumab), and fludarabine (3,45).

Dyspnea, nonproductive cough, and fever are the most common clinical symptoms, and presentation is more fulminant than in HIV patients, with the average interval between symptom onset and diagnosis in non-HIV patients ranging from 5 to 14 days (40,46). The physical exam is often normal, but hypoxemia, which worsens with exercise, is a characteristic finding (47). Radiographs may initially be normal, but the typical appearance is bilateral perihilar symmetric interstitial infiltrates that often progress to fluffy alveolar infiltrates. Solitary and multiple nodules, a miliary pattern, lobar consolidation, thin-walled cysts, cavitary lesions, and pneumothorax have also been described. Pleural effusions and adenopathy are uncommon (48). Findings on high-resolution CT show diffuse or patchy ground glass opacities in a high percentage of cases (Fig. 2) (41). As the organism cannot be cultured, the diagnosis is made by finding the frothy, eosinophilic intra-alveolar exudate filling acini with characteristic troph-ozoite or cyst forms that can be identified by special stains on induced sputum, BAL or lung biopsy (Fig. 1). Stains used are toluidine blue, direct fluorescent antibody, Gomori methenamine silver (GMS) stains, Giemsa, or Giemsa-like rapid stains. Several poly-merase chain reaction (PCR) assays are available and have been more sensitive, but less specific (49). Lung biopsies in non-HIV ICH, compared with HIV-infected patients, show decreased number of organisms, but increased number of neutrophils. Disease is more severe in the non-HIV- versus HIV-infected patients and may progress to respi-ratory failure. Mortality of 35% to 50% is reported (50,51). Use of noninvasive venti-lation has been associated with a high failure rate in this population (51). Identification and prophylaxis of high-risk patients are essential.

B. Bacterial Pneumonia

Pyogenic bacterial pneumonia with gram-positive and gram-negative bacteria is a common cause of pneumonia, particularly in settings of neutropenia, hypo-gammaglobulinemia, or following SOT or HSCT (52,53). It can be community or nosocomially acquired. In one review of 40 neutropenic patients with bacterial pneu-monia and bacteremia, *Pseudomonas aeruginosa* and *Streptococcus pneumoniae* accounted for 72.5% of cases (54). More recently, *Staphylococcus aureus* has also emerged as a pathogen on the rise in neutropenic patients, at least, in part attributable to the widespread use of broad-spectrum antibiotics in this population. Neutropenic pneumonia may present only with fever, and respiratory signs and symptoms can be minimal or absent. Radiographic abnormalities may be subtle because of lack of neu-trophils, but CT imaging is more sensitive (55). It has been noted that infiltrates may become more prominent during the return of the white blood cell count due to an immune reconstitution syndrome.

Legionella spp. are small gram-negative aerobic bacilli that are facultative intra-cellular pathogens. Freshwater sources such as water heaters, air-conditioning units, humidifiers, and nebulizers with contaminated water are potential reservoirs for *Legionella*. Most cases of legionellosis in the ICH are nosocomial. *Legionella pneumophila* is the most common species causing human diseases, particularly serotypes 1, 4, and 5. Other species, including *L. micdadei* and *L. bozemanii*, are also seen. Pneumonia with *Legionella* spp. is common in the general population, but occurs at a higher rate in a setting of defects in cell-mediated immunity (particularly in SOT and HSCT), hairy cell leukemia, or in patients on corticosteroids (56–58). Some SOT centers report that up to 30% of community-acquired and nosocomial pneumonias are due to *Legionella* (59).

The clinical presentation varies from a mild febrile illness to progressive severe pneumonia with respiratory failure and extrapulmonary manifestations, including gastrointestinal symptoms, renal insufficiency, cardiac or pericardial disease, and mental status changes. Fever is present in 90% of patients, with or without respiratory symptoms. One study of Legionnaires' disease in ICH showed fever and malaise in all, with 66% having cough, and 38% hemoptysis (60). Physical exam reveals crackles, and relative bradycardia may be seen in up to 50% of cases. Chest radiographs typically demonstrate alveolar infiltrates that are often unilateral in the lower lobes, but may be segmental, lobar, patchy, diffuse, or appear as a poorly differentiated mass-like opacity. Involvement of other lobes and pleural effusion are common. Cavitation can occur in ICH, with most of the cavities eventually resolving over several months (61). Hyponatremia may also be present. Diagnosis is made both by culture of sputum or other respiratory specimens on selective media and can take several days. Urinary antigen is also helpful for *L. pneumophila* type 1 infection that accounts for a high percentage of community-acquired cases; there is a lower incidence of this species in the ICH (62). The outcome is generally good, if treatment is started early, but one study reported a mortality rate of 31% in cancer patients, with 37% patients requiring prolonged treatment (57,63).

Nocardia spp. belong to the genus *Actinomycetes* and are gram-positive aerobic bacilli that appear as delicate, branching filamentous gram-positive rods on Gram stain (Fig. 1). They are also weakly acid-fast positive. Infection is rare and occurs from inhalation of the organism from the soil and from decaying organic matter, resulting in pneumonia and possible dissemination to the CNS, skin, and subcutaneous tissue (64). Pulmonary involvement occurs in 65% to 85% of cases and may be a pyogenic or granulomatous pneumonia. *Nocardia asteroides* accounts for more than 80% of pulmonary infections that occur predominantly in the ICH with impaired cellular immunity or in individuals on steroids. In SOT, the frequency of infection is 0.7% to 3%, and risk factors include high-dose steroids, history of CMV disease, and high levels of calcineurin inhibitors (65). Presentation can be subacute or chronic with fever, weight loss, and malaise. Cough, dyspnea, chest pain, and hemoptysis have also been reported, although some patients have no respiratory symptoms (65). Chest radiographic studies most commonly show nodules and masses with cavitation in 25% of cases (Fig. 2). Bronchopneumonia and reticulonodular infiltrates occur less commonly. Pleural effusions can be seen in approximately one-third of cases, and adenopathy may be present (66). Diagnosis is made by finding the characteristic organisms in respiratory specimens on direct examination or by culture. The laboratory must be alerted to hold the specimens for 21 days, because cultures may not grow in the typical seven-day culture period. Sputum specimens are positive in only 30% to 40% of cases and, often, invasive procedures are needed to make the diagnosis.

C. Mycobacterial Infections

Cancer patients, particularly those receiving corticosteroid therapy, or with lung cancer, head and neck cancer, lymphoproliferative disorders, and acute leukemia, have an increased risk of developing tuberculosis (67,68). Reactivation is believed to be the main mechanism. In the SOT population, infections typically occur a median of nine months posttransplantation, and most occur within the first year. In one study in this population, approximately half had pulmonary disease, 16% extrapulmonary infection, and one-third had disseminated disease (69). Symptoms are often fever and cough. Chest radiographs show focal infiltrates, a miliary pattern, pleural effusions, diffuse interstitial infiltrates, and cavitary lung disease (68,69).

Lung disease due to nontuberculous mycobacteria (NTM) is increasingly being encountered in immunosuppressed patients, in some cases with dissemination, as well as pneumonia (70,71). Studies indicate that the incidence of NTM in individuals having undergone HSCT ranges from 0.4% to 4.9% (71,72). In SOT recipients, pleuropulmonary disease is most often seen in lung and heart transplants (70). *Mycobacterium avium* is most often associated with pulmonary disease, but *M. kansasii, M. abscessus, M. asiatica* and *M. fortuitum* also are seen (73). Clinical symptoms of NTM lung disease are nonspecific, but patients may experience a chronic or recurring cough. Other manifestations can be fever, malaise, dyspnea, fatigue, chest pain, and weight loss. Radiographic findings include single or multiple pulmonary nodules or masses, thin-walled cavities, pleural involvement, intrathoracic lymphadenopathy, and alveolar infiltrates that may cavitate (70,71).

D. Viral Infections

Community-Acquired Viral Pneumonia

Respiratory viruses are being increasingly detected as a cause of pneumonia (74). The most common viruses are *respiratory syncytial virus* (RSV), *influenza* (A and B), and *parainfluenza virus. Adenovirus* is less frequent, but can cause significant morbidity. Infections occur at the time of community outbreaks, with most cases of RSV and *influenza* occurring in late fall, winter, and spring, while *parainfluenza* and *adenovirus* infections occur year round. Compared with the normal population, infections in ICH tend to be nosocomial, have longer period of viral shedding and a higher incidence of lower respiratory tract involvement (75–77). The prolonged viral shedding without symptoms contributes to the occurrence of nosocomial transmission in the ICH.

RSV presents with upper respiratory symptoms of nasal congestion and rhinitis, as well as pharyngitis, cough, and fever. Wheezing due to the development of bronchiolitis is common. This is a helpful diagnostic finding, since many opportunistic infections, such as *P. jiroveci* and other fungal infections, typically have a normal chest examination. With pneumonia, bilateral infiltrates on chest radiographs are typically seen (78). Morbidity and mortality are associated with progression to pneumonia, which is related to the level of immunosuppression. With RSV infection, pneumonia can develop in 50% of neutropenic leukemic patients and in up to 80% of HSCT recipients early after transplantation. Respiratory failure and death has been reported in two-thirds of severely compromised patients (78–81). Prognosis is much better with lesser degrees of compromise.

Parainfluenza virus causes pulmonary infection predominantly in the transplant populations. From 1.6% to 11.9% of lung transplant recipients have *parainfluenza virus* recovered during routine frequent bronchoscopies, some without symptoms, but others with lower tract infection (82). Cough is the hallmark of infection, and other upper respiratory tract infection symptoms may be absent. Fever is uncommon. Progression to pneumonia varies, but has been reported from 18% to 77% in HSCT (79). There is a significant incidence of coinfection with bacterial or fungal pathogens.

Primary influenza pneumonia predominantly affects those who have undergone allogeneic bone marrow transplantation and SOT (83,84). Symptoms of fever, headache, myalgias, malaise, and cough during an outbreak should suggest influenza infection. Severity of infection is related in part to level of immunosuppression, but prognosis tends to be good. Bacterial pneumonia due to superinfection with *S. aureus* and *S. pneumoniae* is the most common cause of death among influenza patients.

Adenovirus pneumonitis is associated with high mortality in immunocompromised patients, occurring predominantly in SOT or HSCT recipients (85). It may occur as a primary infection or can be reactivated. The most common clinical findings include upper respiratory tract infection, enteritis, hemorrhagic cystitis, and pneumonia. Dissemination can occur even without respiratory tract infection and is associated with high mortality (86).

Human metapneumovirus is a newly discovered ribonucleic acid (RNA) para-myxovirus that can cause both upper and lower respiratory tract infections. More than 70% of individuals harbor antibodies against the virus (87). It has been linked to respiratory failure in HSCT recipients and to idiopathic pneumonia syndrome (5).

Herpesviruses

CMV infection generally occurs in patients following HSCT (10–30%), lung and heart lung transplantation and, rarely, in other ICH (1,88). The virus remains latent following primary infection, and reactivation occurs in the setting of immunosuppression. In HSCT, the median time to occurrence in the preprophylactic period was 44 days, but onset is substantially delayed to more than 100 days with prophylaxis (89). The risk of developing CMV pneumonia is increased by initial seropositive status before trans-plantation, older age, T cell–depleted grafts, or viremia. There is a bimodal distribution with both early and late cases. The highest mortality is seen in seronegative recipients with seropositive grafts (88). In autologous transplants, pneumonia is less common and less severe. In SOT, CMV pneumonia usually occurs in the first three months post-transplantation. The frequency of CMV pneumonia in the transplant populations has been decreased by use of universal prophylaxis for a period of time after engraftment, as well as screening for subclinical viremia using the highly sensitive pp65 antigenemia or PCR assay, with initiation of preemptive therapy if early infection is found (90–93). Diagnosis of CMV pneumonia in the setting of infection requires finding characteristic intranuclear inclusion in epithelial cells, but, often, recovery of the virus or an elevated antigen in the appropriate setting is considered presumptive evidence.

Signs and symptoms of CMV pneumonitis include fever, dyspnea, nonproductive cough, and hypoxemia. Pleurisy is not uncommon. CT most commonly shows patchy or diffuse ground glass attenuation, but focal consolidations, reticular opacities, thickened interlobular septa, and tree-in-bud abnormalities can also be seen. The pattern of diffuse abnormalities with progression to consolidation during treatment has been associated with a poor outcome (94). Mortality is improved using methods for early detection. Significant indirect effects of CMV infection include acute and chronic graft rejection, GVHD, and superinfection with bacteria and fungi.

Herpes simplex virus (HSV) infection causes pneumonia in ICH due to aspiration of organisms from the oropharynx, extension of herpetic tracheobronchitis or hema-togenous dissemination. The incidence has decreased with the widespread use of pro-phylaxis. Pulmonary manifestations include tracheitis, tracheobronchitis, and pneumonia. Wheezing is occasionally heard and herpetic lesions may be detected in the oropharynx. Radiographic findings are most often focal infiltration, but may be diffuse in the setting of hematogenous dissemination (95). The diagnosis of HSV pneumonia usually requires tissue confirmation, and coinfection with other pathogens is not rare. Pneumonia due to varicella infection is fulminant and potentially life threatening. It usually manifests a few days after the onset of the rash and presents with cough, dyspnea, fever, and, occasionally, pleuritic chest pain. Chest radiographs reveal either focal or diffuse nodular infiltrates. *Human herpesvirus* 6 (HHV-6) has been isolated from the respiratory tract of bone marrow transplant recipients with interstitial pneumonitis and high levels of HHV-6 have been found by PCR in lung biopsies in these patients (96,97).

E. Parasites

Strongyloides stercoralis is an intestinal nematode endemic to tropical and subtropical countries, in the Caribbean, Central America, Central Africa, as well as the southeastern United States. The infection is now rare in the United States, with only one infection found per 1000 patients at a major cancer center (98). Initial infection is through the skin, followed by migration to the lung, where transient eosinophilic infiltrates can occur. The larvae are swallowed and reside in the duodenum and jejunum, where the burden of worms can increase with autoinfection. Waxing and waning gastrointestinal, cutaneous, and pulmonary symptoms with eosinophilia are common. Hyperinfection syndrome is rare, but occurs when the larvae penetrate the intestinal wall into the bloodstream associated with widespread dissemination of the parasite, often associated with polymicrobial sepsis. Hyperinfection can occur with cellular immune dysfunction (98,99). Manifestations include fever, wheezing, and respiratory failure. Chest radiographs show infiltrates with foci of hemorrhage, pneumonitis, and edema. Eosinophilia is usually not present. There is a high mortality with pulmonary hyperinfection syndrome, in spite of treatment. Stool examinations or analysis of duodenojejunal aspirates by a string test can be helpful in detecting latent or gastrointestinal infection and should be performed before immunosuppression in any patient with unexplained eosinophilia.

Toxoplasmosis is caused by the intracellular protozoan parasite *Toxoplasma gondii*. The organism may be acquired by vertical transmission from the mother, blood transfusion, organ transplant, or ingesting oocysts from soil contaminated by feline feces. Reactivation of latent infection has been reported in those with HSCT or HIV infection and, rarely, in patients with malignancy, such as Hodgkin's disease, lymphoma and leukemia (100). *T. gondii* seropositivity, a low CD4 count of less than 200 cells/mm^3, fever, and GVHD have been associated with toxoplasmosis during immunosuppressive therapy (100,101). Disseminated disease can also result from new acquisition of the parasite while the patient is immunosuppressed. Toxoplasmosis most commonly presents with neurologic symptoms, such as altered consciousness, motor deficits, seizures, or focal findings on neurologic examination. Myocarditis or retinal involvement may occur (102). *Toxoplasma* pneumonia is manifest by fever, dyspnea, and cough (102). Chest radiographs demonstrate diffuse interstitial disease or patchy infiltrates. Mortality can be high unless it is recognized early, with mortality rates over 90% observed in HSCT patients (103). Monitoring for presence of *T. gondii* DNA by PCR has been helpful in detecting early infection in some cases (101).

V. Diagnostic Approach

The diagnostic approach to evaluation of pulmonary infiltrates in ICH requires the assessment of several factors. The first is assessing the risk profile for the patient, which includes types of immune defects present based on the disease process and treatment given, any community or nosocomial exposures to specific organisms, and prophylactic therapy given. The temporal relationship between pneumonia and the initiation of

Table 2 Common Radiographic Patterns and Presentations of Pulmonary Infections in the ICH

Organisms	Patterns	Presentation
Legionella spp.	Focal/lobar infiltrates Cavitary infiltrates	Acute to subacute
Nocardia spp.	Cavitary or nodular infiltrates	Subacute to chronic
Mycobacteria	Focal infiltrates, cavitary or diffuse interstitial infiltrates	Subacute to chronic
Pyogenic bacteria	Focal/segmental/lobar infiltrates	Acute
Aspergillus	Nodules or nodular infiltrates	Subacute
Mucor	Focal infiltrate/nodules/mass	Acute
Cryptococcus	Focal infiltrate/nodules/mass	Chronic
Pneumocystis jiroveci	Diffuse interstitial	Acute to subacute
CMV	Focal or diffuse infiltrates	Subacute to chronic
RSV	Focal or diffuse infiltrates	Acute
Strongyloides (hyperinfection)	Diffuse infiltrates	Acute
Toxoplasmosis	Diffuse infiltrates	Acute

Abbreviations: ICH, immunocompromised hosts; CMV, *cytomegalovirus*; RSV, *respiratory syncytial virus*.

immunosuppression can be important. In the time period post-HSCT before engraftment, bacterial and fungal pneumonia is common, whereas CMV and *Pneumocystis* tend to be seen in weeks to months following engraftment. The duration of neutropenia is a significant risk factor for *Aspergillus* infection. The rate of onset and progression of symptoms may also be helpful in suggesting diagnostic possibilities, with some infections following a rapid course and others with a subacute or chronic presentation (Table 2). Multiple infections may be present simultaneously, for example, viral and bacterial pneumonia; in addition, many noninfectious etiologies can simulate infections.

A. Noninvasive Diagnostic Tests
Chest Radiography/CT Scans
Chest radiography may be normal in up to 10% of ICH with proven pulmonary disease (104), in part related to a poor inflammatory response. CT is a much more sensitive and specific tool than radiography and is the test of choice when a suspicion of pneumonia exists or in the ICH with unexplained fever. The CT pattern in association with concomitant clinical factors can suggest the diagnosis (Table 2). Cavitary or nodular lesions raise the possibility of *Aspergillus*, *Nocardia*, *Cryptococcus*, mycobacteria, or some pyogenic bacterial infections. Diffuse infiltrates are more common with *Pneumocystis*, CMV, community-acquired viruses, as well noninfectious entities, such as drug toxicity or alveolar hemorrhage.

Nasopharyngeal Swabs or Washes
These are useful for the detection of community acquired viral pathogens such as *influenza, parainfluenza, adenovirus*, and RSV. In addition to culture, rapid assay on these specimens with antigen-capture technology or PCR can give an early answer, allowing appropriate therapy and isolation procedures. Although some reports initially

indicated a lower yield of nasopharyngeal specimens in the ICH compared with normal hosts (105), a recent study found PCR on nasopharyngeal washes or swabs identified 95% of respiratory viruses in ICH (106).

Sputum Analysis

In addition to detection of pyogenic bacteria and mycobacteria, sputum analysis is helpful in identifying some cases of *Legionella*, *Cryptococcus*, and *Nocardia*. Induced sputum using hypertonic saline is useful for identification of *Pneumocystis* and *M. tuberculosis*. The highest diagnostic yield of sputum for *Pneumocystis* is reported in HIV patients, and the sensitivity in non-HIV patients has been variable at different institutions, ranging from 40% to 79% (48,107,108). The significance of sputum cultures may be difficult to interpret with some organisms. For example, *Aspergillus* spp. recovery does not always correlate with disease. The positive predictive value of recovery of *Aspergillus* in respiratory secretions representing invasive disease following HSCT is as high as 80% to 90%, but is lower in other settings (13,109). The recovery of NTM in sputum must also be assessed for clinical significance.

Serologic Markers

Galactomannan (GM) is an *Aspergillus*-specific antigen released by invading hyphae detected by enzyme immunoassay. Using a cutoff index of 0.5 ng/mL, GM has a specificity of greater than 85% for invasive aspergillosis when used for serial screening in high-risk groups (110). Recent studies in a variety of clinical settings found a range of 29% to 100%, with highest sensitivities in neutropenic patients and lower sensitivities in patients with low probability of aspergillosis or prior antifungal treatment (111). False-positive tests in serum may occur with concomitant use of piperacillin-tazobactam and amoxicillin-clavulanate (112,113). GM may also be used to monitor response to therapy, with a decreasing level associated with a good prognosis (114,115). Though still investigational, incorporation of the GM in BAL fluid analysis, in addition to standard cultures and cytology, has improved identification of *Aspergillus* species in BAL fluid (116).

$(1 \rightarrow 3)$-β-D-glucans is a panfungal antigen that may be useful for detecting *Aspergillus* spp. and *Pneumocystis*, but is not useful for Zygomycetes. Detection of *Cryptococcus* is variable (117). In one retrospective review evaluating the performance of $(1 \rightarrow 3)$-β-D-glucans assay for the diagnosis of invasive fungal infections, the assay had a sensitivity of 77.8% and yielded a positive result in 68% of patients with documented invasive pulmonary aspergillosis, 85.2% of patients with fungemia, and in 100% of patients with *P. jiroveci* pneumonia (118). Further studies are needed to determine the future role of this test in the diagnosis of invasive fungal infections.

Cryptococcal antigen can be detected in serum, cerebrospinal fluid (CSF) and pleural effusions. It is usually present in disseminated disease, but may not be found with pneumonia alone. If positive, it can be useful for both diagnosis and disease monitoring.

The pp65 CMV antigen in peripheral blood leukocytes and quantitative PCR of viral DNA/RNA for CMV in serum have sensitivity and specificity for the diagnosis of active infection of more than 80% and can diagnose early infection (119). The urinary antigen test for *Legionella* can rapidly detect antigens of the *L. pneumophila* serogroup 1 with a sensitivity of 70% and a specificity of 100% and can remain positive for weeks (120). Many cases in ICH are not due to this serotype, so a negative test can be seen in *Legionella* pneumonia. PCR is the primary diagnostic tool for toxoplasmosis post-HSCT. It can be used in blood, BAL, and ocular samples. The *B1* gene is commonly amplified to detect the parasite, but other genes are under study (100). It is most commonly performed in the setting of undiagnosed pulmonary or neurologic infection in the ICH and occasionally for surveillance in high-risk seropositive patients post-HSCT.

B. Invasive Diagnostic Tests
Diagnostic Bronchoscopy
Fiberoptic bronchoscopy with BAL and transbronchial biopsy (TBBX) are frequently used to evaluate pulmonary infiltrates in the ICH. In a review of 16 studies of use of BAL in ICH, diagnostic yields ranged from 31% to 74% depending on the type of patient and infections present (121). Similar results were found in HSCT recipients, with diagnostic sensitivities ranging from 31% to 80% (122). The yield was higher for infectious causes compared with noninfectious causes, and BAL was particularly useful for diagnosis of *P. jiroveci* and CMV infection. TBBX has been found to add to the diagnostic yield, particularly for finding noninfectious causes in some studies, but not in all reports (123–126). A study at the Cleveland Clinic in 104 non-HIV-infected ICH with lung infiltrates found an overall diagnostic yield of 56.2% for bronchoscopy, 38% for BAL, and 38% for TBBX and a higher yield when these modalities were combined (125). The complication rate was 21%, with most common complications being minor bleeding (13%) and pneumothorax (4%). The impact of establishing a diagnosis from bronchoscopy on overall survival and outcome is not clearly established.

Fine Needle Aspiration
Transthoracic fine needle aspiration (FNA) can be useful in the setting of focal nodular or infiltrative lesions where thrombocytopenia or other bleeding dyscrasias are not present and the risk of a pneumothorax is acceptable. In one study of 67 patients with a hematologic malignancy or post-HSCT with focal abnormalities, the overall yield of FNA was 56%, with complications in one-quarter of patients, including a 20% incidence of pneumothorax and 8% incidence of bleeding (127). Another study found a yield for fungal infection post-HSCT in nodular lesions to be 67% with complications occurring in 15% (128).

Surgical Lung Biopsy
When a diagnosis cannot be made by other methods, surgical lung biopsy should be considered, depending on the prognosis of the patient. Obtaining a specific diagnosis from video-assisted thoracotomy (VATS) or open biopsy may allow targeted therapy, but a nonspecific answer such as acute lung injury or interstitial fibrosis is less helpful. Specific diagnoses have been reported in 32% to 83% of surgical lung biopsies in various groups of ICH (128–131). One study from Memorial Sloan-Kettering Cancer Center in 63 patients with hematologic malignancies found a specific diagnosis in 62% of patients (including infection, inflammatory disorders, and malignancy), prompting a change in therapy in 57% of all cases and in 69% of those with a specific diagnosis (130). The complication rate was 13%, with one postoperative death. Higher yields for a

specific diagnosis were associated with a focal versus diffuse abnormality, and finding a specific diagnosis was associated with a significant increase in survival at 90 days (95% vs. 62%). Neutropenic patients and those with respiratory failure also had a low likelihood of finding a specific answer on biopsy. Another study in patients with hematologic malignancy or HSCT showed a specific diagnosis in 67%, with a change in therapy in 48% and improvement in survival with a specific diagnosis (131). Those in respiratory failure had a low diagnostic yield, and the complication rate was 11%. Surgical lung biopsy can be carried out with acceptable morbidity in the ICH, and a specific diagnosis may improve outcome in some cases. Selection of patients most likely to benefit from this procedure is still unclear, and risks must be balanced with the prognosis of patient.

VI. Management
In addition to antimicrobial therapy, reduction of immunosuppression is desirable, whenever possible. Therapy should often be empiric, because earlier therapy may improve survival in some cases.

A. Fungal Infections
Voriconazole is recommended for the primary treatment of invasive aspergillosis in most patients (132). It blocks the synthesis of ergosterol, leading to destruction of the fungal cell membrane and is considered fungicidal. It is well-absorbed and widely distributed in body tissues, including the CSF. It is also active against many other fungi, including *Candida* spp., *Cryptococcus neoformans, Trichosporon* spp., filamentous fungi, and dimorphic fungi such as *C. immitis*, *H. capsulatum*, and *Blastomyces dermatitis*, but is not active against zygomycoses. It may have significant drug interactions and can cause hepatic toxicity. Deoxycholate amphotericin B is an alternative for patients in whom voriconazole is contraindicated (133). This broad-spectrum polyene antifungal binds to ergosterol in the cell wall and is fungicidal. Amphotericin preparations have broad coverage of many fungi, with the exception of *Aspergillus terreus* (134). Lipid formulations of amphotericin B (LFABs), including liposomal amphotericin B, amphotericin B lipid complex, and amphotericin B colloidal dispersion, are equally as efficacious, with less risk of nephrotoxicity and systemic infusion side effects, though more expensive. Amphotericin preparations can cause significant electrolyte abnormalities. Salvage therapy can be given with an echinocandin, such as Caspofungin, which inhibits the synthesis of $(1\rightarrow3)$-β-D-glucans in the fungal cell wall and can also be combined with either of the two primary therapies in select cases, although the efficacy of combined therapy is not clearly established (135,136). Echinocandins have a narrow spectrum of activity and are useful for *Aspergillus* or *Candida* spp., but should not be used as sole therapy, if other fungi are possible. Other options include posaconazole and itraconazole, and in cases of endobronchial *Aspergillus*, adjunctive inhaled amphotericin. Surgical resection should be considered in selected circumstances with persistent focal disease or significant hemoptysis from a focal source. Immune enhancement treatments are experimental, but reversal of immunosuppression, if possible, is helpful (137).

    Treatment of Mucorales is usually with LFABs, in attempts to deliver a high dose with limited nephrotoxicity. Surgical debridement should also be carried out where possible. Posaconazole has been shown to be an effective salvage therapy and can be used to complete a course of treatment when amphotericin preparations have been used initially (138). It is an azole similar to voriconazole, but has activity against Zygomycetes. It is only given orally and absorption is variable, with need to give the medication with a high-fat meal. Side effects are similar to voriconazole, with drug interactions being a major concern.

Treatment should be given for all ICH with cryptococcal pneumonia, even if it is asymptomatic and antigen is negative, because of the risk of dissemination to the CNS. Latent CSF infection should be excluded. Treatment is with an amphotericin preparation and flucytosine. Fluconazole has excellent activity and is occasionally used as sole therapy or to complete a course of treatment. A prolonged course of treatment up to 12 months is usually given. In the ICH, maintenance therapy may be needed for the long-term management of coccidioidomycosis.

Pneumocystis is treated with trimethoprim-sulfamethoxazole, if possible. The drug can be given orally or intravenously with good serum levels. Intravenous pentamidine has equivalent efficacy, but higher risk profile, particularly with renal insufficiency. Primaquine plus clindamycin and atovaquone are alternative agents (48). In severe cases, corticosteroids should be given, similar to that for the HIV-infected patient.

B. Bacterial Pneumonias

The treatment of Legionnaires' disease is with a fluoroquinolone or macrolide. Both are effective, but some observational studies suggest a fluoroquinolone may be more effective (139,140). The former may be preferable in the transplant population because of drug interactions with cyclosporine. Duration of treatment may be extended to 21 days in the ICH with severe disease. *Nocardia* spp. have varying sensitivity profiles, and combination therapy is frequently given initially, certainly in patients with severe disease. Most first-line treatment regimens include trimethoprim-sulfamethoxazole (TMP-SMX), if possible. A variety of other antibiotics can be used, including amikacin, imipenem, meropenem, some third-generation cephalosporins, minocycline, extended-spectrum fluoroquinolones, such as moxifloxacin, linezolid, and tigecycline. Prolonged therapy is needed, given risk of relapse in ICH. Maintenance therapy should be considered in those with severe immunosuppression, using TMP-SMX or, if not possible, doxycycline as an alternative. Occasionally, surgery is helpful for resection of a nocardial abscess that is nonresponsive to treatment. Patients should be monitored closely because of the risk of recurrence.

C. Viral Pneumonias

Preemptive treatment is often given in the transplant population when the pp65 CMV antigen becomes positive, or two consecutive positive PCR results are obtained. Intravenous ganciclovir is the first-line drug. Oral ganciclovir has limited availability, but oral valganciclovir, a prodrug that is rapidly metabolized to active ganciclovir in the intestinal wall and liver, has replaced oral ganciclovir for prophylaxis and preemptive therapy in many cases. Other available drugs include foscarnet, which can be associated with renal and neurologic toxicity, as well as electrolyte abnormalities. Cidofovir is limited by poor bioavailability and nephrotoxicity (141). CMV hyperimmunoglobulin is licensed for prophylactic therapy, but has been used as rescue therapy in some patients.

Optimal duration of therapy is unknown, but ganciclovir is usually given for two to three weeks, and longer in some cases. Quantitative CMV DNA levels should be followed and treatment continued for one week after levels become undetectable.

Herpes simplex and varicella zoster can be treated with acyclovir, valacyclovir, or famciclovir. If treatment is needed for RSV, ribavirin is administered by continuous inhalation for seven days. This may be paired with intravenous immunoglobulin or palivizumab. The latter has been mainly studied in pediatric populations (142). Influenza is treated in a similar manner to the nonimmunocompromised patient. Parainfluenza virus has no known effective treatment. Although ribavirin in HSCT has been used, its efficacy is not proven (143).

For *Strongyloides* infection, treatment of choice is ivermectin orally for two days. An alternative is albendazole, but this may be less effective. In the ICH, particularly with hyperinfection syndrome, both drugs are occasionally used and treatment can be continued for a more prolonged period of time, until there is response (144). In cases where the drug cannot be reliably absorbed, it has occasionally been given by other routes, but these are not FDA approved.

Toxoplasmosis is treated with pyrimethamine and sulfadiazine or, if this is not possible, with pyrimethamine and clindamycin. Folinic acid is given for supplementation. Other choices are addition of pyrimethamine combined with either azithromycin or atovaquone. Therapy is usually given for four to six weeks. TMP-SMX may also be an alternative treatment.

VII. Prevention

Approved regimens for prophylaxis are used in select settings and occasionally outside these indications, at the judgment of the clinician (Table 3). Prophylaxis in appropriate populations can considerably reduce the frequency of infection. Notable examples are the reduction of *Pneumocystis* in the transplant population and the reduction of *Herpes simplex* infection in those with hematologic malignancies and in transplant patients. One of the difficulties is establishing the threshold for preventive therapy in some settings, such as *Pneumocystis* in the non-HIV ICH, outside of the transplant population.

VIII. Cases
A. Case 1

A 58-year-old woman with acute myelogenous leukemia had a complicated course postchemotherapy, with bacterial pneumonia and respiratory failure. She recovered, but was left with mild respiratory impairment and chest radiographic scarring. She was able to undergo allogeneic HSCT without complication. At routine follow-up visit at three months, she was well, but chest CT showed a small nodular infiltrate in the right lower lobe. She was asymptomatic and had engrafted with a normal white blood cell count. A course of treatment was given with Zithromax. A repeat scan in two months showed marked progression of the peripheral infiltrates and several new nodular densities (Fig. 3). She was placed on voriconazole, given the nature of the peripheral infiltrates and nodular densities. GM antigen and $(1\rightarrow3)$-β-D-glucans was negative. There was no sputum. Fine needle aspirate showed granulomatous changes with cultures growing *M. kansasii*. She responded well to specific treatment with decreasing infiltrates.

Table 3 Prevention of Pulmonary Infections

Infection	Drug	Indication
Fungal	Posaconazole	Neutropenia with myelodysplastic syndrome or AML Allogeneic HSCT recipients with GVHD
	Itraconazole Voriconazole Posaconazole Amphotericin B products	Prophylaxis could be considered in HSCT patients with neutropenia
HSV	Acyclovir	Neutropenia
VZV[a]	Valacyclovir	HSCT for at least 30 days
	Famciclovir	Following alemtuzumab therapy for minimum of 2 mo or CD4 > 200 cell/mm^3
CMV	Ganciclovir	HSCT for 1–6 mo, GVHD or CD4 <100 cells/mm^3
	Valganciclovir Foscarnet	Alemtuzumab therapy, minimum of 2 mo or CD4 > 100 cell/mm^3
Pneumocystis jiroveci	Trimethoprim sulfamethoxazole	HSCT for at least 180 days
	Dapsone	Acute lymphocytic leukemia during therapy
	Dapsone	Consider in recipients of:
	Aerosolized pentamidine	T-cell depleting agents, e.g., fludarabine
	Atovaquone	Prolonged corticosteroids[b]
		Autologous HSCT
Influenza A and B	Oseltamivir Zanamivir inhalation	During outbreaks in susceptible population
Bacterial	Intravenous immunoglobulin	Hypogammaglobulinemia patients

[a] Doses may be higher for VZV than HSV
[b] Cancer patient receiving >20 mg/day of prednisone for 4 or more weeks.
Abbreviations: AML, acute myeloid leukemia; HSCT, hematopoietic stem cell transplantation; HSV, *herpes simplex virus*; VZV, *Varicella-zoster virus*; GVHD, graft-versus-host disease.
Source: Adapted from Ref. 142.

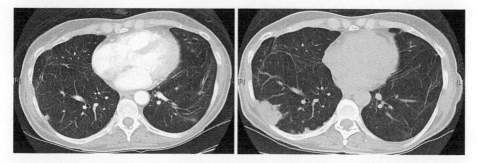

Figure 3 Asymptomatic pulmonary infiltrates post stem cell transplantation (Case 1). (*Left*) Chest CT showed chronic scarring from a previous episode of respiratory failure, with a new small subpleural infiltrate in the right lower lobe at three months posttransplantation. (*Right*) Repeat scan two months later after antibiotic treatment showed a dramatic increase in the nodular density and development of several other small nodules.

This case indicates the important role of CT in early detection of pulmonary disease in high-risk immunosuppressed patients, who may remain asymptomatic for a prolonged period of time. Although CT can suggest a diagnosis, with the pattern in this case being consistent with fungal infection, in atypical situations, such as in this patient who was not neutropenic or on immunosuppression, a firm diagnosis should be established. When it can be performed, FNA has a high yield for focal infiltrates.

B. Case 2

An 83-year-old man was diagnosed with follicular lymphoma, and despite a course of rituximab and fludarabine over 10 months, developed transformation to diffuse large B-cell lymphoma. He also had autoimmune-mediated thrombocytopenia and was treated with high-dose prednisone therapy for six months in the same time period. He was hospitalized with neutropenic fever approximately two weeks following the initiation of salvage chemotherapy. Admission chest radiograph revealed reticulonodular infiltrates in the left mid-to-upper lung field. He defervesced with antibiotics, but had persistent exertional oxygen desaturation. A CT scan revealed no evidence of pulmonary embolism, but showed patchy bilateral ground glass opacities and reticular infiltrates in the left lung. Given the concern for opportunistic infections, especially *P. jiroveci*, in this ICH on chronic steroid therapy with exercise-induced hypoxemia, the patient underwent a diagnostic bronchoscopy with BAL. Specimens were negative for *P. jiroveci*, but the BAL cultures grew HSV. The HSV was treated with a course of acyclovir, with subsequent clinical and radiographic improvement.

This case illustrates the importance of considering multiple etiologies, including more than one infection, in the setting of profound immunosuppression. This patient was neutropenic, on corticosteroids, and had previously used fludarabine, which has prolonged effects on lymphocytes. Early diagnostic bronchoscopy is recommended in the ICH, especially with the presence of diffuse infiltrates. Although the recovery of *Herpes simplex* is not always pathognomonic of infection, this patient had a rapid improvement following initiation of treatment.

References

1. Kotloff RM, Ahya VN, Crawford SW. Pulmonary complications of solid organ and hematopoietic stem cell transplantation. Am J Respir Crit Care Med 2004; 170:22–48.
2. Rano A, Agusti C, Sibila O, et al. Pulmonary infections in non-HIV-immunocompromised patients. Curr Opin Pulm Med 2005; 11:213–217.
3. White DA. Drug-induced pulmonary infection. Clin Chest Med 2004; 25:179–187.
4. Rano A, Agusti C, Jimenez P, et al. Pulmonary infiltrates in non-HIV immunocompromised patients: a diagnostic approach using non-invasive and bronchoscopic procedures. Thorax 2001; 56:379–387.
5. Englund JA, Boeckh M, Kuypers J, et al. Brief communication: fatal human metapneumovirus infection in stem-cell transplant recipients. Ann Intern Med 2006; 144:344–349.
6. Singh N, Paterson DL. Aspergillus infections in transplant recipients. Clin Microbiol Rev 2005; 18:44–69.
7. Walsh TJ, Groll A, Hiemenz J, et al. Infections due to emerging and uncommon medically important fungal pathogens. Clin Microbiol Infect 2004; 10(suppl 1):48–66.
8. Azoulay E, Mokart D, Rabbat A, et al. Diagnostic bronchoscopy in hematology and oncology patients with acute respiratory failure: prospective multicenter data. Crit Care Med 2008; 36:100–107.

9. Roifman CM, Levison H, Gelfand EW. High-dose versus low-dose intravenous immuno-globulin in hypogammaglobulinaemia and chronic lung disease. Lancet 1987; 1:1075–1077.
10. Nucci M, Anaissie E. Emerging fungi. Infect Dis Clin North Am 2006; 20:563–579.
11. Bellocchio S, Bozza S, Montagnoli C, et al. Immunity to Aspergillus fumigatus: the basis for immunotherapy and vaccination. Med Mycol 2005; 43(suppl 1):S181—S188.
12. Lass-Florl C, Griff K, Mayr A, et al. Epidemiology and outcome of infections due to Aspergillus terreus: 10-year single centre experience. Br J Haematol 2005; 131:201–207.
13. Perfect JR, Cox GM, Lee JY, et al. The impact of culture isolation of Aspergillus species: a hospital-based survey of aspergillosis. Clin Infect Dis 2001; 33:1824–1833.
14. Morgan J, Wannemuehler KA, Marr KA, et al. Incidence of invasive aspergillosis following hematopoietic stem cell and solid organ transplantation: interim results of a prospective multicenter surveillance program. Med Mycol 2005; 43(suppl 1):S49–S58.
15. Marr KA, Carter RA, Boeckh M, et al. Invasive aspergillosis in allogeneic stem cell transplant recipients: changes in epidemiology and risk factors. Blood 2002; 100:4358–466.
16. Shaukat A, Bakri F, Young P, et al. Invasive filamentous fungal infections in allogeneic hematopoietic stem cell transplant recipients after recovery from neutropenia: clinical, radiologic, and pathologic characteristics. Mycopathologia 2005; 159:181–188.
17. Cornillet A, Camus C, Nimubona S, et al. Comparison of epidemiological, clinical, and biological features of invasive aspergillosis in neutropenic and nonneutropenic patients: a 6-year survey. Clin Infect Dis 2006; 43:577–584.
18. Pinto PS. The CT Halo Sign. Radiology 2004; 230:109–110.
19. Franquet T, Muller NL, Gimenez A, et al. Spectrum of pulmonary aspergillosis: histologic, clinical, and radiologic findings. Radiographics 2001; 21:825–837.
20. Mehrad B, Paciocco G, Martinez FJ, et al. Spectrum of Aspergillus infection in lung transplant recipients: case series and review of the literature. Chest 2001; 119:169–175.
21. Walsh TJ, Anaissie EJ, Denning DW, et al. Treatment of aspergillosis: clinical practice guidelines of the Infectious Diseases Society of America. Clin Infect Dis 2008; 46:327–360.
22. Marr KA, Carter RA, Crippa F, et al. Epidemiology and outcome of mould infections in hematopoietic stem cell transplant recipients. Clin Infect Dis 2002; 34:909–917.
23. Upton A, Kirby KA, Carpenter P, et al. Invasive aspergillosis following hematopoietic cell transplantation: outcomes and prognostic factors associated with mortality. Clin Infect Dis 2007; 44:531–540.
24. Eucker J, Sezer O, Graf B, et al. Mucormycoses. Mycoses 2001; 44:253–260.
25. Kauffman CA, Malani AN. Zygomycosis: an emerging fungal infection with new options for management. Curr Infect Dis Rep 2007; 9:435–440.
26. Siwek GT, Dodgson KJ, de Magalhaes-Silverman M, et al. Invasive zygomycosis in hematopoietic stem cell transplant recipients receiving voriconazole prophylaxis. Clin Infect Dis 2004; 39:584–587.
27. Bartrum RJ, Jr., Watnick M, Herman PG. Roentgenographic findings in pulmonary mucormycosis. Am J Roentgenol Radium Ther Nucl Med 1973; 117:810–815.
28. Chamilos G, Marom EM, Lewis RE, et al. Predictors of pulmonary zygomycosis versus invasive pulmonary aspergillosis in patients with cancer. Clin Infect Dis 2005; 41:60–66.
29. Pagano L, Ricci P, Tonso A, et al. Mucormycosis in patients with haematological malig-nancies: a retrospective clinical study of 37 cases. GIMEMA Infection Program (Gruppo Italiano Malattie Ematologiche Maligne dell'Adulto). Br J Haematol 1997; 99:331–336.
30. Haron E, Vartivarian S, Anaissie E, et al. Primary Candida pneumonia. Experience at a large cancer center and review of the literature. Medicine (Baltimore) 1993; 72:137–142.
31. Kaplan MH, Rosen PP, Armstrong D. Cryptococcosis in a cancer hospital: clinical and pathological correlates in forty-six patients. Cancer 1977; 39:2265–2274.
32. Aberg JA, Mundy LM, Powderly WG. Pulmonary cryptococcosis in patients without HIV infection. Chest 1999; 115:734–740.

33. Husain S, Wagener MM, Singh N. Cryptococcus neoformans infection in organ transplant recipients: variables influencing clinical characteristics and outcome. Emerg Infect Dis 2001; 7:375–381.

34. Roebuck DJ, Fisher DA, Currie BJ. Cryptococcosis in HIV negative patients: findings on chest radiography. Thorax 1998; 53:554–557.

35. Assi MA, Sandid MS, Baddour LM, et al. Systemic histoplasmosis: a 15-year retrospective institutional review of 111 patients. Medicine (Baltimore) 2007; 86:162–169.

36. Blair JE, Logan JL. Coccidioidomycosis in solid organ transplantation. Clin Infect Dis 2001; 33:1536–1544.

37. Torres HA, Rivero GA, Kontoyiannis DP. Endemic mycoses in a cancer hospital. Medicine (Baltimore) 2002; 81:201–212.

38. Franquet T, Gimenez A, Hidalgo A. Imaging of opportunistic fungal infections in immunocompromised patient. Eur J Radiol 2004; 51:130–138.

39. Yoshino MT, Hillman BJ, Galgiani JN. Coccidioidomycosis in renal dialysis and transplant patients: radiologic findings in 30 patients. AJR Am J Roentgenol 1987; 149:989–992.

40. Overgaard UM, Helweg-Larsen J. Pneumocystis jiroveci pneumonia (PCP) in HIV-1-negative patients: a retrospective study 2002-2004. Scand J Infect Dis 2007; 39:589–595.

41. Bollee G, Sarfati C, Thiery G, et al. Clinical picture of Pneumocystis jiroveci pneumonia in cancer patients. Chest 2007; 132:1305–1310.

42. Mahindra AK, Grossman SA. Pneumocystis carinii pneumonia in HIV negative patients with primary brain tumors. J Neurooncol 2003; 63:263–270.

43. Yale SH, Limper AH. Pneumocystis carinii pneumonia in patients without acquired immunodeficiency syndrome: associated illness and prior corticosteroid therapy. Mayo Clin Proc 1996; 71:5–13.

44. Wu AK, Cheng VC, Tang BS, et al. The unmasking of Pneumocystis jiroveci pneumonia during reversal of immunosuppression: case reports and literature review. BMC Infect Dis 2004; 4:57.

45. Krajicek BJ, Limper AH, Thomas CF, Jr. Advances in the biology, pathogenesis and identification of Pneumocystis pneumonia. Curr Opin Pulm Med 2008; 14:228–234.

46. Baughman RP. The lung in the immunocompromised patient. Infectious complications, Part 1. Respiration 1999; 66:95–109.

47. Stover DE, Greeno RA, Gagliardi AJ. The use of a simple exercise test for the diagnosis of Pneumocystis carinii pneumonia in patients with AIDS. Am Rev Respir Dis 1989; 139:1343–1346.

48. Thomas CF, Jr., Limper AH. Pneumocystis pneumonia. N Engl J Med 2004; 350:2487–2498.

49. Huang L, Morris A, Limper AH, et al. An Official ATS Workshop Summary: Recent advances and future directions in pneumocystis pneumonia (PCP). Proc Am Thorac Soc 2006; 3:655–664.

50. Mikaelsson L, Jacobsson G, Andersson R. Pneumocystis pneumonia–a retrospective study 1991–2001 in Gothenburg, Sweden. J Infect 2006; 53:260–265.

51. Monnet X, Vidal-Petiot E, Osman D, et al. Critical care management and outcome of severe Pneumocystis pneumonia in patients with and without HIV infection. Crit Care 2008; 12:R28.

52. Gasink LB, Blumberg EA. Bacterial and mycobacterial pneumonia in transplant recipients. Clin Chest Med 2005; 26:647–659, vii.

53. Girmenia C, Martino P. Pulmonary infections complicating hematological disorders. Semin Respir Crit Care Med 2005; 26:445–457.

54. Carratala J, Roson B, Fernandez-Sevilla A, et al. Bacteremic pneumonia in neutropenic patients with cancer: causes, empirical antibiotic therapy, and outcome. Arch Intern Med 1998; 158:868–872.

55. Heussel CP, Kauczor HU, Heussel G, et al. Early detection of pneumonia in febrile neutropenic patients: use of thin-section CT. AJR Am J Roentgenol 1997; 169:1347–1353.

56. England AC, III, Fraser DW, Plikaytis BD, et al. Sporadic legionellosis in the United States: the first thousand cases. Ann Intern Med 1981; 94:164–170.
57. Jacobson KL, Miceli MH, Tarrand JJ, et al. Legionella pneumonia in cancer patients. Medicine (Baltimore) 2008; 87:152–159.
58. Singh N, Stout JE, Yu VL. Prevention of Legionnaires' disease in transplant recipients: recommendations for a standardized approach. Transpl Infect Dis 2004; 6:58–62.
59. Muder RR, Stout JE, Yu VL. Nosocomial Legionella micdadei infection in transplant patients: fortune favors the prepared mind. Am J Med 2000; 108:346–348.
60. Saravolatz LD, Burch KH, Fisher E, et al. The compromised host and Legionnaires' disease. Ann Intern Med 1979; 90:533–537.
61. Coletta FS, Fein AM. Radiological manifestations of Legionella/Legionella-like organisms. Semin Respir Infect 1998; 13:109–115.
62. Helbig JH, Uldum SA, Bernander S, et al. Clinical utility of urinary antigen detection for diagnosis of community-acquired, travel-associated, and nosocomial Legionnaires' disease. J Clin Microbiol 2003; 41:838–840.
63. Schlossberg D, Bonoan J. Legionella and immunosuppression. Semin Respir Infect 1998; 13:128–131.
64. Lederman ER, Crum NF. A case series and focused review of nocardiosis: clinical and microbiologic aspects. Medicine (Baltimore) 2004; 83:300–313.
65. Peleg AY, Husain S, Qureshi ZA, et al. Risk factors, clinical characteristics, and outcome of Nocardia infection in organ transplant recipients: a matched case-control study. Clin Infect Dis 2007; 44:1307–1314.
66. Feigin DS. Nocardiosis of the lung: chest radiographic findings in 21 cases. Radiology 1986; 159:9–14.
67. Kamboj M, Sepkowitz KA. The risk of tuberculosis in patients with cancer. Clin Infect Dis 2006; 42:1592–1595.
68. Kaplan MH, Armstrong D, Rosen P. Tuberculosis complicating neoplastic disease. A review of 201 cases. Cancer 1974; 33:850–858.
69. Singh N, Paterson DL. Mycobacterium tuberculosis infection in solid-organ transplant recipients: impact and implications for management. Clin Infect Dis 1998; 27:1266–1277.
70. Doucette K, Fishman JA. Nontuberculous mycobacterial infection in hematopoietic stem cell and solid organ transplant recipients. Clin Infect Dis 2004; 38:1428–1439.
71. Weinstock DM, Feinstein MB, Sepkowitz KA, et al. High rates of infection and colonization by nontuberculous mycobacteria after allogeneic hematopoietic stem cell transplantation. Bone Marrow Transplant 2003; 31:1015–1021.
72. Roy V, Weisdorf D. Mycobacterial infections following bone marrow transplantation: a 20 year retrospective review. Bone Marrow Transplant 1997; 19:467–470.
73. Malouf MA, Glanville AR. The spectrum of mycobacterial infection after lung transplantation. Am J Respir Crit Care Med 1999; 160:1611–1616.
74. Garbino J, Gerbase MW, Wunderli W, et al. Lower respiratory viral illnesses: improved diagnosis by molecular methods and clinical impact. Am J Respir Crit Care Med 2004; 170:1197–1203.
75. Harrington RD, Hooton TM, Hackman RC, et al. An outbreak of respiratory syncytial virus in a bone marrow transplant center. J Infect Dis 1992; 165:987–993.
76. Weinstock DM, Gubareva LV, Zuccotti G. Prolonged shedding of multidrug-resistant influenza A virus in an immunocompromised patient. N Engl J Med 2003; 348:867–868.
77. Whimbey E, Champlin RE, Couch RB, et al. Community respiratory virus infections among hospitalized adult bone marrow transplant recipients. Clin Infect Dis 1996; 22:778–782.
78. Englund JA, Sullivan CJ, Jordan MC, et al. Respiratory syncytial virus infection in immunocompromised adults. Ann Intern Med 1988; 109:203–208.

79. Barton TD, Blumberg EA. Viral pneumonias other than cytomegalovirus in transplant recipients. Clin Chest Med 2005; 26:707–720, viii.

80. Hertz MI, Englund JA, Snover D, et al. Respiratory syncytial virus-induced acute lung injury in adult patients with bone marrow transplants: a clinical approach and review of the literature. Medicine (Baltimore) 1989; 68:269–281.

81. Whimbey E, Couch RB, Englund JA, et al. Respiratory syncytial virus pneumonia in hospitalized adult patients with leukemia. Clin Infect Dis 1995; 21:376–379.

82. Vilchez RA, Dauber J, McCurry K, et al. Parainfluenza virus infection in adult lung transplant recipients: an emergent clinical syndrome with implications on allograft function. Am J Transplant 2003; 3:116–120.

83. Garantziotis S, Howell DN, McAdams HP, et al. Influenza pneumonia in lung transplant recipients: clinical features and association with bronchiolitis obliterans syndrome. Chest 2001; 119:1277–1280.

84. Weinstock DM, Eagan J, Malak SA, et al. Control of influenza A on a bone marrow transplant unit. Infect Control Hosp Epidemiol 2000; 21:730–732.

85. Hierholzer JC. Adenoviruses in the immunocompromised host. Clin Microbiol Rev 1992; 5: 262–274.

86. Raboni SM, Nogueira MB, Tsuchiya LR, et al. Respiratory tract viral infections in bone marrow transplant patients. Transplantation 2003; 76:142–146.

87. Ebihara T, Endo R, Kikuta H, et al. Seroprevalence of human metapneumovirus in Japan. J Med Virol 2003; 70:281–283.

88. Ison MG, Fishman JA. Cytomegalovirus pneumonia in transplant recipients. Clin Chest Med 2005; 26:691–705, viii.

89. Taplitz RA, Jordan MC. Pneumonia caused by herpesviruses in recipients of hematopoietic cell transplants. Semin Respir Infect 2002; 17:121–129.

90. Kalil AC, Levitsky J, Lyden E, et al. Meta-analysis: the efficacy of strategies to prevent organ disease by cytomegalovirus in solid organ transplant recipients. Ann Intern Med 2005; 143:870–880.

91. Kanda Y, Mineishi S, Saito T, et al. Pre-emptive therapy against cytomegalovirus (CMV) disease guided by CMV antigenemia assay after allogeneic hematopoietic stem cell transplantation: a single-center experience in Japan. Bone Marrow Transplant 2001; 27:437–444.

92. Reusser P, Einsele H, Lee J, et al. Randomized multicenter trial of foscarnet versus ganciclovir for preemptive therapy of cytomegalovirus infection after allogeneic stem cell transplantation. Blood 2002; 99:1159–1164.

93. Vij R, Khoury H, Brown R, et al. Low-dose short-course intravenous ganciclovir as pre-emptive therapy for CMV viremia post allo-PBSC transplantation. Bone Marrow Transplant 2003; 32:703–707.

94. Horger MS, Pfannenberg C, Einsele H, et al. Cytomegalovirus pneumonia after stem cell transplantation: correlation of CT findings with clinical outcome in 30 patients. AJR Am J Roentgenol 2006; 187:W636—W643.

95. Umans U, Golding RP, Duraku S, et al. Herpes simplex virus 1 pneumonia: conventional chest radiograph pattern. Eur Radiol 2001; 11:990–994.

96. Carrigan DR, Drobyski WR, Russler SK, et al. Interstitial pneumonitis associated with human herpesvirus-6 infection after marrow transplantation. Lancet 1991; 338:147–149.

97. Cone RW, Hackman RC, Huang ML, et al. Human herpesvirus 6 in lung tissue from patients with pneumonitis after bone marrow transplantation. N Engl J Med 1993; 329: 156–161.

98. Safdar A, Malathum K, Rodriguez SJ, et al. Strongyloidiasis in patients at a comprehensive cancer center in the United States. Cancer 2004; 100:1531–1536.

99. Keiser PB, Nutman TB. Strongyloides stercoralis in the Immunocompromised Population. Clin Microbiol Rev 2004; 17:208–217.

100. Edvinsson B, Lundquist J, Ljungman P, et al. A prospective study of diagnosis of Toxoplasma gondii infection after bone marrow transplantation. APMIS 2008; 116:345–351.
101. Bretagne S, Costa JM, Foulet F, et al. Prospective study of toxoplasma reactivation by polymerase chain reaction in allogeneic stem-cell transplant recipients. Transpl Infect Dis 2000; 2:127–132.
102. Pomeroy C, Filice GA. Pulmonary toxoplasmosis: a review. Clin Infect Dis 1992; 14:863–870.
103. Sing A, Leitritz L, Roggenkamp A, et al. Pulmonary toxoplasmosis in bone marrow transplant recipients: report of two cases and review. Clin Infect Dis 1999; 29:429–433.
104. Franquet T. High-resolution computed tomography (HRCT) of lung infections in non-AIDS immunocompromised patients. Eur Radiol 2006; 16:707–718.
105. Englund JA, Piedra PA, Jewell A, et al. Rapid diagnosis of respiratory syncytial virus infections in immunocompromised adults. J Clin Microbiol 1996; 34:1649–1653.
106. Camps Serra M, Cervera C, Pumarola T, et al. Virological diagnosis in community-acquired pneumonia in immunocompromised patients. Eur Respir J 2008; 31:618–624.
107. Bigby TD, Margolskee D, Curtis JL, et al. The usefulness of induced sputum in the diagnosis of Pneumocystis carinii pneumonia in patients with the acquired immunodeficiency syndrome. Am Rev Respir Dis 1986; 133:515–518.
108. Pitchenik AE, Ganjei P, Torres A, et al. Sputum examination for the diagnosis of Pneumocystis carinii pneumonia in the acquired immunodeficiency syndrome. Am Rev Respir Dis 1986; 133:226–229.
109. Horvath JA, Dummer S. The use of respiratory-tract cultures in the diagnosis of invasive pulmonary aspergillosis. Am J Med 1996; 100:171–178.
110. Maertens J, Theunissen K, Verhoef G, et al. Galactomannan and computed tomography-based preemptive antifungal therapy in neutropenic patients at high risk for invasive fungal infection: a prospective feasibility study. Clin Infect Dis 2005; 41:1242–1250.
111. Pfeiffer CD, Fine JP, Safdar N. Diagnosis of invasive aspergillosis using a galactomannan assay: a meta-analysis. Clin Infect Dis 2006; 42:1417–1427.
112. Adam O, Auperin A, Wilquin F, et al. Treatment with piperacillin-tazobactam and false-positive Aspergillus galactomannan antigen test results for patients with hematological malignancies. Clin Infect Dis 2004; 38:917–920.
113. Viscoli C, Machetti M, Cappellano P, et al. False-positive galactomannan platelia Aspergillus test results for patients receiving piperacillin-tazobactam. Clin Infect Dis 2004; 38: 913–916.
114. Boutboul F, Alberti C, Leblanc T, et al. Invasive aspergillosis in allogeneic stem cell transplant recipients: increasing antigenemia is associated with progressive disease. Clin Infect Dis 2002; 34:939–943.
115. Woods G, Miceli MH, Grazziutti ML, et al. Serum Aspergillus galactomannan antigen values strongly correlate with outcome of invasive aspergillosis: a study of 56 patients with hematologic cancer. Cancer 2007; 110:830–834.
116. Musher B, Fredricks D, Leisenring W, et al. Aspergillus galactomannan enzyme immunoassay and quantitative PCR for diagnosis of invasive aspergillosis with bronchoalveolar lavage fluid. J Clin Microbiol 2004; 42:5517–5522.
117. Odabasi Z, Mattiuzzi G, Estey E, et al. Beta-D-glucan as a diagnostic adjunct for invasive fungal infections: validation, cutoff development, and performance in patients with acute myelogenous leukemia and myelodysplastic syndrome. Clin Infect Dis 2004; 39: 199–205.
118. Persat F, Ranque S, Derouin F, et al. Contribution of the $(1{\to}3)$-beta-D-glucan assay for diagnosis of invasive fungal infections. J Clin Microbiol 2008; 46:1009–1013.
119. Li H, Dummer JS, Estes WR, et al. Measurement of human cytomegalovirus loads by quantitative real-time PCR for monitoring clinical intervention in transplant recipients. J Clin Microbiol 2003; 41:187–191.

120. Plouffe JF, File TM Jr., Breiman RF, et al. Reevaluation of the definition of Legionnaires' disease: use of the urinary antigen assay. Community Based Pneumonia Incidence Study Group. Clin Infect Dis 1995; 20:1286–1291.

121. Ramirez P, Valencia M, Torres A. Bronchoalveolar lavage to diagnose respiratory infections. Semin Respir Crit Care Med 2007; 28:525–533.

122. Feller-Kopman D, Ernst A. The role of bronchoalveolar lavage in the immunocompromised host. Semin Respir Infect 2003; 18:87–94.

123. Cazzadori A, Di Perri G, Todeschini G, et al. Transbronchial biopsy in the diagnosis of pulmonary infiltrates in immunocompromised patients. Chest 1995; 107:101–106.

124. Hsu AA, Allen DM, Yeo CT, et al. Bronchoscopy in immunocompromised host with pulmonary infiltrates. Ann Acad Med Singapore 1996; 25:797–803.

125. Jain P, Sandur S, Meli Y, et al. Role of flexible bronchoscopy in immunocompromised patients with lung infiltrates. Chest 2004; 125:712–722.

126. White P, Bonacum JT, Miller CB. Utility of fiberoptic bronchoscopy in bone marrow transplant patients. Bone Marrow Transplant 1997; 20:681–687.

127. Wong PW, Stefanec T, Brown K, et al. Role of fine-needle aspirates of focal lung lesions in patients with hematologic malignancies. Chest 2002; 121:527–532.

128. Crawford SW, Hackman RC, Clark JG. Biopsy diagnosis and clinical outcome of persistent focal pulmonary lesions after marrow transplantation. Transplantation 1989; 48:266–271.

129. Ellis ME, Spence D, Bouchama A, et al. Open lung biopsy provides a higher and more specific diagnostic yield compared to broncho-alveolar lavage in immunocompromised patients. Fungal Study Group. Scand J Infect Dis 1995; 27:157–162.

130. White DA, Wong PW, Downey R. The utility of open lung biopsy in patients with hematologic malignancies. Am J Respir Crit Care Med 2000; 161:723–729.

131. Zihlif M, Khanchandani G, Ahmed HP, et al. Surgical lung biopsy in patients with hematological malignancy or hematopoietic stem cell transplantation and unexplained pulmonary infiltrates: improved outcome with specific diagnosis. Am J Hematol 2005; 78: 94–99.

132. Herbrecht R, Denning DW, Patterson TF, et al. Voriconazole versus amphotericin B for primary therapy of invasive aspergillosis. N Engl J Med 2002; 347:408–415.

133. Bowden R, Chandrasekar P, White MH, et al. A double-blind, randomized, controlled trial of amphotericin B colloidal dispersion versus amphotericin B for treatment of invasive aspergillosis in immunocompromised patients. Clin Infect Dis 2002; 35:359–366.

134. Walsh TJ, Petraitis V, Petraitiene R, et al. Experimental pulmonary aspergillosis due to Aspergillus terreus: pathogenesis and treatment of an emerging fungal pathogen resistant to amphotericin B. J Infect Dis 2003; 188:305–319.

135. Aliff TB, Maslak PG, Jurcic JG, et al. Refractory Aspergillus pneumonia in patients with acute leukemia: successful therapy with combination caspofungin and liposomal amphotericin. Cancer 2003; 97:1025–1032.

136. Marr K. Combination antifungal therapy: where are we now, and where are we going? Oncology (Williston Park) 2004; 18:24–29.

137. Safdar A. Strategies to enhance immune function in hematopoietic transplantation recipients who have fungal infections. Bone Marrow Transplant 2006; 38:327–337.

138. van Burik JA, Hare RS, Solomon HF, et al. Posaconazole is effective as salvage therapy in zygomycosis: a retrospective summary of 91 cases. Clin Infect Dis 2006; 42:e61–e65.

139. Mykietiuk A, Carratala J, Fernandez-Sabe N, et al. Clinical outcomes for hospitalized patients with Legionella pneumonia in the antigenuria era: the influence of levofloxacin therapy. Clin Infect Dis 2005; 40:794–799.

140. Sabria M, Pedro-Botet ML, Gomez J, et al. Fluoroquinolones vs macrolides in the treatment of Legionnaires disease. Chest 2005; 128:1401–1405.

141. Torres-Madriz G, Boucher HW. Immunocompromised hosts: perspectives in the treatment and prophylaxis of cytomegalovirus disease in solid-organ transplant recipients. Clin Infect Dis 2008; 47:702–711.
142. Segal BH, Freifeld AG, Baden LR, et al. Prevention and treatment of cancer-related infections. J Natl Compr Canc Netw 2008; 6:122–174.
143. Nichols WG, Corey L, Gooley T, et al. Parainfluenza virus infections after hematopoietic stem cell transplantation: risk factors, response to antiviral therapy, and effect on transplant outcome. Blood 2001; 98:573–578.
144. Igual-Adell R, Oltra-Alcaraz C, Soler-Company E, et al. Efficacy and safety of ivermectin and thiabendazole in the treatment of strongyloidiasis. Expert Opin Pharmacother 2004; 5: 2615–2619.

13
Respiratory Infections in HIV-Positive Patients

ROSEMARY BOYTON and CLARE SANDER
National Heart and Lung Institute, Imperial College London, London, U.K.

I. Introduction

The syndrome of human immunodeficiency virus (HIV) is caused by one of two retroviruses of the Lentivirus genera, HIV-1, and HIV-2. HIV-1 accounts for the majority of cases globally, being easier to transmit and progressing more aggressively than HIV-2, which is found predominantly in West Africa. Following initial infection with HIV, individuals may experience a viral type illness. Then there is usually a period of clinical latency when most are unaware of their infection. As the virus replicates, it causes progressive immunosuppression, resulting in opportunistic infections, neoplasms, and other manifestations, which eventually lead to a diagnosis of acquired immunodeficiency syndrome (AIDS). The interval between infection and the development of AIDS is highly variable, but the mean duration is about 10 years in the absence of highly active antiretroviral therapy (HAART). Respiratory infections are a common manifestation of HIV infection and occur at all stages of the syndrome. They are often the first clinical manifestation of HIV infection and sometimes prompt practitioners to make the diagnosis of HIV. It was a cluster of cases of *Pneumocystis jirovecci* pneumonia (PCP) in young homosexual men in New York in 1981 that were among the first cases of HIV to be described.

HIV is an expanding global problem. At the end of 2007, it was estimated that the number of people living with HIV was 33.2 million, of which 30.8 million were adults and 15.4 million were women. In 2007 there were an estimated 2.5 million new infections and 1.7 million AIDS deaths. The largest burden of the HIV/AIDS epidemic is in Sub-Saharan Africa, where an estimated 76% of cases occur, and at least eight southern African countries have prevalence rates exceeding 15%. At the end of 2007, North America had an estimated 1.3 million, with 46,000 new cases per year, and Western Europe had an estimated 760,000 cases with 31,000 new cases per year (1).

HIV is a blood-borne virus transmitted through sexual intercourse, sharing needles, blood transfusions, and perinatally. In Sub-Saharan Africa and Asia, heterosexual transmission is the most frequent route of infection, whereas in the United States transmission between men accounts for 50% of new cases. In the former Soviet Union, two-third of cases are transmitted through intravenous drug use (1). Heterosexual transmission is increasing in many parts of the world, and in 2007 accounted for a third of new cases in the United States and was the most common route of infection in the United Kingdom (2).

Perinatal transmission is declining worldwide, through the use of antiretroviral drugs during pregnancy, and by the use of breast milk alternatives.

HAART consists of various combinations of nucleoside reverse-transcriptase inhibitors (NRTI), nonnucleoside reverse-transcriptase inhibitors (NNRTI), and protease inhibitors (PI), has been widely used in the developed world since 1996, and is increasingly being introduced to the developing world. However, the WHO's target of universal treatment for all by 2010 outlined in the millennium development goals is far from being achieved. The pulmonary manifestations of HIV are influenced by the use of HAART and antibiotic chemoprophylaxis. But, HAART is not available to all, many are unaware of their HIV status, and some lack a sustained response to HAART due to poor adherence, drug toxicity, drug interactions, or drug-resistant strains of HIV-1. Consequently, pulmonary infections including opportunistic infections continue to be seen in HIV-positive individuals in the post-HAART era. In addition, HAART is linked to new pathologies, including immune reconstitution inflammatory syndrome (IRIS), in which the reconstituted immune system responds strongly to the immune stimulus from residual previous infections such as tuberculosis (TB) or PCP (3,4).

The sections below give an overview of the range of respiratory infections seen in HIV-positive individuals and focus on the epidemiology, pathology, diagnosis, management, and prevention of the common respiratory infections.

II. Definition

HIV infection is associated with many respiratory complications, the majority of which are infective in origin. CD4 counts are a reliable predictor of the type and nature of respiratory infection (Table 1). Bacterial infections of the upper and lower respiratory tract, PCP, and TB are the most common respiratory complications in HIV-positive individuals.

Noninfective respiratory complications in HIV-positive individuals include non-Hodgkin's lymphoma, lung cancer, congestive heart failure, emphysema, and lymphocytic or lymphoid interstitial pneumonitis (LIP). Infection may also play a contributory role in the etiology of some classically noninfective complications. For example,

Table 1 CD4 Count and the Type of Pulmonary Infections Seen in HIV-Positive Individuals

CD4 count	Pulmonary infection
>500	Sinusitis
	Bronchitis
	Pharyngitis
<400	Bacterial pneumonia
	Pulmonary *Mycobacterium tuberculosis*
<200	*Pneumocystis jirovecii* pneumonia
	Bacterial sepsis
	Disseminated *M. tuberculosis*
<100	Disseminated *M. avium*
	Cytomegalovirus disease
	Disseminated fungal infections

pulmonary Kaposi sarcoma (KS) has been attributed to infection with human herpes-virus (HHV-8) and pulmonary hypertension, which occurs 1000 times more frequently in HIV-positive individuals than in the general population, may develop as the conse-quence of prior respiratory infection (5,6).

The widespread use of HAART has changed the incidence and presentation of respiratory infection in HIV-positive individuals. IRIS usually occurs within weeks or months of starting HAART, with pulmonary symptoms consistent with an infective or inflammatory syndrome. Other HAART associated complications with respiratory symptoms include the development of nucleoside induced lactic acidosis that presents with tachypnea and dyspnea; abacavir (NRTI)-induced hypersensitivity with fever, rash, myalgia, dyspnea, cough, pharyngitis, and pulmonary infiltrates; and enfuvirtide-associated bacterial pneumonia.

III. Epidemiology

Pulmonary infections are common in HIV infected individuals. Lung complications of HIV were investigated in a prospective multicenter study of 1100 HIV-positive indi-viduals and 167 controls, between 1988 and 1994, pre-HAART but following the introduction of prophylaxis against PCP (7). Infections of both the upper and lower respiratory tracts were more common in the HIV-positive individuals, for all CD4 counts, compared with that in controls. Acute bronchitis was the most common lower airway infection, occurring at all stages of HIV infection and twice as frequently in HIV-positive individuals compared with that in controls. Bacterial pneumonia and PCP were the two most common AIDS defining illnesses. The incidence of both types of pneumonia increases with declining CD4 count. A retrospective study of 18,000 HIV-infected individuals showed that early in HIV disease, respiratory infections are similar to those seen in the general population, while opportunistic infections develop as CD4 counts fall below 200 (8).

The incidence of pulmonary infections has declined following the introduction of HAART, resulting in a reduction in both morbidity and mortality (9,10). There is some evidence to suggest that there has been a greater decline in PCP than bacterial pneu-monia, independent of PCP prophylaxis, although prophylactic antibiotics are beneficial (11–13).

The likelihood of developing a respiratory infection is influenced by the preva-lence and exposure to different infective agents and is influenced by both past and present countries of residence. For example, in Sub-Saharan Africa, there is a prepon-derance of *Mycobacterium tuberculosis* among AIDS patients, whereas in North America more *M. avium* infections are seen (14). Disseminated fungi such as histo-plasmosis and coccidioidomycosis are common infections in AIDS patients living in endemic parts of the United States, but are rarely seen elsewhere.

A. Epidemiology of PCP

Seroepidemiologocal studies suggest that most individuals are exposed to *Pneumocystis* during infancy (15). Asymptomatic colonization with this fungus is well recognized. *Pneumocystis* DNA has been detected in respiratory specimens from different populations, including 20% of oral washes from adults in the general population and sputum/bronchoalveolar lavage (BAL) of the majority (68%) of hospitalized

HIV-infected patients with non-PCP pneumonia (16,17). The natural history of *Pneumocystis* colonization has not been fully elucidated and controversy remains as to whether individuals who develop PCP do so as a result of progression from colonization, with increasing immunosuppression, or infection with a different strain acquired from other individuals.

Colonization with *Pneumocystis* increases with declining CD4 counts and PCP prophylaxis reduces the odds of colonization (17). Because prophylaxis reduces the risk of developing PCP, this provides support for the concept that colonization leads to disease. Molecular genotyping of *Pneumocystis* from PCP cases has shown geographic clustering related to the place of diagnosis rather than the place of birth and that recurrent episodes of PCP are of different genotypes (18,19). Additionally, outbreaks of PCP have been reported from orphanages, hospitals, and in immunocompromised individuals who have prolonged contact with each other.

PCP in HIV-positive individuals in the tropics was in the past thought to be lower than in the industrialized world. This may be partly explained by difficulties in making the diagnosis, but also by the fact that coinfection with other common, virulent pathogens, such as *M. tuberculosis* may be more common in the tropics. A study published in 2003 showed that 80% of infants with HIV in Africa presenting with severe pneumonia had PCP (20).

Risk factors for the development of PCP are CD4 counts of less than 200, previous PCP, oral candidiasis, recurrent bacterial pneumonia, weight loss, smoking, and high viral load. Most cases occur in those unaware of their HIV diagnosis or in those with advanced HIV.

B. Epidemiology of TB

The likelihood of being infected following exposure to *M. tuberculosis* is influenced by the nature of exposure and individual's host defense. The chance of being infected following a significant exposure to *M. tuberculosis* is higher in HIV-positive individuals. This vulnerability is illustrated by the fact that immunosuppressed individuals can be reinfected with *M. tuberculosis* during treatment for active TB as well as years after a previous infection. HIV also increases the probability of those infected with *M. tuberculosis* developing active TB disease. The risk increases to a 10% annual risk in contrast to a 10% lifetime risk, in immunocompetent individuals, and HAART does not completely eradicate this increased susceptibility (21). Being dually infected with HIV and TB worsens outcome from both diseases. TB is the leading cause of death among HIV-positive individuals, accounting for 50% of deaths in those with AIDS (22).

It was estimated that in 2006, 11 million people were living with TB/HIV coinfection, the majority being in Sub-Saharan Africa. In the United Kingdom, TB is currently the second most common opportunistic infection in HIV-positive individuals and in the United States 9% of all TB cases are thought to be coinfected (23,24). Worldwide, HIV infection is the greatest risk factor for the development of active TB (1,25). Diabetes mellitus, silicosis, alcohol excess, extremes of age, recent migration, poor housing, malnutrition, and a smoking history all increase the risk of developing TB disease.

Multidrug resistant TB (MDR-TB), defined as *M. tuberculosis* resistant to at least rifampicin and isoniazid, was first reported in the 1990s, and by 2006 WHO estimated that there were 0.5 million cases globally. Countries in Eastern Europe have reported one-fifth of TB cases as being MDR-TB. Debate is ongoing as to whether HIV infection is an independent risk factor for the development of MDR-TB.

Extremely drug resistant TB (XDR-TB), defined as *M. tuberculosis* resistant to rifampicin, isoniazid, plus any fluoroquinolone, and to at least one of capreomycin, kanamycin, and amikacin, has now been identified in over 41 countries and is associated with high mortality. Outbreaks of XDR-TB in HIV-infected individuals have reported mortality rates of up to 98% within 16 days of diagnosis (26).

C. Epidemiology of Bacterial Pneumonia

It is estimated that the incidence of bacterial pneumonia is increased more than 10-fold in HIV-positive compared with immunocompetent individuals in industrialized and resource poor settings, with surprisingly similar rates in United States, Europe, and Africa. Specific causative agents have been identified in 40% to 75% of HIV adults with bacterial pneumonia. Transmission of these bacteria is thought to occur from person to person through respiratory secretions.

Streptococcus pneumoniae is the most common etiological agent of bacterial pneumonia in HIV. Advanced HIV infection increases the rates of invasive pneumococcal disease by 100-fold. All 91 serotypes of *S. pneumoniae* are able to colonize the nasopharynx, although some are found more frequently, but only 20 serotypes have been found in other body sites. There is evidence supporting the concept that disease develops from a state of colonization. During infancy and childhood, colonization with *S. pneumoniae* is very common, with acquisition of one strain followed by another either sequentially or simultaneously. An individual strain can be carried for weeks or months. Once adulthood is reached, only 10% of the population is colonized (27). Carriage among children is extremely important for whole populations, as evidenced by the reduction in adult disease seen in populations following vaccination of children with polysaccharide conjugate vaccine against *S. pneumoniae* (28).

Haemophilus influenzae (types a–f and nontypeable) account for 10% to 15% cases of bacterial pneumonia and 5% of bacteremias. Colonization with one or more strains from infancy onwards is common, with each strain being present for days to months. Nontypeable *H. influenzae* are present in up to 80% of healthy adults, whereas *H. influenzae* type b is only present in 1% to 4%, depending on the vaccination status of a community.

Staphylococcus aureus and gram-negative bacteria, especially *Pseudomonas aeruginosa*, each account for 5% of pneumonias in HIV-positive individuals, and *Chlamydia pneumonaie* has been detected in up to 16% of cases in intravenous drug users. *Legionella* is thought to be relatively uncommon, although the risk of developing this infection increases 42-fold in AIDS patients compared with the general population.

Bacterial pneumonia can occur earlier than other opportunistic infections, perhaps because encapsulated bacteria are intrinsically more virulent. However, higher rates are seen in those with lower CD4 counts. Risk factors for developing bacterial pneumonias include intravenous drug usage; smoking tobacco, cocaine, crack, and marijuana; alcoholism; cirrhosis; low albumin; asthma; and sickle cell disease. Recent viral infection, including with influenza virus, is a recognized risk as is being of a lower socioeconomic class and having close contact with children. Black adults have an increased risk of invasive pneumococcal disease compared with white adults in United States. Recurrent pneumonia is common, with reports from Kenya of rates as high as 209/1000 person years after a first episode.

It is difficult to compare mortality rates between HIV-infected and non-HIV infected individuals with pneumonia, because of major differences in ages of these groups. There is no increased mortality seen in HIV-infected subjects compared with community controls, but when matching for age, there may be an increase mortality rate in older HIV-infected adults and patients with AIDS.

IV. Etiology

HIV is associated with more than 100 opportunistic infections, many of which infect the lung. Table 2 lists recognized infections pathogens. Multiple respiratory infections can occur simultaneously (29).

Table 2 Lung Infections Associated with HIV Infection

Common	
Bacterial	*Streptococcus pneumoniae*
	Haemophilus influenzae
	No organism isolated, but response to antibiotics
Mycobacterial	*Mycobacterium tuberculosis*
Fungal	*Pneumocystis jirovecii*
Less common	
Bacterial	*Pseudomonas aeruginosa*
	Staphylococcus aureus
	Enterobacteriaceae
	Legionella spp.
	Nocardia spp.
	Rhodococcus equi
Mycobacterial	*Mycobacterium kansasii*
	Mycobacterium avium complex
Fungal	*Cryptococcus neoformans*
	Histoplasma capsulatum
	Coccidoides spp.
	Aspergillus spp.
	Blastomyces dermatitidis
	Penicillum marneffei
Viral	*Influenza*
	Cytomegalovirus
	Herpes simplex virus
	Adenovirus
	Respiratory syncytial virus
	Parainfluenza virus
Parasitic	*Toxoplasma gondii*
	Strongyloides stercoralis
	Microsporidia spp.
	Cyrptosporidium parvum

A. PCP

The genus *Pneumocystis* was classified as a fungus in the late 1980s, supported by genomic sequence analysis of a number of genes, and the presence of a specific factor required for protein synthesis. However, *Pneumocystis* does share many biological characteristics with protozoa and is insensitive to antifungal drugs that target the biosynthesis of ergosterol, as its plasma membranes lack this lipid. The *Pneumocystis* species is host specific, with *P. jirovecii* (known until 1999 as *P. cariini*) being the human isolate and *P. cariini* the rat isolate. The pneumonia caused by *P. jirovecii* continues to be referred to as PCP.

B. Tuberculosis

Mycobacteria are slow growing, facultative intracellular pathogens. Over 91 species of mycobacteria have been identified, the vast majority of which are nonpathogenic. Traditionally classification is based on growth rate, pigmentation, and clinical significance, but more recently, molecular techniques, including sequencing of 16S RNA, are being used to identify different species. *M. tuberculosis* is the most common pathogenic mycobacteria, causing disease in both immunocompetent and immunosuppressed individuals. *M. kansasii* is another virulent mycobacteria infecting individuals with HIV. *M. avium* is present in the environment and can be pathogenic in HIV-positive individuals but causes disease at greater levels of immunosuppression.

C. Bacterial Infections

S. pneumoniae and *H. influenzae* are the most common bacterial pathogens identified in HIV and can cause sinusitis, pharyngitis, bronchitis, and pneumonia (29). The 91 serotypes of *S. pneumoniae* have varying capacities to cause disease, as do the six typeable forms of *H. influenzae*, labeled a to f (27). The latter are distinguished by their antigenically distinct capsular polysaccharides (CPS), with type b being a particularly important invasive pathogen. There are, additionally, nontypeable *H. influenzae* that lack polysaccharide capsules and are consequently nonreactive to typing antisera.

   Mycoplasma, *Chlamydia*, and *Legionella* cause atypical pneumonia. *Rhodococcus equi*, an aerobic, gram-positive, acid-fast bacillus (AFB), can cause focal consolidation, endobronchial lesions, and cavitation in advanced disease. *Pseudomonas aeruginosa* can cause both tracheitis and pneumonia in those with CD4 counts less than 50, in the absence of other risk factors such as neutropenia, steroid use, or hospitalization. *Nocardia asteroides*, an anaerobic soil saprophyte, can cause nodules, consolidation, cavitation, pleural effusions, empyema, and intrathoracic lymphadenopathy.

D. Others

HIV-positive individuals are prone to viral infections, including those affecting the respiratory tract, such as coronavirus, influenza, parainfluenza, and adenoviruses. Although many viruses have the potential to cause pneumonitis, this is rarely seen in HIV-infected individuals. For example, cytomegalovirus (CMV) is often found in BAL without evidence of CMV pneumonitis. The presence of intranuclear or intracytoplasmic inclusion bodies in BAL or in biopsy material and finding CMV at other sites makes a diagnosis of pulmonary CMV infection more likely. Fungal infections, other than PCP, rarely cause respiratory disease in the context of HIV, but *Histoplasmosis*,

Coccidiomycosis, and *Blastomycosis* occurs in certain parts of the United States and *Cryptococcus neoformans* occurs throughout world. Although the latter is mainly associated with meningitis, it can have respiratory manifestations. *Aspergillus* can cause an invasive parenchymal infection usually affecting the upper lobes, causing cavitation and hemoptysis and frequently being fatal, or it can cause bronchial disease with dyspnea and airway obstruction.

V. Pathogenesis
A. Mechanisms Relating to the Pathogen
Destruction of the Immune System by HIV
Many aspects of the host's immune defense, both innate and adaptive, are damaged by HIV infection (30). The hallmark of HIV disease is destruction of CD4 T cells, particularly in mucosal compartments. CD4 T cells are central to adaptive immunity to pathogens, and are critical in orchestrating many other aspects of the immune response and protecting against a range of opportunistic infections. HIV also impairs the functioning of monocyte/macrophages, natural killer (NK) cells, neutrophils, CD8+ T cells, and B cells.

Pneumocystis Pathogenesis
Pneumocystis is inhaled, escapes the defenses of the upper respiratory tract, and is deposited in alveoli. It attaches to the type 1 alveolar cell, through opposition of its cell surface to that of the alveolar cell, without fusing. The major surface glycoproteins (MSG), a family of highly immunogenic antigens on the surface of the *Pneumocystis* are involved, adhering to extracellular matrix glycoproteins such as fibronectin. Organisms exist within the alveoli and obtain essential nutrients from alveolar fluid and living cells. *Pneumocystis* utilizes antigenic variation of the MSGs to evade host immunity. There are multiple genes encoding this family of proteins, clustered at the end of chromosomes, but transcription of these genes only takes place at a single expression site, the upstream conserved sequence (UCS). Only one isoform of MSG is expressed on the surface of *Pneumocystis* at any one time, but gene conversion and recombination at the UCS can result in antigenic variation (31).

Mycobacterium tuberculosis Pathogenesis
Inhaled mycobacteria that are not cleared by the mucociliary system lodge themselves in alveoli and establish foci of infection. They are phagocytosed by macrophages through their interaction with mannose, complement and other receptors. Normally, bacteria containing phagosomes are acidified by fusing with lysosomes. This enables bacterial degradation, releasing peptides to be presented to T cells. However, mycobacteria subvert this process by inhibiting the fusion of phagosomes to lysosomes. Consequently mycobacteria escape the bactericidal activity of these acids and other products such as nitric oxide (NO). The phagosome is inefficient at antigen processing, because mycobacteria block HLA class II molecule presentation at the cell surface, thereby preventing mycobacterial products from entering antigen-processing pathways. Other immune evasion strategies include countering microbicidal products such as reactive oxygen intermediates (ROI), inhibiting interleukin (IL)-12 and interferon (IFN)-γ, and making macrophages refractory to IFN-γ activation.

Role of Bacteria in Pathogenesis

There are some common pathogenic mechanisms shared between different species of bacteria, as well as some unique methods of evading immune defense. The development of disease depends in part on the virulence factors produced by bacteria. Because disease does not usually promote transmission for most bacteria, the aim of many virulence factors is to promote persistence. Variation in transcription, translation, and post-translational modification of virulence factors at different times enables some colonizing bacteria to invade, although this process is poorly understood.

S. pneumoniae are highly adaptable bacteria, they have retained an enormous capacity to colonize and yet continue to have the potential to be virulent. Disease caused by *S. pneumoniae* is the consequence of bacteria accessing the usually sterile lower respiratory tract and causing inflammation. A number of virulence factors are involved in pneumococcal infection and the role of each depends on the location of bacteria. Bacterial capsules consist of polysaccharides covalently attached to outer cell wall peptidoglycan. They are negatively charged and consequently reduce bacterial entrapment in mucus and allow access to nasal epithelial cells. Phase variation results in the expression of capsules of varying thickness. Thinner capsules promote binding to epithelium, whereas thicker ones aid mucus transit, resist opsonophagocytic killing, complement attack, and are selected for transition from mucosa to bloodstream. Capsules have varying affinities for SIGN-1, a C-type lectin expressed on macrophages in the marginal zone of spleen. This influences phagocytosis and bacterial clearance by the spleen and results in differing capacities of various capsular serotypes to cause disease.

There are numerous protein virulence factors, for example, pneumolysin. This multifunctional protein creates pores in cells through the creation of oligomers within cell membranes and results in cytolysis. It also activates epithelial cells to secrete chemokines and attract neutrophils. Promoting an inflammatory response can aid transmission but at the expense of bacterial clearance. Pneumolysin inhibits a number of host defense mechanisms, such as ciliary beating, phagocytic respiratory burst, cytokine synthesis, CD4 T-cell chemotaxis, and classical complement pathway activation.

A number of pneumococcal cell surface proteins act as virulence factors. These include choline-binding proteins (ChoP), pneumococcal surface protein (Psp)A, PspC, and autolysin (LytA). ChoP is a bacterial adhesin, present on many bacteria including *H. influenzae*. It plays an important role in airway colonization. The ChoP from *S. pneumoniae* mediates adherence to the platelet-activating factor (PAF) receptor, which is widely distributed on nasopharyngeal epithelium. Bacteria can mimic PAF in activating these receptors and triggering host cell signaling. Both PspA and PspC inhibit complement-mediated opsonization, whereas autolysin causes bacterial disintegration and release of pneumolysin.

Other virulence factors include zinc metalloproteases secreted by *S. pneumoniae* that inactivate mucosal IgA by cleaving Fab fragments from Fc regions. There is competition within the pharynx between the excess of 700 microbial species that reside there, and induction of the innate immune system by one species can result in the clearance of others. Evidence for competition between different pneumoccocal strains, is demonstrated by serotype replacement following the introduction of the pneumococcal capsular polysaccharide conjugate vaccine. However, bacterial fitness can be increased by this co-colonization. For example, *S. pneumoniae* can incorporate exogenous DNA from closely related oral *Streptococci* to increase virulence.

H. influenzae is both an extracellular and intracellular pathogen, sharing some virulence factors with *S. pneumoniae*. It binds to mucin and adheres to epithelial cells in the airway lumen and is found within the interstitium of the submucosa and within cells of respiratory tract. It colonizes the upper respiratory tract using a variety of adhesion molecules, including ChoP, each with their own specificity for host receptors. The prevalence and distribution of adhesins vary among nontypeable *H. influenzae*, and this affects their pathogenic potential. An example of one of these virulence factors is outer membrane protein P2, a major porin protein that undergoes point mutations to evade the host immune response. *H. influenzae* type b is able to gain access to blood, wheareas nontypeable strains only cause local mucosal invasion.

B. Mechanisms Relating to Host Defense

Pathogenesis of PCP

The host immune response to *Pneumocystis* is incompletely understood, but the complex defects in defense induced by HIV leads to its unchecked replication. Alveolar macrophages provide the first line of defense against *Pneumocystis* and can clear organisms from the lung, if activated by CD4 T cells. *Pneumocystis* is ingested, degraded, and killed by macrophages through the release of tumor necrosis factor (TNF), eicosanoids, and reactive oxidants. The organisms use MSG and B-glucan to adhere to extracellular matrix, surfactant proteins, and mannose and Fc receptors on cells. HIV downregulates mannose receptor expression on alveolar macrophages, thereby impairing the phagocytosis of *Pneumocystis*. This is further exacerbated by the fact that *Pneumocystis* itself promotes the shedding of the mannose receptor.

The fact that the incidence of PCP increases dramatically when CD4 cell counts fall below 200 emphasizes the importance of CD4 T cells in host defense. A compromised immune defense enables *Pneumocystis* to proliferate and leads to the filling of alveolar lumens with a foamy, eosinophilic exudate. As the severity of the infection increases, hyaline membrane formation, interstitial fibrosis, and edema occur. The clinical severity of infection correlates more closely with the inflammatory response than with fungal burden.

HIV and *Pneumocystis* can be reciprocally detrimental. It has been demonstrated that BAL from HIV patients with PCP has lower levels of β-chemokines, RANTES (regulated on activation normal T cell expressed and secreted), macrophage inflammatory protein (MIP-1α and MIP-1β compared with those without PCP. This together with the imbalance of cytokines may contribute to increased lung viral load and the more rapid HIV progression seen in those with PCP (32).

Pathogenesis of TB

Genetic factors play an important role in susceptibility to *M. tuberculosis*, with high concordance seen among monozygotic twins, and certain ethnic groups showing particular vulnerability to disease. Rare mutations in the IFN-γ and IL-12, signaling pathway increase susceptibility (33,34). Further associations have been made between susceptibility to *M. tuberculosis* and vitamin D receptor, natural resistance–associated macrophage protein (NRAMP1), HLA alleles, and mannose-binding lectin (MBL). Inhaled mycobacteria activate macrophages directly by interacting with Toll-like receptors (TLR) 2 and 4 or through the effects of IFN-γ and TNF-α. These macrophages provide the link between the innate and adaptive immune response, through the induction and activation of CD4 and CD8 T cells that can induce apoptosis of infected macrophages resulting in mycobacterial death. In immunocompetent individuals, granulomas form at sites of infection, in addition to draining lymph nodes. They consist of a central core, containing mycobacteria, and macrophages some of which merge to form multinuclear giant cells, surrounded by a zone of lymphocytes, including αβ γδ T, and NK cells. If macrophages remain inactivated, they can be parasitized by mycobacteria, resulting in bacilli residing and replicating within them and leading to latent infection. However, the majority of mycobacteria within granulomas are killed by activated macrophages, partly through the induction of apoptosis but also by a process of autophagy leading to the development of central necrosis, known as caseous necrosis.

Latent disease is defined as the state in which mycobacteria are viable but in a poorly understood state of dormancy. Little is known about the location of these bacilli or whether they are nonreplicating or slowly replicating. These mycobacteria have the capability to cause disease at a later time-point. Viable mycobacteria and *M. tuberculosis* DNA have been detected in lungs from post mortem specimens, both in granulomatous lesions but also in apparently normal lung tissue. In immunocompetent individuals, 15% of TB cases are in extrapulmonary locations probably resulting from direct reactivation of TB foci in these sites. In HIV-infected individuals, there is more extrapulmonary TB compared with immunocompetent individuals. Post mortem examinations of TB/HIV coinfected individuals revealed higher bacterial loads, loss of granuloma formation, and loss of macrophage function associated with falling CD4 T-cell counts (35).

When immune control is lost, granulomas are destroyed by liquefaction, resulting in cavity formation and facilitating the transmission of mycobacteria. The cavities provide a highly permissive environment for extracellular *M. tuberculosis* growth that is difficult for the cellular immune response to reach. Less cavitary lung disease is seen in HIV-infected individuals, probably as a result of the impaired immune response to mycobacteria.

The increased rates of TB disease seen in the context of HIV infection illustrates the essential role that T cells, particularly CD4 T cells, play in host resistance (22,36). Different experimental models have been used to study the role of CD4 and CD8 T cells in primary host defense against mycobacterial infection. In addition to human and murine studies, TB/HIV coinfection has been studied in the macaque simian immunodeficiency virus (SIV)–*M. tuberculosis* model. These studies demonstrate the critical role of CD4 T cells in host defense against mycobacterial infections, whereas the role of CD8 T cells is less clear-cut but seems to be important in preventing reactivation from the latent state (37).

IFN-γ is important to host defense against mycobacterial infection as evidenced by the increased susceptibility to atypical mycobacterial infection in individuals with IFN-γ receptors abnormalities and in IFN-γ knockout mice (33). Activated macrophages and lymphocytes expressing αβ-, γδ-, and NK-associated markers are all able to produce IFN-γ, although CD4 T cells are the primary producers following mycobacterial infection. IFN-γ activates macrophages to enzymatically synthesize reactive nitrogen intermediates that are toxic to intracellular mycobacteria. Additionally IFN-γ sensitizes macrophages to TNF-α, facilitates the acidification of mycobacterial vacuoles and limits early granulocyte accumulation at inflammatory sites. There are also synergistic effects of the cytokines IFN-γ and TNF-α together they augment IL-12 production from human monocytes and increase NO production in mice.

TNF-α strongly promotes a granulomatous response leading to consolidation in tissues but in excess can be tissue damaging. Although predominantly secreted by monocytes and macrophages, it is also secreted by dendritic, NK, and T cells. The increased risk of TB reactivation seen in individuals who are being treated with anti-TNF treatments such as infliximab and etanercept indicates the importance of this cytokine in maintaining latency. Studies of human granulomas demonstrate an association of TNF-α with necrotic lesions, suggesting that TNF-α has a role in granuloma formation and maintenance.

Pathogenesis of Bacterial Pneumonia

Colonization of the upper respiratory tract with bacteria, including *S. pneumoniae* and *H. influenzae*, activates both innate and adaptaive immunity.

Activation of the innate system results in deposition of opsonins, complement, C-reactive protein (CRP), lectins, and IgM directed against carbohydrate on bacteria. Toll like receptors, such as TLR2, recognize lipoteichoic acid and/or lipoproteins of *S. pneumoniae*, and are important at initiating inflammation. Neutrophils influx early in infection, attracted by chemokines, but are often ineffective at clearing bacteria. Multiple cell types infiltrate sites of infection and secrete both pro and anti-inflammatory cytokines. A cascade of inflammation is triggered, since autolysis of pneumococci result in the production of more proinflammatory cytokines and leads to the development of immunopathology. The strength and quality of the adaptive response are influenced by the innate response and the balance of production of different cytokines.

Strain and type specific mucosal and systemic antibodies directed against capsular polysaccharides develop during colonization, but their role in bacterial clearance is uncertain. During adulthood, the clearance of *S. pneumoniae* does not develop in a serotype-specific manner. Capsular antibodies are restricted to IgM and IgG2 in humans, and multiple exposures do not yield an anamnestic response. As a consequence, antibody levels do not boost as polysacchardies do not recruit CD4 T-cell help. Antibodies to major cell surface proteins, such as PspA, also develop and levels of these antibodies correlate with susceptibility to pneumococcal carriage.

There is evidence to support a role for T cells in host defense against *S. pneumoniae*. HIV-1 infected patients with lower CD4 are more likely to be persistent pneumococcal carriers compared with those with higher CD4 counts and those with AIDS develop more severe pneumoccocal infections. Additionally, CD4 counts are suppressed during the acute stage of pneumonia, but lymphopenia recovers when acute infection resolves suggesting that such cells are involved in the immune response. The exact effector function of CD4 T cells that abrogates colonization have not been identified, although proliferative CD4 T-cell responses have been associated with clearing of pneumoccoci from the nasopharynx.

Understanding of immunity to typeable and nontypeable *H. influenzae* is incomplete. Infection with *H. influenzae* type b results in antibody responses to lipooligosaccharide and outer membrane proteins. These antibodies activate complement and have been shown to mediate bacteriocidal and opsonic activity in vitro and mediate protective immunity against systemic infections. Nontypeable *H. influenzae* induce antibodies directed against strain specific determinants, such as the outer membrane protein P2, however these do not prevent recurrent infections.

There is no doubt that the immune response to bacterial infection plays an important role in disease pathogenesis. Furthermore, having had bacterial pneumonia accelerates HIV disease progression and is an independent predictor of progression to AIDs and mortality in HIV (38).

VI. Diagnostic Approach
A. Clinical Assessment

Respiratory illness may be the first manifestion of HIV infection that brings an individual to medical attention. Therefore confirming a diagnosis of HIV may be important acutely as it may influence the diagnoses being considered and consequently may affect immediate and subsequent management (Table 3).

PCP presents with dyspnea, fever, and dry cough, rarely there can be sputum production, hemoptysis, and chest pain. Symptoms may take weeks or months to develop. Clinical signs may be absent, dry crackles can sometimes be heard, but it may require the patient to exercise for them to be audible. Oxygen desaturation with exercise is indicative of abnormal A-a gradient but is not specific for PCP (39). The magnitude of hypoxemia or the alveolar-oxygen gradient has been used as a marker of disease severity and to monitor progression (9). The clinical presentation of TB will depend on the degree of immunosuppression. Pulmonary TB tends to occur in individuals with milder immunosuppression, presenting with similar symptoms and signs to immunocompetent individuals. More atypical clinical presentations occur as CD4 counts fall, with extrapulmonary involvement, including pleural disease, lymphadenopathy, gastrointestinal, and bone marrow pathology (36,40). A short history of fever, sputum production with or without pleuritic pain for days, and focal signs on chest examination is suggestive of bacterial pneumonia.

As shown in Table 1, some infections occur only below a certain level of immunosuppression. So for example, sinusitis, bronchitis, and pharyngitis can occur at all stages of HIV disease, whereas PCP tends to occur when the CD4 count falls to less than 200. Other clues toward a diagnosis of PCP are the presence of oral candidiasis and weight loss (9,41,42). At severe levels of immunosuppression, HIV-infected individuals are susceptible to all types of infection characteristic of AIDS.

A full drug history is important, including whether an individual is taking HAART and/or PCP prophylaxis and the degree of compliance, as this will clearly influence the type and nature of infection. Knowledge of prior opportunistic infections is also useful. An individual is more prone to PCP if they have already had it, especially if they are not taking chemoprophylaxis or are not on HAART. Some individuals are particularly susceptible to encapsulated bacteria such as *S. pneumonaie* and *H. influenzae*. Such individuals may have presented with previous bacterial pneumonia, otitis media, bronchitis, and other bacterial respiratory infections and seem to have prominent B-cell dysfunction. Intravenous drug users are more prone to invasive bacterial infection than other groups (43).

Knowledge of past and present residence and travel history is important, as the prevalence of TB varies markedly across the world, and exposure to *M. tuberculosis* will have a strong influence on the likelihood of an individual being infected or developing active TB (44). Fungal infections such as histoplasmosis, coccidiodomycosis, and blastomycosis are location specific.

Table 3 Clinical Features of the Most Common Lung Manifestations of HIV Infection

	PCP	Bacterial pneumonia	Pulmonary TB
Symptoms	Developing over few weeks: Fever Dry cough Dyspnea Weight loss	Developing over few days: Fever Productive cough Dyspnea Possible pleuritic pain	Developing over weeks and months: Fever Night sweats Cough Weight loss
Past history	May have had PCP in past	May have had previous *S. pneumoniae* or *H. influenzae* infections of ears, sinuses, or chest	May be known to be latently infected with *M. tuberculosis*
Drug history	Not on PCP prophylaxis or poor compliance	IV drug user	
Past and present residence/travel/ social history			From or travelled to TB endemic areas
Signs	None or dry crackles Hypoxia especially after exertion Oral candidiasis	May be focal signs of consolidation	None or signs of consolidation
CD4 count	<200	<400	<400 for pulmonary TB, if disseminated TB <200
Radiology CXR essential	Perihilar diffuse interstitial infiltrates Cyst formation	Focal consolidation	Upper lobe consolidation/cavitation Diffuse infiltration, miliary patterns and intrathoracic lymphadenopathy in advanced disease
Essential blood tests CBC LDH Blood cultures Arterial blood gas	LDH linked to severity Hypoxia linked to severity	May be neutrophilia Need to cover *Pseudomonas aeruginosa* if neutropenic Blood cultures +ve in 60% with *S. pneumoniae*	
Essential sputum test	Induced sputum or BAL for staining or immunofluorescence	Gram stain and culture	AFB stain (auramine or Ziehl–Neelsen) and culture May need induced sputum or BAL

Abbreviations: TB, tuberculosis; PCP, *Pneumocystis jirovecii* pneumonia; CXR, chest X ray; AFB, acid-fast bacillus; CBC, complete blood count; LDH, lactic acid dehydrogenase; BAL, bronchoalveolar lavage.

B. Diagnostic Tests

Radiological examination can show characteristic changes. Focal consolidation on chest X ray (CXR) strongly suggests bacterial pneumonia, while diffuse interstitial infiltrates emanating from the hila in a butterfly pattern suggests PCP. However, these findings are not specific and can be misleading (45). For example, bacterial pneumonia caused by *H. influenzae* can present with diffuse infiltrates. PCP can produce almost any CXR appearance including nodules, asymmetric disease, cysts, and pneumothorax. The other important differential for cystic abnormalities and spontaneous pneumothorax is TB. About 10% of cases with confirmed PCP or TB present with a normal CXR. Radiological abnormalities caused by TB in advanced immunosuppression include diffuse infiltrates, miliary patterns, and intrathoracic lymphadenopathy.

A total blood count and differential may indicate a bacterial infection or a hypersensitivity reaction. Serum lactic dehydrogenase (LDH) levels, which reflect lung injury, can rise in PCP and decline with successful therapy; however, these changes are nonspecific. Duplicate blood cultures should be obtained. In 60% of individuals with HIV and pneumococcal pneumonia, blood cultures are positive for the pneumococcus. Sputum should be obtained for Gram stain, culture, and AFB staining with either auramine/phenol or Ziehl–Neelsen. Although there is high concordance between these tests, the former immunofluorescent test demonstrates higher sensitivity. Ideally, sputum should also be obtained for mycobacterial culture.

Often, empiric antibiotic treatment is started, and if this results in a prompt clinical response, a diagnosis of HIV-related pneumonia is likely. PCP treatment can also be started empirically, but should be followed up with attempts to confirm the diagnosis. Detection rates are lower if either chemoprophylaxis, especially with nebulized pentamidine, or empiric treatment has been given. However, since the fungal burden is higher in HIV-positive individuals compared to other forms of immunosuppression, *Pneumocystis* can still be detected several days after initiation of therapy.

C. Special Investigations

Pneumocystis cannot be cultured in vitro and consequently histopathological demonstration of the organism is required for diagnosis. If an individual presents with a characteristic clinical picture, a diagnostic test is required. Induced sputum, using hypertonic saline can be performed. This simple, noninvasive test does require use of a negative pressure room and dedicated trained staff. Detection rates for PCP of between 50% and 90% have been achieved but depend on the expertise of those performing the procedure (46). Samples can also be sent for bacterial culture and mycobacterial staining and culture.

Fiberoptic bronchoscopy is invasive but has detection rates of up to 90% for PCP (46). BAL is more sensitive with lower morbidity than washings and brushings. The diagnostic yield can be increased by sampling multiple lobes or targeting the site of greatest disease. BAL is also useful to determine the fungal burden, investigate for other infections, and investigate the host inflammatory response (47). Transbronchial biopsies increase the diagnostic yield for PCP to 95% to 100% but are associated with relatively high complication rates. Consequently, the main indication for undertaking these would be a high probability of an additional and/or alternative diagnosis, such as

CMV, aspergillus, LIP, and malignancy other than KS. Open lung biopsies are infrequently required, but they do detect PCP in 95% to 100% of cases and provide tissue for investigating other conditions such as KS. However, if tissue is required it is now more common to perform video-assisted thoracoscopic surgery (VATS) or minithoracotomy.

Experienced microscopists do multiple stains for *Pneumocystis*. They include cyst wall stains such as toluidine blue and stains such as Giemsa that reveal multiple developmental stages of *Pneumocystis* but do not stain the cell wall (46,48). The most widely used immunological technique for diagnosing *Pneumocystis* is immunofluorescence. This is more sensitive than histological staining but requires commercial antibody kits and specialized facilities. Other immunological techniques include immunohistochemistry of tissue sections and immunoblotting, which detects the *Pneumocystis* antigen. PCR has the advantage of increased sensitivity but the disadvantage of being unable to differentiate between live and dead organisms. PCR results are often difficult to interpret as recent anti-*Pneumocystis* drugs, subclinical infection, or colonization can all give false positives.

Several algorithms have been established to aid the diagnosis of PCP in HIV-positive individuals with a normal CXR. PCP is ruled out in individuals with normal, unchanged, or equivocal CXRs and either a high-resolution CT (HRCT) scan of the chest without ground glass or a carbon monoxide diffusing capacity (DLCO) measurement of greater than 75% predicted (49). Although HRCT, pulmonary function tests, and exercise oximetry all have strong negative predictive values, they do not have high specificity for PCP. Algorithims and simple diagnostic techniques to diagnose PCP are used in resource poor settings and when trying to decrease costs. The problem with such algorithms is that they fail to distinguish PCP from other causes of pulmonary infiltrates in HIV (46,48,50). Use of empiric therapy for PCP is often undertaken in such settings, but results in higher mortality rates compared to patients who have undergone bronchoscopy. Empiric treatment can impair later attempts to establish a specific diagnosis. It is known that 13% to 18% of individuals with documented PCP have another cause of respiratory dysfunction, such as TB, KS, or bacterial pneumonia (50).

Confirming a diagnosis of TB is more difficult in HIV positive compared with HIV negative individuals. Obtaining sputum, induced sputum, BAL, or tissue biopsies from infected sites for mycobacterial culture is important for confirming the diagnosis, identifying species and also assessing drug sensitivities. Mycobacterial blood cultures are useful in immunosuppressed individuals and have been found to be positive in 10% to 23% with confirmed TB infection. Molecular diagnostics can be helpful in speeding up the diagnosis of mycobacterial infection and speciation but are less sensitive and should not be done as an alternative to culture. These techniques can also rapidly detect rifampicin resistance.

Serological and urinary antigen testing for *S. pneumoniae, Legionella pneumophilia*, and *Histoplasmosis* (in endemic areas) can be useful in making a diagnosis of bacterial or fungal pneumonia. Cryptococcal pneumonia is rare and is diagnosed by visualizing cryptococci in sputum, BAL, pleural fluid, or lung biopsies. Serum cryptococcal antigen testing is 100% sensitive in the context of disseminated disease. To diagnose CMV pneumonitis, BAL staining with anti-CMV antibodies and lung biopsy findings of cytomegalic cells and inclusion bodies associated with inflammatory reactions and tissue destruction are required.

VII. Management

A. Antimicrobial Treatment

It is not uncommon for HIV-positive individuals to present with acute respiratory failure, requiring empiric treatment for multiple infections, including PCP and bacterial pneumonia. Initial investigations should be performed before commencing therapy, and further investigations performed, as necessary, once treatment has been commenced to confirm diagnoses.

Antimicrobial Therapy for Treating PCP

A number of treatment options are available for treating PCP both in hospital and in an outpatient setting (Table 4).

Antimicrobial Therapy for Treatment of TB

Management of TB in the context of HIV uses similar principles to those used for managing TB in the HIV uninfected, for example optimal regimens should contain rifampicin and isoniazid. The complexity of safely combining medications to treat both conditions necessitates multidisciplinary input with expertise in both HIV and TB.

Ideally the aim should be for every individual to be given daily therapy with antituberculous drugs; however, supervised therapy administered five days per week is also acceptable. Intermittent therapy using three times a week regimens with directly observed treatment short course (DOTS) is not a method of choice but can be used if essential. Therapy administered any less frequently, particularly in those with CD4 less than 100, results in unacceptable relapse rates.

It is recommended that a standard six months of therapy be administered, except in central nervous system infection, when 12 months' treatment is advised. Nine months' treatment is recommended when pyrazinamide is not used, cavities are present, and if an individual remains sputum-culture positive at two months. Quadruple therapy using rifampicin, isoniazid, ethambutol, and pyrazinamide is advised as the optimal initial treatment but can be reduced to rifampicin and isoniazid after two months, if drug susceptibility testing confirms sensitivity.

The major challenge of treating TB/HIV coinfection is the problem of drug interactions and toxicities (Table 5).

Many drugs used to treat these two diseases share the same methods of metabolism, with some drugs inducing enzymes, while others inhibit them (67). For example, cytochrome P4503A4 metabolizes PIs and NNRTIs and is powerfully induced by rifampicin. The induction of this enzyme takes two weeks to be maximal and persists for at least two weeks once therapy is stopped. Predicting drug levels can be further complicated, since rifampicin also increases the activity of multidrug transporter P-glycoprotein (P-gp) that contributes to elimination of PI. Nonetheless rifampicin is the drug of choice where possible.

As a general rule, modifying HAART is preferable to modifying TB treatment, except when a patient is intolerant, has severe drug toxicity, or has genotypic resistance to HIV drugs. If there is intolerance, toxicity, or resistance to HIV drugs, then TB treatment may need to be prolonged. Rifabutin, also from the rifamycin group, can be used as an alternative to rifampicin causing less induction of cytochrome P4503A4 (68,69). In general, NRTIs do not have any major interactions with rifampicin, unlike

Table 4 Treatment of PCP

Drug	Duration of treatment	Side effects	Comment
First line Trimethoprim-sulfamethoxazole (TMP-SMX) 15–20 mg/kg of TMP and 75–100 mg/kg of SMX in 2–4 divided doses Oral and parenteral forms available Inhibits folic acid metabolism (51)	21 days (52)	>80% have some adverse reaction, higher frequency than in HIV negative Skin rash (mild to life threatening, e.g., toxic epidermal necrolysis and Stevens–Johnson), fever, cytopenias, nausea and vomiting, hepatitis, pancreatitis, nephritis, hyperkalemia, metabolic acidosis, CNS manifestations, and anaphylactoid reaction (51,53). Probably caused by the sulfonamide element, except hyperkalemia caused by the potassium sparing diuretic effect of trimethoprim (54).	20 years of use with high success rates (55,56) Dose adjustment may be effective and can minimize side effects (53,55,57). Steroids can be helpful for skin reactions (58). Evidence for cautiously desensitizing those who have had mild to moderate reactions (59). Treat those who have been on Septrin prophylaxis in the same way and for the same length of time.
Second line Trimethoprim and dapsone (51) TMP (15–20 mg/kg/day) oral or parental Dapsone 100 mg/day Oral only	21 days	Adverse reactions to dapsone are methemoglobinemia, rash, fever, nausea and vomiting, and hemolysis in those with G6PD deficiency.	As effective as TMP-SMX, fewer side effects but more pills (60) Use with caution in those who have been intolerant of sulfonamides. Activity against *Pneumocystis* decreased when used with DDI (dideoxyinosine), possibly related to decreased absorption of dapsone

(Continued)

Table 4 Treatment of PCP (*Continued*)

Drug	Duration of treatment	Side effects	Comment
Clindamycin and primaquine Clindamycin (600 mg every 6 hr IV or 300–450 mg every 6 hr orally) and primaquine (15–30 mg/day orally)	21 days	Skin rash, fever, neutropenia, gastrointestinal side effects, and methemoglobinemia. Primaquine can cause hemolysis in G6PD deficiency (60)	Comparable efficacy with TMP-SMX and TMP and dapsone *Clostridium difficile* diarrhea associated with clindamycin use Caution using primaquine in G6PD deficiency
Atovaquone (750 mg b.i.d.) (61)	21 days	Skin rash, fever, gastrointestinal side effects, abnormal liver function tests	Less effective than TMP-SMX but as effective as pentamidine but better tolerated. Consider using with IV pentamidine
Pentamidine isethionate 4 mg/kg/day IV	21 days	Adverse reactions in at least 80%, severe enough to discontinue in 50% Hypotension, cardiac arrythmias, azotemia, pancreatitis, dysglycemia, high K, low Mg, low Ca, neutropenia, hepatic disturbance, bronchospasm, and muscle necrosis at injection sites	Major alternatives to TMP-SMX for moderate-severe hospitalized patients (51) As effective as TMP-SMX, but single daily dose (55,56,62) Administer over 1 hr with patient lying flat, monitoring BP, BMs closely Not recommended to be given by aerosol because less effective and associated with more relapses (63–65)
Trimetrexate 45 mg/ IV and folinic acid 80 mg/m²	21 days	Bone marrow suppression, diarrhea, vomiting, oral and gastrointestinal ulceration, fever, and confusion	Alternative to TMP-SMX and pentamidine Less effective but better tolerated than TMP-SMX (55). Use with folinic acid (for 72 hr after last dose), to prevent bone marrow suppression Useful as salvage therapy (51)

Note: Please refer to the British National Formulary (bnf.org) for up-to-date information on drug therapy.

Table 5 Drug Interactions to Consider when Treating TB in the Context of HIV-Infected Individuals on HAART

Antiretroviral	Rifampicin	Rifabutin	Isoniazid Pyrazinamide Streptomycin Amikacin Azithromycin Ofloxacin Ciprofloxacin	Clarithromycin
NRTI				
Abacavir (ABC)	⊕	⊕	⊕	⊕
Didanosine EC capsules only (DDI)	⊕	⊕	⊕	⊕
Lamivudine (3TC)	⊕	⊕	⊕	⊕
Stavudine (D4T)	⊕	⊕	⊕	⊕
Zalcitabine (DDC)	⊕	⊕	⊕	⊕
Zidovudine (AZT)	⊕	⊕	⊕	⊕
NNRTI				
Tenofovir	⊕	⊕	⊕	⊕
Delaviridine	⊗ 96% reduction in delaviridine AUC, but no change in rifampicin	⊗ 80% reduction in delaviridine AUC and highly significant changes in rifabutin	⊕	⊕
Efavirenz	Ø Increase dose of efavirenz to 800 mg/day.	Ø Reduction in AUC of rifabutin. Consider increasing dose of rifabutin by 50% (450 mg)	⊕	Ø 39% reduction in clarithromycin AUC. 11% reduction in efavirenz AUC
	No dose adjustment for rifampicin	No effect on efavirenz		No dose adjustment required. Increased risk of drug rash, consider alternative of azithromycin

(Continued)

Table 5 Drug Interactions to Consider when Treating TB in the Context of HIV-Infected Individuals on HAART (*Continued*)

Antiretroviral	Rifampicin	Rifabutin	Isoniazid Pyrazinamide Streptomycin Amikacin Azithromycin Ofloxacin Ciprofloxacin	Clarithromycin
Protease inhibitors (PI)				
Nevirapine	⊗ 58% reduction in nevirapine AUC, but no change in rifampicin	∅ Dose both as normal 12% increase in AUC with rifabutin, no significant changes to active metabolite of rifabutin	⊕	∅ 30% reduction in clarithromycin AUC 26% increase in nevirapine AUC No dose adjustment required
Amprenavir	⊗ 82% reduction in amprenavir AUC.	∅ Reduce dose of rifabutin to half (150 mg o.d.) Monitor for signs of neutropenia	⊕	⊕
Indinavir	⊗ 89% reduction in indinavir AUC	⊗ 33% reduction in indinavir AUC 204% increase in rifabutin AUC	⊕	⊕

Kaletra	⊗ Reduction in kaletra AUC	⊕ Reduce dose of rifabutin to 150 mg 3×/wk	Ø Reduce dose of clarithromycin in renal impairment	⊕
Nelfinavir	⊗ 82% reduction in nelfinavir AUC.	⊕	Ø 77% increase in clarithromycin AUC, only reduce dose in renal impairment	⊕
Ritonavir	⊗ 35% reduction in ritonavir AUC	⊕	Ø 34% increase in Clarithromycin AUC	⊕
Saquinavir	⊗ 70% reduction in Fortovase AUC, 80% reduction in Invirase AUC	⊕	177% increase in Saquinavir AUC. Ø No dose adjustment necessary	⊕
Boosted PI	⊗	Ø Little information. Consider using rifabutin 150mg 3×/wk	Ø No information but based on single proteases and kaletra should be safe	⊕

⊕, no interaction, dose as normal; ⊗, definite interaction, do not combine; Ø, potential interaction, see advice.
Source: Adapted from Ref. 66.

NNRTIs and PIs. PIs should not be used with rifampicin because concentrations of PIs are reduced so dramatically that it would encourage the development of drug resistance. PIs are also not generally recommended with rifabutin since concentrations of the latter are increased so much that they can become toxic. Drug interactions are potentially so complex, that detailed guidelines have been created to highlight the main interactions [see Table 5, adapted from BHIVA (British HIV Association) guidelines (66)]. Impaired drug absorption can also be problematic and means that therapeutic drug-level monitoring is often necessary (66,70). Monodrug resistance to isoniazid can be managed using other first line drugs. Resistance to rifampicin requires use of either a fluoroquinolone or injectable agents such as amikacin or capreomycin. Management of MDR and XDR-TB requires expertise and needs individualized treatment plans. Thioacetazone should not be administered to HIV-positive individuals because this has been associated with an increased risk of severe and, sometimes fatal, skin reactions.

Another challenge of treating TB/HIV coinfection is that several drugs have overlapping toxicity profiles. For example, both stavudine and isoniazid can cause peripheral neuropathy, and both rifampicin and NNRTIs can cause rash. Not only can this result in more severe pathology but it also can cause difficulties when trying to attribute causation to a particular drug. The rifamycin drugs are so important for successful treatment of TB that omission of these drugs should only be contemplated when serious toxicity has been experienced.

It is important that TB/HIV patients are monitored regularly with clinical, bacteriological, laboratory (including liver function tests), and radiographic studies. The recommended frequency of performing these investigations varies (66,71–73). Increasing efforts are being made to link up TB and HIV control programs in resource poor settings (74). It is important for both the individual and the community to ensure that therapy is working and that any serious adverse reactions are detected early. There are many reasons why treatment might be interrupted, including problems associated with multiple therapies, intercurrent illness, and social factors, but there are little data to guide management if and when this occurs. It has been recommended that if treatment is interrupted for at least 14 days during the initial phase of treatment or less than 80% of treatment has been taken and treatment lapse lasts for at least three months, then treatment should be restarted. If a treatment lapse is less than three months, then treatment should be continued to ensure a full treatment course, in terms of total number of doses administered (66).

Antimicrobial Therapy for Bacterial Pneumonia

Bacterial pneumonia should be managed in a similar way to that in patients not infected by HIV, although treatment for PCP will often be started together. Risk stratification can be performed using one of the severity index scores, such as the "pneumonia severity score" or the CURB-65 score (75), although some HIV-specific scoring systems have also been developed (76,77). It is important that antibiotics are started promptly, as this is associated with reduced mortality. Recommended antibiotic therapy varies between guidelines, influenced by importance of geographic area, antibiotic resistance, and antibiotic licensing. Therapy should be rationalized once the causative organism has been identified. In North America, macrolides and quinolones are used more frequently first line than in Europe, where there is greater use of β-lactam antibiotics. A prospective, multicenter, international study of patients with pneumococcal bacteremia (mainly due to pneumonia) showed no difference in mortality between HIV-positive and negative patients but did show benefit from the use of combination antibiotics in the critically ill group (78).

B. HAART

There are no randomized control trials to show that early introduction of HAART in the context of acute opportunistic respiratory infection changes outcome. Balancing the relative merits of when to start HAART is challenging. Improving immune function should result in more rapid resolution of respiratory infection, and HAART should reduce the risk of developing a second opportunistic infection. But, these advantages must be weighed against the increased risk of drug toxicities and potential for drug interactions, particularly with TB therapy. Because of the shared metabolic pathways of PIs, NNRTIs, and many antimicrobials, it is often hard to obtain appropriate serum concentrations of either concurrent drugs or HAART. Also, introducing HAART early increases the risk of developing IRIS. BHIVA and CDC (Centers for Disease Control and Prevention) recommend delaying HAART until after the intensive phase of TB treatment in those with CD4 counts between 100 and 200 (66,73). There are no data for those with CD4 less than 100, but it is recommended that such patients either be entered into clinical trials or treatment be commenced as soon as feasible (66).

C. Other Treatment
Respiratory Isolation

HIV-positive patients with respiratory infection may need respiratory isolation, if TB is a diagnostic possibility. In the past, infection control guidelines have not recommended isolation of individuals infected with *Pneumocystis*, since PCP was thought to be the result of reactivation of latent infection. However, opinion is currently shifting since outbreaks and clusters of cases, and the CDC now recommends isolation from other immunocompromised hosts (79,80).

Corticosteroids

The prognosis of PCP relates to hypoxemia at presentation. It is recommended those with moderate to severe hypoxemia (defined as a PaO_2 <70 mmHg or an A-a gradient of >35 mm Hg on room air) should be treated with corticosteroids within 72 hours of starting PCP therapy (81–83). The rationale is that clinical deterioration often occurs in the first few days after starting therapy. It remains unclear whether steroids have a role after this initial 72-hour period. However, most regimens recommend oral prednisolone 40 mg twice a day on days 1 to 5, followed by 40 mg a day on days 6 to 10 and then 20 mg on days 11 to 21 (81,84). Corticosteroids are usually well tolerated, the most frequent side effects being candidiasis, mucocutaneous herpes simplex, and hyperglycemia. An increased frequency of CMV, other fungi, and mycobacterial infections has not been seen (84,85). However, corticosteroids have been shown to increase the morbidity from pneumothorax, hence the need for careful patient selection (86).

Respiratory Support

Noninvasive respiratory support, intubation, mechanical ventilation, and positive end-expiratory pressure should be offered to HIV-positive individuals presenting with respiratory failure because long-term survival is possible. The rate of response to PCP treatment is variable and depends on the antimicrobial therapy used; the number of previous episodes, severity, and degree of immunodeficiency; and the timing of the initiation of therapy (87). Survival is estimated to be approximately 40% in those that require mechanical ventilation (88–90). Survival is better in milder (HIV) disease or those who are on concurrent HAART treatment (90).

Management of Complications

An individual recovered from PCP is at risk of recurrent episodes if immunosuppression persists (88,91). Recurrences of PCP are frequent and are likely to represent relapse if they occur within six months of previous infection. After this, they are more likely to be the result of new infection. Outcomes are similar for recurrent episodes. Pneumothorax is a recognized complication for those recovering from PCP, with use of nebulized pentamidine and cigarette smoking being recognized risk factors (42,86). Pneumoatoceles, pneumomediastinum, and subcutaneous emphysema can also occur. Management of these complications needs to be individualized, but may include chest drain, chemical, and surgical pleurodesis, VATS, and stapling. Complications of pneumonia and TB should be managed similarly to non-HIV patients, with drainage of empyemas, consideration for surgery for lung abscesses and physiotherapy and antibiotics for bronchiectasis.

VIII. Case Study

A 35-year-old Ugandan-born female nurse with no past medical history presents to a U.K. emergency department with four weeks' history of increasing shortness of breath on exertion and nonproductive cough. She was working until one week before presentation. On examination, she has a low-grade pyrexia, oral candidiasis, tachycardia, and is hypoxic, with oxygen saturations on room air of 90%. A CXR showed mild diffuse interstitial shadowing.

1. What is the differential diagnosis? This woman may have underlying immunosuppression secondary to HIV infection given her oral candidiasis. The differential diagnosis is as follows: (*i*) PCP: features found to be independent predictors of PCP are diffuse infiltrates on CXR, oral candidiasis, low CD4 count, perihilar infiltrates, oral hairy leuokoplakia, LDH more than 220 IU and an ESR more than 50 mm/hr, and absence of purulent sputum; (*ii*) *M. tuberculosis*: Uganda is a country of high TB endemicity; (*iii*) atypical pneumonia; (*iv*) CMV; (*v*) coccidiodomycosis; (*vi*) histoplasmosis; (*vii*) *M. avium* complex; and (*viii*) LIP can give interstitial reticular and reticulo-nodular infiltrates. If this woman is not immunosuppressed the differential diagnosis is wide and includes interstitial lung disease.

2. What initial investigations would you like to carry out? Complete blood count, renal and liver function tests, LDH, ESR, CRP, arterial blood gas, HIV test, blood cultures, sputum sample for Gram stain, culture, and AFB stain, and culture.

3. What is your immediate management strategy? Administering controlled oxygen therapy and assessing the severity of respiratory failure. Consider the need for respiratory support, such as continuous positive airway pressure

(CPAP) or bilevel positive airway pressure (BiPAP). Commence on high-dose oral TMP-SMX at a dose of 15 to 20 mg/kg of TMP and 75 to 100 mg/kg of SMX in two to four divided doses. If the PaO_2 is less than 70 mm Hg commence oral prednisolone at a dose of 40 mg b.i.d. Treat with broad-spectrum antibiotics against bacterial pneumonia, including an atypical infection.

4. She becomes more breathless, and her oxygen saturations fall despite oxygen therapy. What would you do next? Perform a full clinical review and repeat arterial blood gases. Check the results of the HIV test and CD4 count. The critical care team should be involved as early as possible to assess the need for additional ventilatory support using noninvasive ventilation and/or intubation and mechanical ventilation. Consider adding IV gancyclovir, since there is evidence to suggest that CMV may worsen outcome from PCP.

5. How would you make the diagnosis? Fiberoptic bronchoscopy with BAL would be the best option. Samples will need to be sent for tests to specifically look for pneumocystis. BAL fluid should also be sent for culture and sensitivities, AFB culture, viral studies (CMV), diagnostic PCR, and fungal culture.

IX. Prevention

Primary prevention aims to prevent first infection with an opportunistic infection, whereas secondary prevention aims to prevent recurrent episodes of infection.

A. Prevention Using HAART

There has been a decline in opportunistic infections since the introduction of HAART. In respiratory infection, HAART is associated with a dramatic reduction in the incidence of PCP, *M. tuberculosis*, and bacterial pneumonia.

B. Lifestyle Modification

There are lifestyle modifications that reduce the risk of opportunistic infection. For example, avoidance of high-risk occupations such as working in certain health care settings or with the homeless and avoidance of close contact with individuals with PCP may reduce the chance of developing TB and PCP. Smoking cessation and recreational drug use reduce susceptibility to respiratory infection.

C. Prevention with Prophylactic Medication

Several factors influence the decision to start chemoprophylaxis. These include, incidence of infection in a given population, effectiveness of drug, safety, ease of administration, and cost.

PCP

The USPHS and IDSA recommend primary and secondary PCP chemoprophylaxis for any HIV-positive adults, adolescents, and pregnant women with a CD4 less than 200 or a history of oropharyngeal candidiasis. Lifelong PCP prophylaxis is recommended when used as secondary chemoprophylaxis (79). BHIVA does not currently have any guidelines on PCP prophylaxis.

TMP-SMX is recommended as first-line PCP prophylaxis as it is very effective, and if compliance is good, breakthrough infections are rare. It also reduces the incidence of bacterial pneumonia and protects against *Toxoplasma gondii*, but increases colonization by drug resistant bacteria, especially pneumococci (29,92,93). It is recommended that a dose of 160 mg TMP and 800 mg SMX per day is used. However, 80 mg/400 mg TMP/SMX per day, or 160/800 every other day is also acceptable, the latter regimen being associated with fewer side effects (79). Atovaquone, dapsone with or without pyrimethamine, and folinic acid and aerosolized pentamidine can be used, but are associated with more treatment failures (92,94–96). Pentamidine should be administered at a dose of 300 mg/wk using a Respirgard nebulizer. It is less effective, more expensive, but better tolerated than TMP-SMX. The major side effects are cough and bronchospasm, although these symptoms can be reduced with β-agonist use. It should be administered in negative pressure rooms and pulmonary TB is a contraindication to its use.

Overall, 20% of patients fail PCP chemoprophylaxis (97). Those at most risk have very low CD4 counts (94,97). These breakthrough infections have atypical manifestations, especially if pentamidine has been used as the prophylactic agent, for example upper lobe disease, pneumothorax, extrapulmonary disease, and pyrexia of unknown origin (98). There is some resistance to TMP-SMX especially in areas where chemoprophylaxis is being extensively used (99).

None of the drugs are lethal to *Pneumocystis*; therefore, treatment needs to be continued for the duration of immunosuppression. However, it is safe to discontinue primary and secondary prophylaxis in patients whose response to antiretroviral therapy has resulted in CD4 cell counts increasing to greater than 200 cells for at least three months (79). An exception is in patients who have developed prior episodes of PCP with CD4 cell levels of greater than 200 cells, they should remain on secondary prophylaxis for life (79).

Tuberculosis

In HIV-positive patients latently infected with TB (LTBI), there is a 10% annual risk of reactivation. The recommended approach to screening for LTBI and for administering chemoprophylaxis varies worldwide, being influenced in part by the underlying prevalence of TB. The NIH and CDC recommend that all patients are screened for latent tuberculosis and suggest that repeat testing should be considered in those with initial negative results but who have high exposure to TB (100). The recommended tests are the tuberculin skin test (TST) or one of the new IFN-γ release assays (IGRAs) that assess IFN-γ production to specific mycobacterial antigens using ELISA or ELISpot. The TST lacks specificity because of cross-reactivity with bacillus Calmette–Guérin (BCG) and environmental mycobacteria and lacks the ability to distinguish LTBI from active infection or past from current infection. It also has reduced sensitivity in those with HIV. The sensitivity of the IGRAs is higher compared with that of TST in the context of HIV, but they are also unable to differentiate infection from disease (101,102). Screening for latent infection is not recommended by BHIVA and is not routinely performed in South Africa, where most patients would be expected to have a positive skin test. The NIH and CDC recommend those with positive TST or IGRA and with no evidence of active TB on the basis of clinical assessment, and CXR should be treated for LTBI (100). They recommend isoniazid daily or twice weekly for nine months, or rifampicin or rifabutin daily for four months. Therapy with either rifampicin or rifabutin together with pyrazinamide is not recommended as this regimen has been associated with fatal and severe liver injury (100). BHIVA does not recommend TB chemoprophylaxis routinely in HIV-positive patients, but suggests that chemoprophylaxis can be considered in at risk groups such as immigrants until their CD4 count increases to above 200 to 300 (66). In South Africa isoniazid is given to all adults when the CD4 count is equal to or less than 300, with evidence that this approach is beneficial in both adults and children (103).

Bacterial Pneumonia

Studies investigating prophylactic regimens in the pre-HAART era, which included TMP-SMX for PCP, and azithromycin with or without rifabutin for *M. avium* complex, showed a fall in the rates of bacterial pneumonia by 50% to 75% (29,92,104,105). Overall, the evidence seems to suggest that prophylactic antibiotics lower rates of bacterial pneumonia in patients with advanced HIV disease but have no role in preventing bacteremia. Of note, prophylactic antibiotics used against PCP such as TMP-SMX have been associated with increased antimicrobial resistance (106,107). There are issues about long-term tolerability, particularly since drug reactions are common in HIV infection, although doses and schedules can be modified. African studies show decreased mortality in those given antimicrobial prophylaxis and the WHO/UNAIDS recommend chronic TMP-SMX in adults with symptomatic HIV infection and in those with asymptomatic HIV infection and a CD4 count less than 500 (108). It is likely that some benefit is achieved by reducing the mortality from bacterial infections, as well as PCP.

D. Prevention with Vaccination

Vaccinations are likely to be most effective at developing strong memory responses if administered early in HIV disease.

PCP

There is currently no vaccine against PCP infection. MSG would be a good candidate antigen for such a vaccine.

BCG

In the past, WHO recommended that single BCG vaccine should be given to healthy infants in countries with a high burden of tuberculosis as close to birth as possible, unless the infant had symptomatic HIV infection (109). Recent evidence shows that HIV-positive infants, even if healthy when BCG vaccinated are at increased risk of developing disseminated BCG disease, and this risk outweighs any advantage achieved in preventing TB (110). WHO now recommends not vaccinating HIV-positive infants.

Streptococcus pneumoniae

The 23-valent capsular polysaccharide vaccine includes 81% to 90% of the pneumococcal serotypes that cause invasive disease in United States and 64% to 91% of those in Africa (111–115). USPHS and IDSA recommend that this vaccine be given as a single dose to those with a CD4 count greater than 200 and who have not been vaccinated in the previous five years (79). However, it is underused with an uptake of between 26% and 85% in the United States (116). The vaccine elicits capsule-specific antibodies in HIV-infected individuals but with a lower magnitude than in those not infected with

HIV. There is no difference in magnitude of antibody response at different CD4 counts, but the functional quality of the antibody response is more robust in those with a CD4 count greater than 500 or soon after seroconversion (117). HAART makes no difference to the immunogenicity of this vaccine. Efficacy studies in industrialized countries have given mixed results. There appears to be modest efficacy against laboratory confirmed pneumococcal disease, but not pneumonia, in those with higher CD4 counts, who are white and HIV positive in United States. Unfortunately, the vaccine is poorly efficacious in Africa (117).

The pneumococcal 7-valent conjugate vaccine contains serotypes that cause 44% to 66% of HIV-associated invasive pneumoccocal infection in the United States and 36% in Africa (117). Because there are currently no efficacy studies, this vaccine is not recommended for routine use. Use of this vaccine in young children may protect HIV-positive parents by increasing herd immunity as long as uptake in a given population is sufficient to achieve this (117).

Haemophilus influenzae
Although *H. influenzae* type b vaccine is available, its use is limited in HIV-positive patients. This is because most infections are caused by strains that cannot be typed, and there is relatively low incidence of invasive Hib disease in HIV-infected individuals (117).

Influenza
Vaccination against influenza is recommended (118,119).

References
1. UNAIDS. 2007 AIDS epidemic update. Available at: http://www.unaids.org/en/Knowledge Centre/HIVData/EpiUpdate/EpiUpdArchive/2007/default.asp. Accessed on October 2009.
2. AVERT. HIV & AIDS statistics from around the world. Available at: http://www.avert.org/ aids-statistics.htm. Accessed on October 2009.
3. Narita M, Ashkin D, Hollender ES, et al. Paradoxical worsening of tuberculosis following antiretroviral therapy in patients with AIDS. Am J Respir Crit Care Med 1998; 158(1): 157–161.
4. Wislez M, Bergot E, Antoine M, et al. Acute respiratory failure following HAART introduction in patients treated for *Pneumocystis carinii* pneumonia. Am J Respir Crit Care Med 2001; 164(5):847–851.
5. Kanmogne GD. Noninfectious pulmonary complications of HIV/AIDS. Curr Opin Pulm Med 2005; 11(3):208–212.
6. Mehta NJ, Khan IA, Mehta RN, et al. HIV-Related pulmonary hypertension: analytic review of 131 cases. Chest 2000; 118(4):1133–1141.
7. Wallace JM, Hansen NI, Lavange L, et al. Respiratory disease trends in the Pulmonary Complications of HIV Infection Study cohort. Pulmonary Complications of HIV Infection Study Group. Am J Respir Crit Care Med 1997; 155(1):72–80.
8. Hanson DL, Chu SY, Farizo KM, et al. Distribution of CD4+ T lymphocytes at diagnosis of acquired immunodeficiency syndrome-defining and other human immunodeficiency virus-related illnesses. The Adult and Adolescent Spectrum of HIV Disease Project Group. Arch Intern Med 1995; 155(14):1537–1542.
9. Phair J, Muñoz A, Detels R, et al. The risk of *Pneumocystis carinii* pneumonia among men infected with human immunodeficiency virus type 1. Multicenter AIDS Cohort Study Group. N Engl J Med 1990; 322(3):161–165.

10. Furrer H, Egger M, Opravil M, et al. Discontinuation of primary prophylaxis against *Pneumocystis carinii* pneumonia in HIV-1-infected adults treated with combination anti-retroviral therapy. Swiss HIV Cohort Study. N Engl J Med 1999; 340(17):1301–1306.
11. Sullivan JH, Moore RD, Keruly JC, et al. Effect of antiretroviral therapy on the incidence of bacterial pneumonia in patients with advanced HIV infection. Am J Respir Crit Care Med 2000; 162(1):64–67.
12. Palella FJ Jr., Delaney KM, Moorman AC, et al. Declining morbidity and mortality among patients with advanced human immunodeficiency virus infection. HIV Outpatient Study Investigators. N Engl J Med 1998; 338(13):853–860.
13. Graham NM, Zeger SL, Park LP, et al. Effect of zidovudine and *Pneumocystis carinii* pneumonia prophylaxis on progression of HIV-1 infection to AIDS. The Multicenter AIDS Cohort Study. Lancet 1991; 338(8762):265–269.
14. Chaisson RE, Moore RD, Richman DD, et al. Incidence and natural history of *Mycobacterium avium* complex infections in patients with advanced human immunodeficiency virus disease treated with zidovudine. The Zidovudine Epidemiology Study Group. Am Rev Respir Dis 1992; 146(2):285–289.
15. Vargas SL, Hughes WT, Santolaya ME, et al. Search for primary infection by *Pneumocystis carinii* in a cohort of normal, healthy infants. Clin Infect Dis 2001; 32(6):855–861.
16. Medrano FJ, Montes-Cano M, Conde M, et al. *Pneumocystis jirovecii* in general population. Emerg Infect Dis 2005; 11(2):245–250.
17. Davis JL, Welsh DA, Beard CB, et al. Pneumocystis colonisation is common among hospitalised HIV infected patients with non-Pneumocystis pneumonia. Thorax 2008; 63(4): 329–334.
18. Dohn MN, White ML, Vigdorth EM, et al. Geographic clustering of *Pneumocystis carinii* pneumonia in patients with HIV infection. Am J Respir Crit Care Med 2000; 162(5):1617–1621.
19. Morris AM, Swanson M, Ha H, et al. Geographic distribution of human immunodeficiency virus-associated *Pneumocystis carinii* pneumonia in San Francisco. Am J Respir Crit Care Med 2000; 162(5):1622–1626.
20. Fisk DT, Meshnick S, Kazanjian PH. *Pneumocystis carinii* pneumonia in patients in the developing world who have acquired immunodeficiency syndrome. Clin Infect Dis 2003; 36(1):70–78.
21. Rieder HL, Cauthen CM, Comstock GW, et al. Epidemiology of tuberculosis in the United States. Epidemiol Rev 1989; 11:79–98.
22. Grant AD, Djomand G, De Cock KM. Natural history and spectrum of disease in adults with HIV/AIDS in Africa. AIDS 1997; 11(suppl B):S43–S54.
23. Rose AM, Sinka K, Watson JM, et al. An estimate of the contribution of HIV infection to the recent rise in tuberculosis in England and Wales. Thorax 2002; 57(5):442–445.
24. Centers for Disease Control and Prevention (CDC). Reported HIV status of tuberculosis patients- United States, 1993-2005. MMWR 2007; 56:1103–1106.
25. Corbett EL, Watt CJ, Walker N, et al. The growing burden of tuberculosis: global trends and interactions with the HIV epidemic. Arch Intern Med 2003; 163(9):1009–1021.
26. Gandhi NR, Moll A, Sturm AW, et al. Extensively drug-resistant tuberculosis as a cause of death in patients co-infected with tuberculosis and HIV in a rural area of South Africa. Lancet 2006; 368(9547):1575–1580.
27. Kadioglu A, Weiser JN, Paton JC, et al. The role of *Streptococcus pneumoniae* virulence factors in host respiratory colonization and disease. Nat Rev Microbiol 2008; 6(4):288–301.
28. Lexau CA, Lynfield R, Danila R, et al. Changing epidemiology of invasive pneumococcal disease among older adults in the era of pediatric pneumococcal conjugate vaccine. JAMA 2005; 294(16):2043–2051.
29. Hirschtick RE, Glassroth J, Jordan MC, et al. Bacterial pneumonia in persons infected with the human immunodeficiency virus. Pulmonary Complications of HIV Infection Study Group. N Engl J Med 1995; 333(13):845–851.

30. Douek DC, Roederer M, Koup RA. Emerging concepts in the immunopathogenesis of AIDS. Annu Rev Med 2009; 60:471–484.
31. Stringer JR, Keely SP. Genetics of surface antigen expression in Pneumocystis carinii. Infect Immun 2001; 69(2):627–639.
32. Koziel H, Kim S, Reardon C, et al. Enhanced in vivo human immunodeficiency virus-1 replication in the lungs of human immunodeficiency virus-infected persons with *Pneumocystis carinii* pneumonia. Am J Respir Crit Care Med 1999; 160(6):2048–2055.
33. Newport MJ, Huxley CM, Huston S, et al. A mutation in the interferon-gamma-receptor gene and susceptibility to mycobacterial infection. N Engl J Med 1996; 335(26):1941–1949.
34. Altare F, et al. Impairment of mycobacterial immunity in human interleukin-12 receptor deficiency. Science 1998; 280(5368):1432–1435.
35. Lucas SB, Nelson AM. Pathogenesis of tuberculosis in human immunodeficiency virus-infected people. Tuberculosis: Pathogenesis, Protection and Control, 1994:503.
36. Jones BE, Young SM, Antoniskis D, et al. Relationship of the manifestations of tuberculosis to CD4 cell counts in patients with human immunodeficiency virus infection. Am Rev Respir Dis 1993; 148(5):1292–1297.
37. Mogues T, Goodrich ME, Ryan L, et al. The relative importance of T cell subsets in immunity and immunopathology of airborne Mycobacterium tuberculosis infection in mice. J Exp Med 2001; 193(3):271–280.
38. Kohli R, Lo Y, Homel P, et al. Bacterial pneumonia, HIV therapy, and disease progression among HIV-infected women in the HIV epidemiologic research (HER) study. Clin Infect Dis 2006; 43(1):90–98.
39. Smith DE, McLuckie A, Wyatt J, et al. Severe exercise hypoxaemia with normal or near normal X-rays: a feature of *Pneumocystis carinii* infection. Lancet 1988; 2(8619): 1049–1051.
40. Perlman DC, el-Sadr WM, Nelson ET, et al. Variation of chest radiographic patterns in pulmonary tuberculosis by degree of human immunodeficiency virus-related immunosuppression. The Terry Beirn Community Programs for Clinical Research on AIDS (CPCRA). The AIDS Clinical Trials Group (ACTG). Clin Infect Dis 1997; 25(2):242–246.
41. Hoover DR, Saah AJ, Bacellar H, et al. Clinical manifestations of AIDS in the era of pneumocystis prophylaxis. Multicenter AIDS Cohort Study. N Engl J Med 1993; 329(26): 1922–1926.
42. Stansell JD, Osmond DH, Charlebois E, et al. Predictors of *Pneumocystis carinii* pneumonia in HIV-infected persons. Pulmonary Complications of HIV Infection Study Group. Am J Respir Crit Care Med 1997; 155(1):60–66.
43. Afessa B, Green B. Clinical course, prognostic factors, and outcome prediction for HIV patients in the ICU. The PIP (Pulmonary complications, ICU support, and prognostic factors in hospitalized patients with HIV) study. Chest 2000; 118(1):138–145.
44. Recommendations for prevention and control of tuberculosis among foreign-born persons. Report of the Working Group on Tuberculosis among Foreign-Born Persons. Centers for Disease Control and Prevention. MMWR Recomm Rep 1998; 47(RR-16):1–29.
45. Crans CA Jr., Boiselle PM. Imaging features of *Pneumocystis carinii* pneumonia. Crit Rev Diagn Imaging 1999; 40(4):251–284.
46. Kroe DM, Kirsch CM, Jensen WA. Diagnostic strategies for *Pneumocystis carinii* pneumonia. Semin Respir Infect 1997; 12(2):70–78.
47. Huang L, et al. Suspected *Pneumocystis carinii* pneumonia with a negative induced sputum examination. Is early bronchoscopy useful? Am J Respir Crit Care Med 1995; 151(6): 1866–1871.
48. Montaner JS, Zala C. The role of the laboratory in the diagnosis and management of AIDS-related *Pneumocystis carinii* pneumonia. In: Sattler FR, Walzer PD (eds.). Pneumocystis carinii. London: Bailliére Tindall, 1995:471–485.

49. Huang L, Stansell J, Osmond D, et al. Performance of an algorithm to detect *Pneumocystis carinii* pneumonia in symptomatic HIV-infected persons. Pulmonary Complications of HIV Infection Study Group. Chest 1999; 115(4):1025–1032.
50. Baughman RP, Dohn MN, Frame PT. The continuing utility of bronchoalveolar lavage to diagnose opportunistic infection in AIDS patients. Am J Med 1994; 97(6):515–522.
51. Barry SM, Johnson MA. *Pneumocystis carinii* pneumonia: a review of current issues in diagnosis and management. HIV Med 2001; 2(2):123–132.
52. Kovacs JA, Hiemenz JW, Macher AM, et al. *Pneumocystis carinii* pneumonia: a comparison between patients with the acquired immunodeficiency syndrome and patients with other immunodeficiencies. Ann Intern Med 1984; 100(5):663–671.
53. Stein DS, Stevens R. Treatment-associated toxicities: incidence and mechanisms. In: Sattler FR, Walzer PD (eds.). Pneumocystis carinii. London: Bailliére Tindall, 1995:505–530.
54. Velazquez H, Perazella MA, Wright FS, et al. Renal mechanism of trimethoprim-induced hyperkalemia. Ann Intern Med 1993; 119(4):296–301.
55. Sattler FR, Cowan R, Nielsen DM, et al. Trimethoprim-sulfamethoxazole compared with pentamidine for treatment of *Pneumocystis carinii* pneumonia in the acquired immunodeficiency syndrome. A prospective, noncrossover study. Ann Intern Med 1988; 109(4):280–287.
56. Wharton JM, Coleman DL, Wofsy CB, et al. Trimethoprim-sulfamethoxazole or pentamidine for *Pneumocystis carinii* pneumonia in the acquired immunodeficiency syndrome. A prospective randomized trial. Ann Intern Med 1986; 105(1):37–44.
57. Joos B, Blaser J, Opravil M, et al. Monitoring of co-trimoxazole concentrations in serum during treatment of *Pneumocystis carinii* pneumonia. Antimicrob Agents Chemother 1995; 39(12):2661–2666.
58. Caumes E, Roudier C, Rogeaux O, et al. Effect of corticosteroids on the incidence of adverse cutaneous reactions to trimethoprim-sulfamethoxazole during treatment of AIDS-associated *Pneumocystis carinii* pneumonia. Clin Infect Dis 1994; 18(3):319–323.
59. Leoung GS, Stanford JF, Giordano MF, et al. Trimethoprim-sulfamethoxazole (TMP-SMZ) dose escalation versus direct rechallenge for *Pneumocystis carinii* pneumonia prophylaxis in human immunodeficiency virus-infected patients with previous adverse reaction to TMP-SMZ. J Infect Dis 2001; 184(8):992–997.
60. Safrin S, Finkelstein DM, Feinberg J, et al. Comparison of three regimens for treatment of mild to moderate *Pneumocystis carinii* pneumonia in patients with AIDS. A double-blind, randomized, trial of oral trimethoprim-sulfamethoxazole, dapsone-trimethoprim, and clindamycin-primaquine. ACTG 108 Study Group. Ann Intern Med 1996; 124(9):792–802.
61. Rosenberg DM, McCarthy W, Slavinsky J, et al. Atovaquone suspension for treatment of *Pneumocystis carinii* pneumonia in HIV-infected patients. AIDS 2001; 15(2):211–214.
62. Hughes WT, Kuhn S, Chaudhary S, et al. Successful chemoprophylaxis for *Pneumocystis carinii* pneumonitis. N Engl J Med 1977; 297(26):1419–1426.
63. Conte JE Jr., Chernoff D, Feigal DW Jr., et al. Intravenous or inhaled pentamidine for treating *Pneumocystis carinii* pneumonia in AIDS. A randomized trial. Ann Intern Med 1990; 113(3):203–209.
64. Montgomery AB, Feigal DW Jr., Sattler F, et al. Pentamidine aerosol versus trimethoprim-sulfamethoxazole for *Pneumocystis carinii* in acquired immune deficiency syndrome. Am J Respir Crit Care Med 1995; 151(4):1068–1074.
65. Soo Hoo GW, Mohsenifar Z, Meyer RD. Inhaled or intravenous pentamidine therapy for *Pneumocystis carinii* pneumonia in AIDS. A randomized trial. Ann Intern Med 1990; 113(3):195–202.
66. Pozniak AL, M.R., Lipman MCI, Freedman AR, et al., on behalf of the BHIVA guidelines writing committee. BHIVA treatment guidelines on TB/HIV infection. 2005. Available at: http://www.bhiva.org/files/file1001577.pdf.

67. Burman WJ, Gallicano K, Peloquin C. Therapeutic implications of drug interactions in the treatment of human immunodeficiency virus-related tuberculosis. Clin Infect Dis 1999; 28(3): 419–429; quiz 430.
68. McGregor MM, Olliaro P, Wolmarans L, et al. Efficacy and safety of rifabutin in the treatment of patients with newly diagnosed pulmonary tuberculosis. Am J Respir Crit Care Med 1996; 154(5):1462–1467.
69. Schwander S, Rüsch-Gerdes S, Mateega A, et al. A pilot study of antituberculosis combinations comparing rifabutin with rifampicin in the treatment of HIV-1 associated tuberculosis. A single-blind randomized evaluation in Ugandan patients with HIV-1 infection and pulmonary tuberculosis. Tuber Lung Dis 1995; 76(3):210–218.
70. CDC. Managing drug interactions in the treatment of HIV related tuberculosis. 2007. Available at: http://www.cdc.gov/tb/publications/guidelines/TB_HIV_Drugs/default.htm. Accessed on October 2009.
71. NICE. Tuberculosis. Clinical diagnosis and management of tuberculosis, and measures for its prevention and control. 2006. Available at: http://www.nice.org.uk/nicemedia/pdf/CG033niceguideline.pdf. Accessed on October 2009.
72. Chemotherapy and management of tuberculosis in the United Kingdom: recommendations 1998. Joint Tuberculosis Committee of the British Thoracic Society. Thorax 1998; 53(7): 536–548.
73. Treatment of tuberculosis. MMWR Recomm Rep 2003; 52(RR-11):1–77.
74. WHO. Joint tuberculosis/HIV interventions. 2008. Available at: http://www.who.int/hiv/topics/tb/tuberculosis/en/. Accessed on October 2009.
75. Armitage K, Woodhead M. New guidelines for the management of adult community-acquired pneumonia. Curr Opin Infect Dis 2007; 20(2):170–176.
76. Arozullah AM, Yarnold PR, Weinstein RA, et al. A new preadmission staging system for predicting inpatient mortality from HIV-associated *Pneumocystis carinii* pneumonia in the early highly active antiretroviral therapy (HAART) era. Am J Respir Crit Care Med 2000; 161(4 pt 1):1081–1086.
77. Arozullah AM, Parada J, Bennett CL, et al. A rapid staging system for predicting mortality from HIV-associated community-acquired pneumonia. Chest 2003; 123(4):1151–1160.
78. Baddour LM, Yu VL, Klugman KP, et al. Combination antibiotic therapy lowers mortality among severely ill patients with pneumococcal bacteremia. Am J Respir Crit Care Med 2004; 170(4):440–444.
79. US Public Health Service (USPHS), Infectious Diseases Society of America (IDSA), USPHS/IDSA Prevention of Opportunistic Infections Working Group. 2001 USPHS/IDSA guidelines for the prevention of opportunistic infections in persons infected with human immunodeficiency virus. HIV Clin Trials 2001; 2(6):493–554.
80. Garner JS. Guideline for isolation precautions in hospitals. Part I. Evolution of isolation practices, Hospital Infection Control Practices Advisory Committee. Am J Infect Control 1996; 24(1):24–31.
81. Consensus statement on the use of corticosteroids as adjunctive therapy for pneumocystis pneumonia in the acquired immunodeficiency syndrome. The National Institutes of Health-University of California Expert Panel for Corticosteroids as Adjunctive Therapy for Pneumocystis Pneumonia. N Engl J Med 1990; 323(21):1500–1504.
82. Bozzette SA, Sattler FR, Chiu J, et al. A controlled trial of early adjunctive treatment with corticosteroids for *Pneumocystis carinii* pneumonia in the acquired immunodeficiency syndrome. California Collaborative Treatment Group. N Engl J Med 1990; 323(21):1451–1457.
83. Gallant JE, Chaisson RE, Moore RD. The effect of adjunctive corticosteroids for the treatment of *Pneumocystis carinii* pneumonia on mortality and subsequent complications. Chest 1998; 114(5):1258–1263.

84. Bozzette SA, Morton SC. Reconsidering the use of adjunctive corticosteroids in Pneumocystis pneumonia? J Acquir Immune Defic Syndr Hum Retrovirol 1995; 8(4):345–347.
85. Walmsley S, Levinton C, Brunton J, et al. A multicenter randomized double-blind placebo-controlled trial of adjunctive corticosteroids in the treatment of *Pneumocystis carinii* pneumonia complicating the acquired immune deficiency syndrome. J Acquir Immune Defic Syndr Hum Retrovirol 1995; 8(4):348–357.
86. Metersky ML, Colt HG, Olson LK, et al. AIDS-related spontaneous pneumothorax. Risk factors and treatment. Chest 1995; 108(4):946–951.
87. Boyton RJ, Mitchell DM, Kon OM. The pulmonary physician in critical care: HIV associated pneumonia. Thorax 2003; 58:721–725.
88. Curtis JR, Yarnold PR, Schwartz DN, et al. Improvements in outcomes of acute respiratory failure for patients with human immunodeficiency virus-related *Pneumocystis carinii* pneumonia. Am J Respir Crit Care Med 2000 162(2 pt 1):393–398.
89. Dworkin MS, Hanson DL, Navin TR. Survival of patients with AIDS, after diagnosis of *Pneumocystis carinii* pneumonia, in the United States. J Infect Dis 2001; 183(9):1409–1412.
90. Morris A, Wachter RM, Luce J, et al. Improved survival with highly active antiretroviral therapy in HIV-infected patients with severe *Pneumocystis carinii* pneumonia. AIDS 2003; 17(1):73–80.
91. Mansharamani NG, Garland R, Delaney D, et al. Management and outcome patterns for adult *Pneumocystis carinii* pneumonia, 1985 to 1995: comparison of HIV-associated cases to other immunocompromised states. Chest 2000; 118(3):704–711.
92. Hardy WD, Feinberg J, Finkelstein DM, et al. A controlled trial of trimethoprim-sulfamethoxazole or aerosolized pentamidine for secondary prophylaxis of *Pneumocystis carinii* pneumonia in patients with the acquired immunodeficiency syndrome. AIDS Clinical Trials Group Protocol 021. N Engl J Med 1992; 327(26):1842–1848.
93. Mayer HB, Rose DN, Cohen S, et al. The effect of *Pneumocystis carinii* pneumonia prophylaxis regimens on the incidence of bacterial infections in HIV-infected patients. AIDS 1993, 7(12):1687–1689.
94. Bozzette SA, Finkelstein DM, Spector SA, et al. A randomized trial of three anti-pneumocystis agents in patients with advanced human immunodeficiency virus infection. NIAID AIDS Clinical Trials Group. N Engl J Med 1995; 332(11):693–699.
95. Chan C, Montaner J, Lefebre EA, et al. Atovaquone suspension compared with aerosolized pentamidine for prevention of *Pneumocystis carinii* pneumonia in human immunodeficiency virus-infected subjects intolerant of trimethoprim or sulfonamides. J Infect Dis 1999; 180(2):369–376.
96. Torres RA, Barr M, Thorn M, et al. Randomized trial of dapsone and aerosolized pentamidine for the prophylaxis of *Pneumocystis carinii* pneumonia and toxoplasmic encephalitis. Am J Med 1993; 95(6):573–583.
97. Saah AJ, Hoover DR, Peng Y, et al. Predictors for failure of *Pneumocystis carinii* pneumonia prophylaxis. Multicenter AIDS Cohort Study. JAMA 1995; 273(15):1197–1202.
98. Sepkowitz KA. Effect of prophylaxis on the clinical manifestations of AIDS-related opportunistic infections. Clin Infect Dis 1998; 26(4):806–810.
99. Kazanjian PH, Fisk D, Armstrong W, et al. Increase in prevalence of *Pneumocystis carinii* mutations in patients with AIDS and *P. carinii* pneumonia, in the United States and China. J Infect Dis 2004; 189(9):1684–1687.
100. Kaplan JE, Benson C, Holmes KH, et al. Guidelines for the prevention and treatment of opportunistic infections in HIV-infected adults and adolescents: recommendations from CDC, National Institutes of Health, and the HIV Medicine Association of the Infectious Diseases Society of America. MMWR Recomm Rep; 58(RR-4):1–207; quiz CE1-4. Available at: http://aidsinfo.nih.gov/contentfiles/Adult_OI.pdf. Accessed on October 2009.

101. Vincenti D, Carrara S, Butera O, et al. Response to region of difference 1 (RD1) epitopes in human immunodeficiency virus (HIV)-infected individuals enrolled with suspected active tuberculosis: a pilot study. Clin Exp Immunol 2007; 150(1):91–98.

102. Karam F, Mbow F, Fletcher H, et al. Sensitivity of IFN-gamma release assay to detect latent tuberculosis infection is retained in HIV-infected patients but dependent on HIV/AIDS progression. PLoS One 2008; 3(1):e1441.

103. Colebunders R, Apers L, Dieltiens G, et al. Tuberculosis in resource poor countries. BMJ 2007; 334(7585):105–106.

104. Havlir DV, Dubé MP, Sattler FR, et al. Prophylaxis against disseminated *Mycobacterium avium* complex with weekly azithromycin, daily rifabutin, or both. California Collaborative Treatment Group. N Engl J Med 1996; 335(6):392–398.

105. Oldfield EC 3rd, Fessel WJ, Dunne MW, et al. Once weekly azithromycin therapy for prevention of Mycobacterium avium complex infection in patients with AIDS: a randomized, double-blind, placebo-controlled multicenter trial. Clin Infect Dis 1998; 26(3):611–619.

106. Edge MD, Rimland D. Community-acquired bacteremia in HIV-positive patients: protective benefit of co-trimoxazole. AIDS 1996; 10(14):1635–1639.

107. Martin JN, Rose DA, Hadley WK, et al. Emergence of trimethoprim-sulfamethoxazole resistance in the AIDS era. J Infect Dis 1999; 180(6):1809–1818.

108. WHO/UNAIDS. Recommendations on the use of cotrimoxazole prophlaxis in adults and children living with HIV/AIDS in Africa. 2000. Available at: http://data.unaids.org/publications/IRC-pub04/recommendation_en.pdf. Accessed on October 2009.

109. Folb PI, Bernatowska E, Chen R, et al. A global perspective on vaccine safety and public health: the Global Advisory Committee on Vaccine Safety. Am J Public Health 2004; 94(11): 1926–1931.

110. Hesseling AC, Cotton MF, Fordham von Reyn C, et al. The risk of disseminated Bacille Calmette-Guerin (BCG) disease in HIV-infected children. Vaccine 2007; 25(1):14–18.

111. Frankel RE, Virata M, Hardalo C, et al. Invasive pneumococcal disease: clinical features, serotypes, and antimicrobial resistance patterns in cases involving patients with and without human immunodeficiency virus infection. Clin Infect Dis 1996; 23(3):577–584.

112. Fry AM, Facklam RR, Whitney CG, et al. Multistate evaluation of invasive pneumococcal diseases in adults with human immunodeficiency virus infection: serotype and antimicrobial resistance patterns in the United States. J Infect Dis 2003; 188(5):643–652.

113. Gilks CF, Ojoo SA, Ojoo JC, et al. Invasive pneumococcal disease in a cohort of predominantly HIV-1 infected female sex-workers in Nairobi, Kenya. Lancet 1996; 347(9003): 718–723.

114. French N, Nakiyingi J, Carpenter LM, et al. 23-valent pneumococcal polysaccharide vaccine in HIV-1-infected Ugandan adults: double-blind, randomised and placebo controlled trial. Lancet 2000; 355(9221):2106–2111.

115. Boyton RJ. Infectious lung complications in patients with HIV/AIDS. Curr Opin Pulm Med 2005; 11:203–207.

116. McNaghten AD, Hanson DL, Jones JL, et al. Effects of antiretroviral therapy and opportunistic illness primary chemoprophylaxis on survival after AIDS diagnosis. Adult/Adolescent Spectrum of Disease Group. AIDS 1999; 13(13):1687–1695.

117. Feikin DR, Feldman C, Schuchat A, et al. Global strategies to prevent bacterial pneumonia in adults with HIV disease. Lancet Infect Dis 2004; 4(7):445–455.

118. Anema A, Mills E, Montaner J, et al. Efficacy of influenza vaccination in HIV-positive patients: a systematic review and meta-analysis. HIV Med 2008; 9(1):57–61.

119. Fiore AE, Shay DK, Broder K, et al. Prevention and control of influenza. Recommendations of the Advisory Committee on Immunization Practices (ACIP), 2007. MMWR Recomm Rep 2007; 56(RR-6):1–54.

14
Tuberculosis

CHI-CHIU LEUNG
Tuberculosis and Chest Service, Department of Health, Hong Kong, China
WING-WAI YEW
Grantham Hospital, Hong Kong, China

I. Introduction

Tuberculosis (TB) is an old disease. Fragments of the spinal column from Egyptian mummies show evidence of TB over 4000 years ago. Large-scale epidemics of this disease have occurred in the recent centuries. With the advent of short-course chemotherapy, the global TB situation improved during 1970s to 1980s. However, since 1990s, TB has resurged alongside rampant drug resistance and HIV coinfection.

II. Definition

TB refers to the disease caused by the *Mycobacterium tuberculosis* complex, which includes *M. tuberculosis, M. bovis, M. africanum, M. microti,* and *M. canetti. M. microti* is a rodent pathogen.

III. Epidemiology

Approximately one-third of the world's population, or 2 billion people, are estimated to have latent infection with *M. tuberculosis*. About 33 million people are estimated to be living with HIV/AIDS worldwide (1). HIV/TB coinfected persons have up to 100 times greater risk of developing active TB disease compared with people not infected with HIV (2). In 2006, there were an estimated 9.2 million new TB cases, and a total of 1.7 million people died of TB, including 0.2 million patients coinfected with HIV (1). Gross disparities occur with respect to disease risk in different parts of the world, and 80% of estimated TB cases are concentrated in 22 high-burden countries (1). With social inequity and poor health care infrastructure in many of the worst-affected areas, drug resistance is an increasing concern.

Almost half a million cases of multidrug-resistant TB (MDR-TB) with bacillary resistance to at least isoniazid and rifampin are estimated to emerge every year worldwide, with China and India together carrying approximately 50% of this global burden and the Russian Federation a further 7% (3). Extensively drug-resistant TB (XDR-TB), recently emerging, is defined as MDR-TB with additional resistance to fluoroquinolones and one or more of the three injectable drugs—kanamycin, amikacin, and capreomycin. It has been reported in 45 countries (3). The problem is likely to be more serious in countries with high prevalence of MDR-TB, and around 40,000 cases are estimated to emerge globally every year (3). In former Soviet Union countries, proportions of XDR-TB among MDR-TB range from 4% in Armenia to almost 24% in Estonia (3).

IV. Etiology

The identification of the tubercle bacillus in 1882 firmly indicated the infectious nature of the disease. *M. tuberculosis* is transmitted by small droplet nuclei through air, a fact established by Riley's classical experiments using guinea pigs in the mid-20th century (4). The chances of exposure to these infectious droplets vary with the incidence of infectious cases and their duration of infectiousness. The likelihood of infection depends largely on the concentration of the infectious agent and the duration of exposure, as well as host factors. Inhalation and implantation of tubercle bacilli in lungs of the host lead to the following outcomes: (*i*) uneventful clearance of the microbe, (*ii*) chronic or latent bacillary infection, (*iii*) rapidly progressive disease (primary disease), and (*iv*) active disease years after the infection (reactivation disease). The disease risk is modified by many sociodemographic, constitutional, and immune factors of the host (2,5,6) (Table 1),

Table 1 Incidence/Relative Risk of Tuberculosis Disease for Selected Risk Factors

	Incidence of disease among tuberculin-positive subjects (per 1000 person-years)	Relative disease risk
Recent TB infection		
Infection <1 yr past	12.9	
Infection 1–7 yr past	1.6	
Old TB scar	2.0–13.6	
HIV infection	35.0–162	
Injection drug use		
HIV seropositive	76.0	
Other	10.0	
Smoking		
Current smokers		2.63
Ex-smokers		1.41
Never smokers		Reference
Body Mass Index		
≥30		0.38
25–<30		0.58
23–<25		0.74
18.5–<23		Reference
<18.5		2.11
Silicosis	68	30
Diabetes mellitus		2.0–4.1
Chronic renal failure		10.0–25.3
Gastrectomy		2–5
Jejunoileal bypass		27–63
Solid organ transplant		
Renal		37
Cardiac		20–74
Head and neck carcinoma		16

apart from virulence and infecting dose of the etiologic agent. On average, only one out of 10 infected people will develop active TB in their lifetimes (2). The disease risk appears to be highest for those infected below one year of age (50%) and lowest among those infected between 5 and 10 years (2%) (7). Disseminated forms of disease and TB meningitis are much more common in young children (7).

V. Pathogenesis
A. Microbiology
One distinguishing feature of the genus *Mycobacterium* is presence of a cell envelope comprising peptidoglycan, arabinogalactan, mycolic acids, and lipoarabinomannan (8). These components confer an array of characteristics including the "acid-fast" staining property. Trehalose dimycolate can elicit cording and granuloma formation (9), and lipoarabinomannan can serve as a scavenger for reactive oxygen intermediates and an inducer for some cytokines (10). Modern genetic approaches have enabled identification of candidate effector molecules specific to *M. tuberculosis* in association with pathogenicity, such as the mycobacterium cell entry protein (Mcep) encoded by *mce1A* (11). Disruption of the *mce1* operon rendered the mutant hypervirulent in BALB/c mice (12). Another important feature of *M. tuberculosis* pathogenesis is the ability to establish a latent infection state (13–16). This is likely to involve a complex microbial adaptive mechanism, with homeostatic "cross-talk" between the microorganism and the host's innate and adaptive immune responses. Animal and in vitro models have been designed to explore such latency and is now thought to be associated with a hypoxic state inside the host. Using whole genome microarray, a large number of genes that are induced under defined hypoxic conditions were identified (17). One of these genes (*dosR*) is believed to be a transcriptional regulator involved in the induction of an α-crystallin-like heat shock protein (18,19). Whether this gene is essential for establishment of latent infection or is merely a "housekeeping" stress response regulator has yet to be unraveled.

B. Immunology
In the last decade, a family of transmembrane proteins in mammalian cells, the Toll-like receptors (TLR), that mediate immune response against infectious pathogens, as well as proinflammatory changes, have been described (20). These receptors recognize pathogen-associated molecular patterns, with TLR2 and TLR4 particularly important for *M. tuberculosis* products (21). *M. tuberculosis* is killed by activation of the TLR2 by mycobacterial lipoprotein, and such killing, largely inside macrophages, is partially dependent on the nitric oxide pathway and the vitamin D receptor—cathelicidin mechanism (22,23). TLR2 and TLR4 partly utilize MyD88, an intracellular adaptor protein required for inducing early innate immune response to pathogens (24,25). Macrophages, dendritic cells, natural killer cells, γδT cells, and CD1-restricted T cells are involved in this initial response to *M. tuberculosis*, which determine the local outgrowth/dissemination of the organism, or containment of infection. If mycobacteria are destroyed immediately, there would be minimal adaptive T-cell response. Some of the mechanisms that are thought to contribute to mycobacterial evasion of macrophage killing include (*i*) resistance to reactive oxygen intermediates (10,26), (*ii*) inhibition of phagosome-lysosome fusion (27), and (*iii*) inhibition of phagosome acidification (28).

Antigens of *M. tuberculosis* are taken up and processed by antigen-presenting cells, such as dendritic cells. Antigens within phagosomes are presented by major histocompatibility complex (MHC) class II molecules to CD4+ T cells that activate macrophages through elaboration of cytokines particularly interferon-γ. *M. tuberculosis* is also known to interfere with antigen presentation, which is important for priming CD4+ T cells (29). Interferon-γ is a potent stimulus for nitric oxide synthase in mice resulting in bacillary control by reactive nitrogen intermediates (30,31). Human macrophages do not express this enzyme when exposed to interferon-γ. However, alveolar macrophages of patients with TB could have expression of nitric oxide synthase (32). Coadministration of interferon-γ and calcitriol (the most active metabolite of vitamin D) has been shown to kill *M. tuberculosis* intracellularly (33). Calcitriol also independently stimulates nitric oxide synthase production and suppresses mycobacterial growth (34). Antigens present in the cytoplasm are presented by MHC class I molecules to CD8+ cells which lyse cells expressing that antigen through a degranulation pathway with perforin and granzymes, and a Fas-Fas-dependent pathway that induces apoptosis of the target cell (35).

T helper (Th) cells, generally CD4+ cells, mature into two functionally different phenotypes, often termed "Th1" and "Th2" cells. The former secrete principally interleukin-2 and interferon-γ, while the latter secrete or induce largely interleukin-4, interleukin-5, interleukin-6, and interleukin-10. Interleukin-12, produced by macrophages, expands the Th1 population and upregulates its functions, and counteracts the downregulatory effects of the anti-inflammatory cytokine interleukin-10. Cell-mediated protective immunity appears to be associated with a Th1 response because genetic defects in signaling by interferon-γ or interleukin-12 increase the susceptibility to development of active TB (36). Superimposed Th2 response would result in tissue necrotizing delayed hypersensitivity. Tumor necrosis factor (TNF)-α, released largely from macrophages, contributes to protect the host by promoting granuloma formation. Antagonism of TNF-α may lead to reactivation/progression of disease from latent TB infection (37). However, TNF-α also causes tissue necrosis under subversive T-cell influences. There is growing evidence on the sabotage role of interleukin-4, in the absence of the counterbalancing activity of its splice variant: interleukin-4δ2 (38). This interleukin-4 overactivity potentially attenuates the Th1-mediated immunity and predisposes to mycobacterial growth, toxicity of TNF-α, immunopathogenicity in the form of tissue necrosis, and subsequent fibrosis. Figure 1 summarizes the immunopathogenesis of TB.

Among the 10% of infected persons who develop disease, approximately one-half will do so within the first two years. This evolution is referred to as rapidly progressive or primary disease, which is manifested as a small nodular granulomatous focus in the lung, alongside hilar lymphadenopathy. The whole pathology is called the Ghon complex. The patient may have constitutional and respiratory symptoms. If mycobacterial growth continues unchecked, the bacilli may spread hematogenously to produce miliary TB with disease in the lungs and other organs like the liver, spleen, and the central nervous system.

Postprimary TB can arise from reactivation or exogenous reinfection, and its course varies greatly. At one extreme, a patient can have marked clinical symptoms and abruptly poor general health. The pathology is in the form of acute/subacute cavitation. There may also be symptoms related to disease complications such as pleural effusion, empyema, laryngitis, and endobronchial involvement. At the other extreme, a patient can have mild symptoms and chronic ill health. The pathology then takes the form of

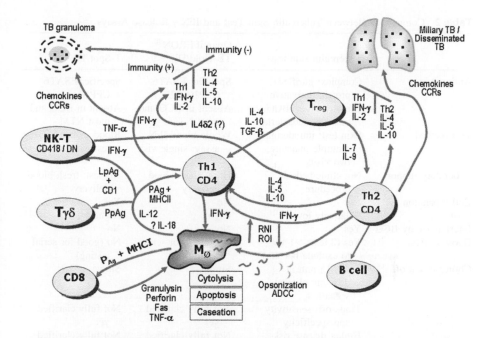

Figure 1 Immunopathogenesis of tuberculosis. *Abbreviations*: ADCC, antibody-dependent cell-mediated cytotoxicity; CCR, chemokine receptor; DN, double negative; Fas, cell receptor inducing apoptosis; IFN-γ, interferon-gamma; IL, interleukin; LpAg, lipopolysaccharide antigen; MHCI, major histocompatibility antigen 1; MHC2, major histocompatibility antigen 2; NK-T, natural killer cell; PAg, peptide antigen; PpAg, phospho-antigen; RNI, reactive nitrogen intermediates; ROI, reactive oxygen intermediates; TGF-β, transforming growth factor-beta; Th, T helper; TNF-α, tumor necrosis factor-alpha; Treg, T regulator lymphocytes.

fibrocaseation. A small proportion of patients can even mount sufficient immunity to contain the disease. The pathology then becomes fibrocalcification.

VI. Diagnostic Approach
A. TB Infection
In the absence of clinical manifestations, the diagnosis of latent TB infection (LTBI) involves measurement of the specific host immune responses to the pathogen, either with the traditional tuberculin skin test (TST) or the newer interferon-γ release assay (IGRA) (39,40). Table 2 summarizes the comparison between these tests (39–43). Serological tests have not yet been shown to be useful for such diagnosis (44).

Diagnosis and treatment of LTBI helps prevent development of the disease. However, all existing tests for LTBI measure the host immune responses rather than microbial pathogenicity, and none of them can accurately differentiate between recent and remote infections. The host immune responses may be affected by many factors, and their time pattern is not necessarily in phase with the activity of the infecting pathogen. Using development of disease as the end point, the positive predictive values of these

Table 2 Comparison Between Tuberculin Skin Test and IFN-γ Release Assays

	Tuberculin skin test	QuantiFERON® TB-Gold/IT	T-Spot.TB
Antigens	Complex: purified protein derivative	Specific: ESAT6, CFP10, TB7.7	Specific: ESAT6, CFP10
	Cross-reaction: BCG, other mycobacteria	Absent in BCG and most NTM	Absent in BCG and most NTM
Test method	Skin test: intradermal/ multiple puncture; two visits	Whole blood IFN assay; single visit	Blood monocyte spot test; single visit
Laboratory support	No; clinic/bedside procedure	High; fresh blood delivery	Highest; fresh blood delivery
Cell separation	No	No	Yes
Cost	Relatively low	High	Highest
Interference by BCG	Yes	No	No
Booster effect	Yes (2 tests >1 wk to exclude booster)	No (good for serial testing)	No (good for serial testing)
Choice of cut-off	5, 10, 15 mm in different clinical scenarios	Single	Single
	Trade-off: sensitivity and specificity	Not fully clarified yet	Not fully clarified yet
	Higher disease risk with larger induration	Not fully clarified yet	Not fully clarified yet
Conversion	Criterion established for recent conversion	Not fully clarified yet	Not fully clarified yet
Infection or disease	Do not distinguish	Do not distinguish	Do not distinguish
Recent vs. remote	Do not distinguish	Do not distinguish adequately	Do not distinguish adequately
Exposure correlation	Some	Higher	Higher/highest
Immune compromise	Affected significantly	Less affected	Least affected
Advance age	Significantly affected	Less affected	Less affected
Proxy sensitivity[a]	65–74%	70–83%	81–95%
Proxy specificity[b]	46–86%; affected by BCG and cut-off	96–99%	86–99%
Longitudinal data	Abundant	Scanty or absent	Scanty or absent

[a]Positive rate among patients with culture-confirmed tuberculosis
[b]Negative rate among low-risk individuals

tests are necessarily low. A highly targeted approach must therefore be employed in the screening and treatment of LTBI to maximize its cost-effectiveness (2).

B. TB Disease

Prudent suspicion of the disease by virtue of clinical and epidemiological evidences is highly warranted. The diagnosis is often made on clinical grounds, together with compatible chest radiograph findings. In 15% to 20% of cases, bacteriologic confirmation is never established (45). Although TB disease must be preceded by infection, the sensitivity and specificity of existing tests for LTBI are not adequate to rule in or rule out active disease (41). Their roles may be further limited in areas or population segments (such as the elderly) with a high background prevalence of LTBI. Therefore, they can only play an adjunctive role in the diagnosis of active TB disease, and the overall clinical picture, including the results of other tests, must be taken into account in reaching a sensible diagnosis.

Radiological Examinations

In postprimary TB, radiological abnormalities can usually be found at the apical and/or posterior segment of the right upper lobe, apicoposterior segment of the left upper lobe, or the apical segments of the lower lobes. Cavitation may be found. Patchy bronchopneumonic shadows may result from bronchogenic spread, while hematogenous dissemination leads to a radiological miliary pattern. Endobronchial TB may cause lung collapse. Computed tomography is more sensitive than the chest radiograph, but the radiation dose is much higher (46). Magnetic resonance imaging is particularly helpful for skeletal and intracranial TB. Radiological changes are however, not entirely specific and atypical presentation may occur, especially among elderly and immunocompromised subjects. Serial assessment may also be necessary to establish the activity of fibrocalcified or other more indolent lesions.

Microbiological Tests

The detection of acid-fast bacilli (AFB) in stained smears (Ziehl–Neelsen and fluorochrome methods) microscopically among symptomatic patients usually means the presence of *M. tuberculosis* (>5000—10,000/mL) (47,48) and implies infectiousness, especially in communities with high TB prevalence. Culture is considerably more sensitive, requiring 10 to 100 AFB per milliliter only (47,48). Conventional culture using solid media usually requires 4 to 10 weeks. Using automated commercial broth systems and microscopic-observation drug-susceptibility (MODS) assay, the turnaround time has been shortened to one to three weeks (49). Subsequent characterization of mycobacteria can be performed by biochemical, nucleic acid hybridization or high-performance liquid chromatography techniques.

Nucleic acid amplification (NAA) techniques, such as polymerase chain reaction (PCR), as applied to sputum specimens, are much faster in detecting *M. tuberculosis*. Specificity is 95% or above, while sensitivity is 95% for smear-positive cases, and 48% to 53% for smear-negative but culture-positive cases (45). Apart from the high cost, they cannot differentiate dead from live bacilli.

Histology and Other Markers

Tissue biopsy may help in the diagnosis of TB and exclude other differential diagnoses, especially for sites accessible either percutaneously (e.g., lymph nodes or pleural effusion) or through a bronchoscope (endobronchial or pulmonary lesions). It may be the only definitive diagnostic test for some extrapulmonary involvement, for example, bone marrow and abdominal disease. Typical histological features pertain to caseating granuloma with multinucleated Langhan's giant cells. Presence of AFB helps to confirm the diagnosis. Biochemical and immunological markers like adenosine deaminase and interferon-γ are useful for the diagnosis of TB pleurisy (50), while other mycobacterial markers may also help in the diagnosis of TB meningitis.

VII. Management

A. Antimicrobial Treatment

Latent Tuberculosis Infection

Isoniazid monotherapy, either daily or twice weekly, for nine months is currently the recommended regimen for treatment of LTBI (2). Treatment with rifampin for four months is an acceptable alternative (2). While this regimen appears to be well tolerated (51,52), relatively limited evidence is currently available on its efficacy. A high rate of hepatotoxicity was reported with two-month treatment with rifampin and pyrazinamide (53,54), and such regimen should generally not be offered to persons with LTBI (55).

Smear-Positive Pulmonary Tuberculosis

The standard short-course chemotherapy regimen comprises two months of rifampin, isoniazid, and pyrazinamide with or without ethambutol (or streptomycin), followed by four months of rifampin and isoniazid (56). The relapse rates are generally less than 5% up to 30 months after stopping treatment. Administration of pyrazinamide beyond two months has not been shown to be advantageous (57). However, for individual cases with extensive disease and slow sputum bacteriologic conversion, prolonging the administration of pyrazinamide and ethambutol/streptomycin beyond two months may be acceptable. Prolonging the total duration of treatment can also be considered on a case-by-case basis. Cavitation and positive sputum culture after two months of treatment have been found to be associated with increased risk of failure/relapse and may justify prolongation of therapy to nine months (58). Regimens based predominantly on isoniazid and rifampin are only good for pansusceptible TB and have to be continued for nine months. They may be more suitable for patients who cannot tolerate pyrazinamide. Intermittent regimens with two drugs given three times or twice weekly in the continuation phase, following an intensive phase of four drugs given on a daily basis, have been shown to be highly effective. The World Health Organization (WHO), however, does not generally recommend twice-weekly treatment because of the higher risk of failure with missed doses (56). A more recent analysis has also raised concerns on the efficacy of three-times weekly six-month regimens in preventing disease relapse in the presence of cavitation (59).

Rifapentine, a long-acting cyclopentyl rifamycin, has been shown to yield rather encouraging activity, when given with isoniazid in a once-weekly dosing schedule during the continuation treatment phase of pulmonary TB among HIV-uninfected subjects, though a failure/relapse rate of around 10% still appears high (60). Such scheduling does not appear suitable for HIV-related TB because of unfavorable treatment outcome and the risk of emergence of rifamycin resistance (61). Indeed, intermittent therapy with other common rifamycins such as rifabutin and rifampin was also found to be associated with higher risk of relapse and acquired rifamycin resistance (62–64). Further exploration of the optimal dosing and scheduling of rifapentine might be warranted (65,66).

For smear-positive pulmonary TB with previous history of treatment, an eight-month regimen is recommended, comprising five first-line drugs (streptomycin, isoniazid, rifampin, pyrazinamide, and ethambutol) for two months, followed by the standard four oral drugs for one month, and then rifampin, isoniazid, and ethambutol for another five months (56). Bacillary drug susceptibilities in vitro can help to guide modification of this regimen as required.

Fixed-dose drug-combination formulations comprising two, three, and even four drugs can enhance the ease of prescription, reduce medication errors, simplify drug pro-curement, and promote adherence by patients (67). When used properly, these combina-tion tablets should decrease the risk of development of MDR-TB (68). The main concern is the quality and bioavailability of their component drugs, especially rifampin (67).

Drug-resistant TB usually results from poor patient adherence and other aspects of failure in the implementation of an effectively functioning TB control program (69). A few decades ago, directly observed treatment (DOT) was shown to be highly efficacious in ensuring patient adherence in Chennai and Hong Kong (70). The short-course regi-men also successfully reduced the treatment duration to six months. In 1993, the WHO officially announced the new global strategy for TB control known as directly observed therapy, short-course (DOTS) (69). DOTS maximizes treatment success and markedly curtails the chance of developing drug resistance and should be regarded as the most cost-effective intervention in the control of TB. It should be viewed as an integral part of a comprehensive service that also includes elements of education, enablers, incentives, and holistic care that are conducive to success. Resolution of social disadvantage, especially poverty, is also of great importance.

Smear-Negative Pulmonary Tuberculosis

In many countries, nearly 50% of patients are diagnosed as having pulmonary TB on clinical and radiographic grounds, without immediate bacteriologic confirmation. In the first smear-negative study in Hong Kong, it was subsequently found that 36% of these patients had one or more initial sputum cultures positive for *M. tuberculosis*. When patients were observed until the appearance of radiographic and/or bacteriologic evi-dence for active disease, 57% of this control group required chemotherapy within 60 months (71).

The WHO currently recommends the use of six-month regimens—isoniazid, rifampin, and pyrazinamide daily for two months followed by isoniazid and rifampin daily or three-times weekly for another four months in the treatment of new smear-negative pulmonary TB (56). For patients living in areas with high levels of initial resistance to isoniazid and/or having extensive disease, or are HIV infected, ethambutol should be added as a component to the initial two months of treatment.

Multidrug-Resistant Pulmonary Tuberculosis

The standard short-course regimen under DOTS is generally regarded as insufficient for controlling established MDR-TB, with a cure rate less than or equal to 60% (72), and recurrence rate greater than or equal to 28% (73). The WHO has recommended a three-pronged approach called "DOTS-Plus" to manage MDR-TB, including widespread implementation of DOTS, improved drug susceptibility testing, and careful use of sec-ond-line anti-TB drugs after sound evaluation of cost, effectiveness, and feasibility (74).

Treatment with appropriate drugs (largely second-line agents) (Table 3) has been shown to improve the outcome of patients with MDR-TB. The typical regimen should contain at least four, preferably five, or even six drugs, with either certain or almost certain efficacy based on drug-susceptibility testing results and/or patient's treatment history (75). An injectable second-line agent (aminoglycosides/capreomycin) and a fluoroquinolone should generally be included. For example, a combination such as

Table 3 Adverse Reactions to Antituberculosis Drugs

Drug	Reactions		
	Common	Uncommon	Rare
Drugs commonly used in conventional therapy			
Isoniazid		Hepatitis cutaneous hypersensitivity	Dizziness
		Peripheral neuropathy	Seizure
			Optic neuritis
			Mental symptoms
			Hemolytic anemia
			Aplastic anemia
			Lupoid reactions
			Arthralgia
			Gynecomastia
Rifampin		Hepatitis	Shortness of breath
		Cutaneous hypersensitivity	Shock
		Gastrointestinal reactions	Hemolytic anemia
		Thrombocytopenic purpura	Acute renal failure
		Febrile reactions	
		"Flu syndrome"	
Pyrazinamide	Anorexia	Hepatitis	Sideroblastic anemia
	Nausea	Vomiting	Gout
	Flushing	Arthralgia	
	Photosensitization	Cutaneous reaction	
Ethambutol		Retrobulbar neuritis	Hepatitis
		Arthralgia	Cutaneous reaction
			Peripheral neuropathy
Streptomycin	Cutaneous hypersensitivity	Vertigo	Renal damage
	Dizziness	Ataxia	Aplastic anemia
	Numbness	Deafness	
	Tinnitus	Deranged renal function tests	
Drugs commonly used in therapy for MDR-TB			
Amikacin Kanamycin Capreomycin	Ototoxicity: hearing damage, vestibular disturbance Nephrotoxicity: deranged renal function test	Clinical renal failure	
Ofloxacin / Levofloxacin[a] Ciprofloxacin Moxifloxacin[b]	Gastrointestinal reactions Insomnia	Anxiety Dizziness Headache Tremor	Seizure Hemolysis
Ethionamide Prothionamide	Gastrointestinal reactions	Hepatitis Cutaneous reactions Peripheral neuropathy	Seizure Depression Impotence Gynecomastia

Table 3 Adverse Reactions to Antituberculosis Drugs (*Continued*)

Drug	Reactions		
	Common	Uncommon	Rare
Cycloserine	Dizziness Headache Depression Memory loss	Psychosis Seizure	Sideroblastic anemia
Para-aminosalicylic acid	Gastrointestinal reactions	Hepatitis Drug fever	Hypothyroidism Hematologic disorders Metabolic acidosis Sodium overload
Clofazimine[c]	Photosensitization Hyperpigmentation Cutaneous reactions	Gastrointestinal reactions Retinopathy	Intestinal obstruction
Amoxicillin-clavulanate[c]	Gastrointestinal reactions Cutaneous hypersensitivity	Headache Hematologic reactions Vasculitis	Hepatitis Colitis Steven–Johnson syndrome Seizure
Linezolid[c,d]	Diarrhea Dyspepsia Headache	Thrombocytopenia Aplastic anemia	Colitis Peripheral and optic neuropathies

[a]Levofloxacin is better tolerated than ofloxacin.
[b]Experience on moxifloxacin tolerance is accumulating.
[c]Role in treatment of MDR-TB not fully delineated.
[d]Toxic effects appear common with long-term use.

kanamycin-fluoroquinolone-cthambutol-pyrazinamide-ethionamide/prothionamide can be used for MDR-TB with bacillary resistance to isoniazid and rifampin only, but recourse to a regimen containing kanamycin–fluoroquinolone–para-aminosalicylic acid–cycloserine–ethionamide/prothionamide is required for bacillary resistance to isoniazid, rifampin, ethambutol, and pyrazinamide, with or without streptomycin. The duration of aminoglycoside is generally six months in total, with lengthening or shortening permitted for difficult disease or drug intolerance, respectively on a case-by-case basis (75). Intermittent treatment can be used to lower the risk of aminoglycoside toxicity. The WHO has recommended treatment duration of at least 18 months after smear conversion, even for HIV-negative patients (76). However, there is some preliminary evidence that at least a proportion of immunocompetent patients who manage to achieve sustained sputum culture conversion to negativity early in the treatment course could be adequately treated with 12-month fluoroquinolone-containing regimens (77). Second-line (reserve) drugs for treating MDR-TB are generally more toxic and difficult to tolerate. About 40% of such patients experienced adverse drug reactions of varying severity in a study in Hong Kong (77). However, only half of them required modification of drug regimens. These adverse reactions are summarized, alongside those of first-line agents, in Table 3.

Development of New Drugs

The development of new anti-TB drugs is required to (*i*) shorten duration and/or improve intermittency of current short-course chemotherapy, (*ii*) improve treatment of MDR-TB and XDR-TB, and (*iii*) provide more effective treatment for LTBI. A number of new drugs are under various phases of clinical development. The most conspicuous examples include moxifloxacin (a 8-methoxyfluoroquinolone) (78), TMC207 (a diarylquinoline) (79), PA-824 (a nitroimidazopyran) (80), OPC-67683 (a nitroimidazo-oxazole) (81), LL-3858 (a pyrrole) (82), and SQ109 (an ethylene diamine) (83).

B. Other Modalities of Treatment

Surgery

The global resurgence of TB, concomitant HIV epidemic, and emergency of MDR-TB/XDR-TB underscore renewed interest on surgical management of pleuropulmonary TB. Broadly speaking, the role of surgery resides in three major areas: (*i*) establishment of definitive diagnosis, after failed attempts with less invasive investigations, (*ii*) treatment of MDR-TB, TB empyema, and other complications of active TB, and (*iii*) treatment of complications representing sequelae of previous TB. The three basic selective criteria for adjunctive surgery in MDR-TB patients include (*i*) profound drug resistance so that there is a high probability of failure or relapse with medical therapy alone, (*ii*) sufficiently localized disease so that the bulk of radiographically discernible disease can be resected with adequate cardiopulmonary capacity postsurgery, and (*iii*) drug activity is enough to diminish the mycobacterial burden to facilitate healing of the bronchial stump after lung resection (84). In general, patients should receive chemotherapy prior to surgery for at least three months (85), and if possible, rendered sputum culture negative before lung resection. However, this may not always occur. In some cases, bacteriologic conversion only occurs following a prolonged course of chemotherapy after surgery. In experienced hands, the outcome of lung resection has been found to be quite rewarding, with cure rates often reaching greater than or equal to 90% (75). In a large series of MDR-TB patients in the United States, surgical resection and medical therapy inclusive of fluoroquinolones were associated with improved outcomes after adjusting for other variables (86). For debilitated patients with apicocavitary TB, failing medical treatment, thoracoplasty, and other forms of collapse therapy can be considered (85). Complications of surgical resection mainly include respiratory failure, bronchopleural fistula, lung and other infections, empyema, wound bleeding, and/or breakdown, as well as recurrent laryngeal nerve injury.

Immunotherapy

In humans, the cell-mediated immunity against *M. tuberculosis* infection/disease is based on macrophage activation and granuloma formation that require cytokines, especially interferon-γ and TNF-α. Cytokine therapy was thus thought to be promising as adjunctive therapy in mycobacterial diseases, including MDR-TB. Some anecdotal reports on interferon-γ, interleukin-2, and interferon-α have shown promising results, but not others (75,87,88). Preliminary data on heat-killed *M. vaccae* have suggested possible efficacy in patients with MDR-TB (75). However, limited sample sizes, together with the often-uncontrolled experimental design, leave much uncertainty regarding the definitive role of these forms of immunotherapy (75).

VIII. Clinical Scenarios

A. Case 1

A 70-year-old man presented with unremitting fever for one month, associated with night sweats and weight loss. Physical examination was uninformative. Blood tests revealed anemia and a leucoerythroblastic picture. Bone marrow biopsy confirmed myelodysplastic syndrome with blastic transformation. While his chest radiograph was essentially normal, his whole-body positron emission tomograph/computed tomograph revealed a hypermetabolic nodule in the superior segment of left lower lobe and hypermetabolic lymph nodes in the right supraclavicular fossa and mediastinum. Aspirate from the supraclavicular lymph node revealed granulomatous inflammation and stainable AFB on direct microscopy. Its culture, as well as that of sputum and urine, subsequently grew *M. tuberculosis.*

Thus, this immunocompromised patient had disseminated TB with some respiratory symptoms and signs. The persistent fever provided a clue to search for an infective cause. The new imaging modalities helped to locate the lesions, and histological and microbiological investigations finally established the diagnosis.

B. Case 2

A 67-year-old woman had persistent fever for one month. She had atrial fibrillation, diabetes mellitus, dyslipidemia, and a previous episode of ischemic stroke. Chest radiograph only showed fibrocalcific changes in the right lung apex and ipsilateral pleural thickening. ESR was 35 mm/hr. Computed tomograph of thorax and abdomen revealed a cystic lesion in the head of pancreas. She underwent a needle aspiration of the pancreatic lesion and excision biopsy of a small but progressively enlarging left cervical lymph node. The latter revealed granulomatous inflammation with AFB on histological section. The pancreatic aspirate grew *M. tuberculosis* subsequently.

This case demonstrated the frequently encountered difficulty in diagnosing extrapulmonary TB, which commonly requires a constellation of investigative modalities.

C. Case 3

A 62-year-old occasional beer drinker with smear-positive pulmonary TB was started on isoniazid, rifampin, ethambutol, and pyrazinamide. After two days of treatment, he developed severe vomiting. Serum bilirubin rose to 2.5 times the upper limit of normal, and serum alanine aminotransferase to three times the upper limit of normal. Hepatitis B virus DNA was found to be present in great abundance in serum. After partial normalization of his liver chemistry, streptomycin, ethambutol, and levofloxacin were administered and tolerated, followed by sequential addition of isoniazid and rifampin. Levofloxacin was finally removed from the drug regimen when coadministration of isonaizid and rifampin could be tolerated.

This case demonstrated the development of drug-induced hepatitis following administration of anti-TB drugs in a patient with chronic hepatitis B infection. Other known risk factors include chronic hepatitis C infection, HIV infection, alcoholism, malnutrition, and old age. Streptomycin, ethambutol, and levofloxacin are potentially less hepatotoxic than isoniazid, rifampin, and pyrazinamide and could find a role in the management of TB patients with drug-induced hepatitis.

D. Case 4

A 35-year-old man presented with history of progressive weight loss and malaise following anti-TB treatment for several months. He had smear-negative pulmonary TB initially and was prescribed a self-administered regimen that was comprised isoniazid, rifampin, and pyrazinamide only, despite a chest radiograph showing a cavitary lesion in the right upper lobe. He was found to have abundant AFB on sputum examination by direct microscopy on admission to the hospital, and MDR-TB was suspected. He was thus given second-line anti-TB drugs comprising kanamycin, levofloxacin, prothionamide, ethambutol, and pyrazinamide. After about two months of such treatment, his sputum smear converted to negativity. Subsequently, his sputum culture grew *M. tuberculosis* resistant to isoniazid and rifampin in vitro.

This case illustrated the most important determinants for development of drug-resistant TB, namely prescription of inadequate drug regimen and poor treatment adherence. In a community where the rate of resistance of *M. tuberculosis* strains to isoniazid is high ($\geq$4%), a fourth drug, ethambutol or less preferably streptomycin, should be added, especially when the disease is multibacillary and/or extensive. Directly observed therapy still provides the best guarantee on patient's adherence.

IX. Prevention

Stopping the disease at source is the key strategy in TB control. Early diagnosis and effective treatment of TB patients by DOTS (and DOTS-Plus) rapidly reduces the number of infectious sources in the community (56,89). Health education, proper health care infrastructure, and community support are essential for promotion of passive case-finding and adherence to treatment.

In view of the airborne nature of the pathogen (4), a hierarchy of administrative, environmental, and personal protective measures is recommended to contain the infectious sources, reduce the environmental pathogen level, and protect those at risk of exposure in health care settings and other high-risk environments (90). Targeted screening and treatment of LTBI help to reduce the risk of developing disease among recent contacts and other at-risk groups (2). It may also have the potential to reduce the incidence of disease arising from endogenous reactivation of remote infection.

Bacille Calmette–Guérin (BCG) vaccine is probably one of the most widely used and safest vaccines. Meta-analyses of previous studies support a protective efficacy of around 80% against the more serious forms of childhood TB, especially miliary TB and TB meningitis (91,92). The protection against adult pulmonary TB is controversial, with efficacy ranging from 0% to 80% (93,94). Revaccination does not offer additional protection (95). Disseminated BCGosis is rare and only occurs in patients with impaired immunity. As a live vaccine, it is contraindicated in pregnancy. In view of the possibility of disseminated disease, WHO no longer recommends BCG vaccination in asymptomatic HIV-infected children, even in areas with high incidence of TB (96). The relatively poor protection of BCG against the infectious adult form of TB has greatly limited its role in the overall control of the disease, in sharp contrast to the pivotal roles of other childhood vaccines (e.g., poliomyelitis and measles vaccines). The deciphering of the *M. tuberculosis* and BCG genome has provided important information to guide the development of new TB vaccines (97,98).

References

1. World Health Organization. Global tuberculosis control: surveillance, planning, financing. WHO Report 2008. Geneva, Switzerland: WHO, 2008. [WHO/HTM/TB/2008.393].

2. Centers for Disease Control and Prevention. Targeted tuberculin skin testing and treatment of latent tuberculosis infection. MMWR Recomm Rep 2000; 49(RR-6):1–51.

3. World Health Organization. Anti-tuberculosis drug resistance in the world. Fourth global report. The WHO/IUATLD global project on antituberculosis drug resistance surveillance. Geneva, Switzerland: WHO, 2008. [WHO/HTM/TB/2008.394].

4. Riley RL, Wells W, Mills C. Air Hygiene in tuberculosis: quantitative studies of infectivity and control in a pilot ward. Am Rev Tuberc Pulm Dis 1957; 75:420–430.

5. Leung CC, Li T, Lam TH, et al. Smoking and tuberculosis among the elderly in Hong Kong. Am J Respir Crit Care Med 2004; 170:1027–1033.

6. Leung CC, Lam TH, Chan WM, et al. Lower risk of tuberculosis in obesity. Arch Intern Med 2007; 167:1297–1304.

7. Marais BJ, Gie RP, Schaaf HS, et al. The natural history of childhood intra-thoracic tuberculosis: a critical review of literature from the pre-chemotherapy era. Int J Tuberc Lung Dis 2004; 8:392–402.

8. McNeil MR, Brennan PJ. Structure, function, and biogenesis of the cell envelope of mycobacteria in relation to bacterial physiology, pathogenesis, and drug resistance: some thoughts and possibilities arising from recent structural information. Res Microbiol 1991; 142:451–463.

9. Crowe LM, Spargo BJ, Ioneda T, et al. Interaction of cord factor (alpha, alpha'-trehalose-6,6'-dimycolate) with phospholipids. Biochim Biophys Acta 1994; 1194:53–60.

10. Chan J, Fan XD, Hunter SW, et al. Lipoarabinomannan, a possible virulence factor involved in persistence of Mycobacterium tuberculosis within macrophages. Infect Immun 1991; 59.1755–1761.

11. Arruda S, Bomfim G, Knights R, et al. Cloning of an M. tuberculosis DNA fragment associated with entry and survival inside cells. Science 1993; 261:1454–1457.

12. Shimono N, Morici L, Casali N, et al. Hypervirulent mutant of Mycobacterium tuberculosis resulting from disruption of the mce1 operon. Proc Natl Acad Sci U S A 2003; 100: 15918–15923.

13. McCune RM, Feldmann FM, Lambert HP, et al. Microbial persistence I. The capacity of tubercle bacilli to survive sterilization in mouse tissues. J Exp Med 1966; 123:445–468.

14. McCune RM, Feldmann FM, McDermott W. Microbial persistence II. Characteristics of the sterile state of tubercle bacilli. J Exp Med 1966; 123:469–486.

15. Scanga CA, Mohan VP, Joseph H, et al. Reactivation of latent tuberculosis: variations on the Cornell murine model. Infect Immun 1999; 67:4531–4538.

16. DeMaio J, Zhang Y, Ko C, et al. A stationary-phase stress-response sigma factor from Mycobacterium tuberculosis. Proc Natl Acad Sci U S A 1996; 93:2790–2794.

17. Sherman DR, Voskuil M, Schnappinger D, et al. Regulation of the Mycobacterium tuberculosis hypoxic response gene encoding alpha-crystallin. Proc Natl Acad Sci U S A 2001; 98:7534–7539.

18. Park HD, Guinn KM, Harrell MI, et al. Rv3133c/dosR is a transcription factor that mediates the hypoxic response of *Mycobacterium tuberculosis*. Mol Microbiol 2003; 48:833–843.

19. Wisedchaisri G, Wu M, Rice AE, et al. Structures of *Mycobacterium tuberculosis* DosR and DosR-DNA complex involved in gene activation during adaptation to hypoxic latency. J Mol Biol 2005; 354:630–641.

20. Medzhitov R, Preston-Hurlburt P, Janeway CA Jr. A human homologue of the Drosophila Toll protein signals activation of adaptive immunity. Nature 1997; 388:394–397.

21. Underhill DM, Ozinsky A, Smith KD, et al. Toll-like receptor-2 mediates mycobacteria-induced proinflammatory signaling in macrophages. Proc Natl Acad Sci U S A 1999; 96:14459–14463.

22. Thoma-Uszynski S, Stenger S, Takeuchi O, et al. Induction of direct antimicrobial activity through mammalian toll-like receptors. Science 2001; 291:1544–1547.

23. Liu PT, Stenger S, Li H, et al. Toll-like receptor triggering of a vitamin-D mediated human antimicrobial response. Science 2006; 311:1770–1773.

24. Takeda K, Kaisho T, Akira S. Toll-like receptors. Annu Rev Immunol 2003; 21:335–376.

25. Sugawara I, Yamada H, Mizuno S, et al. Mycobacterial infection in MyD88-deficient mice. Microbiol Immunol 2003; 47:841–847.

26. Yuan Y, Lee RE, Besra GS, et al. Identification of a gene involved in the biosynthesis of cyclopropanated mycolic acids in *Mycobacterium tuberculosis*. Proc Natl Acad Sci U S A 1995; 92:6630–6634.

27. Goren MB, D'Arcy Hart P, Young MR, et al. Prevention of phagosome-lysosome fusion in cultured macrophages by sulfatides of *Mycobacterium tuberculosis*. Proc Natl Acad Sci U S A 1976; 73:2510–2514.

28. Xu S, Cooper A, Sturgill-Koszycki S, et al. Intracellular trafficking in *Mycobacterium tuberculosis* and *Mycobacterium avium*–infected macrophages. J Immunol 1994; 153:2568–2578.

29. Pancholi P, Mirza A, Schauf V, et al. Presentation of mycobacterial antigens by human dendritic cells: lack of transfer from infected macrophages. Infect Immun 1993; 61:5326–5332.

30. MacMicking JD, North RJ, LaCourse R, et al. Identification of nitric oxide synthase as a protective locus against tuberculosis. Proc Natl Acad Sci U S A 1997; 94:5243–5248.

31. Cooper AM, Dalton DK, Steward TA, et al. Disseminated tuberculosis in interferon-gamma gene-disrupted mice. J Exp Med 1993; 178:2243–2247.

32. Wang CH, Liu CY, Lin HC, et al. Increased exhaled nitric oxide in active pulmonary tuberculosis due to inducible NO synthase upregulation in alveolar macrophages. Eur Respir J 1998; 11:809–815.

33. Poulter LW, Rook GA, Steele J, et al. Influence of 1,25-(OH)2 vitamin D3 and gamma interferon on the phenotype of human peripheral blood monocyte-derived macrophages. Infect Immun 1987; 55:2017–2020.

34. Rockett KA, Brookes R, Udalova I, et al. 1,25-Dihydroxyvitamin D3 induces nitric oxide synthase and suppresses Mycobacterium tuberculosis in human macrophage-like cell line. Infect Immun 1998; 66:5314–5321.

35. Lowin B, Hahne M, Mattmann C, et al. Cytotoxic T-cell cytotoxicity is mediated through perforin and Fas lytic pathways. Nature 1994; 370:650–652.

36. Jouanguy E, Doffinger R, Dupuis S, et al. IL-12 and IFN-gamma in host defense against mycobacteria and salmonella in mice and men. Curr Opin Immunol 1999; 11:346–351.

37. Keane J, Gershon S, Wise RP, et al. Tuberculosis associated with infliximab, a tumor necrosis factor alpha-neutralizing agent. N Engl J Med 2001; 345:1098–1104.

38. Rook GA. Th2 cytokines in susceptibility to tuberculosis. Curr Mol Med 2007; 7:327–337.

39. Ewer K, Deeks J, Alvarez L, et al. Comparison of T-cell-based assay with tuberculin skin test for diagnosis of Mycobacterium tuberculosis infection in a school tuberculosis outbreak. Lancet 2003; 361:1168–1173.

40. Ferrara G, Losi M, D'Amico R, et al. Use in routine clinical practice of two commercial blood tests for diagnosis of infection with Mycobacterium tuberculosis: a prospective study. Lancet 2006; 367:1328–1334.

41. Menzies D, Pai M, Comstock G. Meta-analysis: new tests for the diagnosis of latent tuberculosis infection: areas of uncertainty and recommendations for research. Ann Intern Med. 2007; 146:340–354.

42. Leung CC, Yew WW, Chang KC, et al. Risk of active tuberculosis among schoolchildren in Hong Kong. Arch Pediatr Adolesc Med 2006; 160:247–251.
43. Leung CC, Yam WC, Yew WW, et al. Comparison of T-Spot.TB and tuberculin skin test among silicotic patients. Eur Respir J 2008; 31:266–272.
44. Abebe F, Holm-Hansen C, Wiker HG, et al. Progress in serodiagnosis of Mycobacterium tuberculosis infection. Scand J Immunol 2007; 66:176–191.
45. American Thoracic Society. Diagnostic standards and classification of tuberculosis in adults and children. Am J Respir Crit Care Med 2000; 161:1376–1395.
46. Im JG, Itoh H, Shim YS. Pulmonary tuberculosis: CT findings-early active disease and sequential change with antituberculosis therapy. Radiology 1993; 186:653–660.
47. Yeager HJ, Lacy J, Smith L, et al. Quantititaive studies of mycobacterial population in sputum and saliva. Am Rev Respir Dis 1967; 95:998–1004.
48. Hobby GL, Holman AP, Iseman MD, et al. Enumeration of tubercle bacilli in sputum of patients with pulmonary tuberculosis. Antimicrob Agents Chemother 1973; 4:94–104.
49. Moore DA, Evans CA, Gilman RH, et al. Microscopic observation drug-susceptibility assay for the diagnosis of TB. N Engl J Med 2006; 355:1539–1550.
50. Villegas MV, Labrada LA, Saravia NG. Evaluation of polymerase chain reaction, adenosine deaminase, and interferon-gamma in pleural fluid for the differential diagnosis of pleural tuberculosis. Chest 2000; 118:1355–1364.
51. Hong Kong Chest Service, Tuberculosis Research Centre, Madras, British Medical Research Council. A double-blind placebo-controlled clinical trial of three anti-tuberculosis chemo-prophylaxis regimens in patients with silicosis in Hong Kong. Am Rev Respir Dis 1992; 145:36–41.
52. Menzies D, Dion MJ, Rabinovitch B, et al. Treatment completion and costs of a randomized trial of rifampin for 4 months versus isoniazid for 9 months. Am J Respir Crit Care Med 2004; 170:445–449.
53. Leung CC, Law WS, Chang KC, et al. Initial experience on rifampin and pyrazinamide vs isoniazid in the treatment of latent tuberculosis infection among patients with silicosis in Hong Kong. Chest 2003; 124:2112–2118.
54. Blumberg HM, Leonard MK Jr., Jasmer RM. Update on the treatment of tuberculosis and latent tuberculosis infection. JAMA 2005; 293:2776–2784.
55. Centers for Disease Control and Prevention, American Thoracic Society. Update: adverse event data and revised American Thoracic Society/CDC recommendations against the use of rifampin and pyrazinamide for treatment of latent tuberculosis infection—United States, 2003. MMWR 2003; 52:735–739.
56. World Health Organization. Treatment of tuberculosis. Guidelines for National Programmes. Geneva, Switzerland: WHO, 2003:27–38. [WHO/CDS/TB/2003.313].
57. Hong Kong Chest Service, British Medical Research Council. Controlled trial of 2, 4, and 6 months of pyrazinamide in 6-month three-times weekly regimens for smear-positive pulmonary tuberculosis, including an assessment of a combined preparation of isoniazid, rifampin and pyrazinamide. Results at 30 months. Am Rev Respir Dis 1991; 143:700–706.
58. American Thoracic Society, Centers for Disease Control and Prevention, Infections Diseases Society of America. Treatment of tuberculosis. Am J Respir Crit Care Med 2003; 167: 603–662.
59. Chang KC, Leung CC, Yew WW, et al. A nested case-control study on treatment-related risk factors for early relapse of tuberculosis. Am J Respir Crit Care Med 2004; 170:1124–1130.
60. Tam CM, Chan SL, Kam KM, et al. Rifapentine and isoniazid in the continuation phase of a 6-month regimen. Final report at 5 years: prognostic value of various measures. Int J Tuberc Lung Dis 2002; 6:3–10.

61. Vernon AA, Burman W, Benator D, et al. Tuberculosis Trials Consortium. Acquired rifamycin monoresistance in patients with HIV-related tuberculosis treated with once-weekly rifapentine and isoniazid. Lancet 1999; 353:1843–1847.

62. Li J, Munsiff SS, Driver CR, et al. Relapse and acquired rifampin resistance in HIV-infected patients with tuberculosis treated with rifampin- or rifabutin-based regimens in New York City, 1997–2000. Clin Infect Dis 2005; 41:83–91.

63. Burman W, Benator D, Vernon A, et al. Tuberculosis Trials Consortium. Acquired rifamycin resistance with twice-weekly treatment of HIV-related tuberculosis. Am J Respir Crit Care Med 2006; 173:350–356.

64. Nahid P, Gonzalez LC, Rudoy I, et al. Treatment outcomes of patients with HIV and tuberculosis. Am J Respir Crit Care Med 2007; 175:1199–1206.

65. Bock NN, Sterling TR, Hamilton CD, et al. Tuberculosis Trials Consortium, Centers for Disease Control and Prevention. A prospective, randomized double-blind study of the tolerability of rifapentine 600, 900, 1200 mg plus isoniazid in the continuation phase of tuberculosis treatment. Am J Respir Crit Care Med 2002; 165:1526–1530.

66. Sirgel FA, Fourie PB, Donald PR, et al. The early bactericidal activities of rifampin and rifapentine in pulmonary tuberculosis. Am J Respir Crit Care Med 2005; 172:128–135.

67. Sbarbaro J, Blomberg B, Chaulet P. Fixed-dose combination formulations for tuberculosis treatment. Int J Tuberc Lung Dis 1999; 3:S286–S288.

68. Moulding TS, Le HQ, Rikleen D, et al. Preventing drug-resistant tuberculosis with a fixed dose combination of isoniazid and rifampin. Int J Tuberc Lung Dis 2004; 8:743–748.

69. Yew WW. Directly observed therapy, short-course: the best way to prevent multidrug-resistant tuberculosis. Chemotherapy 1999; 45:S26–S33.

70. Bayer R, Wilkinson D. Directly observed therapy for tuberculosis: history of an idea. Lancet 1995; 345:1545–1548.

71. Hong Kong Chest Service, Tuberculosis Research Centre, Madras, British Medical Research Council. A controlled trial of 2-month, 3-month and 12-month regimens of chemotherapy for sputum smear-negative pulmonary tuberculosis. Results at 60 months. Am Rev Respir Dis 1984; 130:23–28.

72. Espinal MA, Kim SJ, Suarez PG, et al. Standard short-course chemotherapy for drug-resistant tuberculosis: treatment outcomes in 6 countries. JAMA 2000; 283:2537–2545.

73. Migliori GB, Espinal M, Danilova ID, et al. Frequency of recurrence among MDR-TB cases 'successfully' treated with standardised short-course chemotherapy. Int J Tuberc Lung Dis 2002; 6:858–864.

74. Dye C, Williams BG, Espinal MA, et al. Erasing the world's slow stain: strategies to beat multidrug-resistant tuberculosis. Science 2002; 295:2042–2046.

75. Yew WW, Leung CC. Management of multidrug-resistant tuberculosis: update 2007. Respirology 2008; 13(1):21–46.

76. World Health Organization. Guidelines for the programmatic management of drug-resistant tuberculosis. Geneva, Switzerland: WHO, 2006:38–92. [WHO/HTM/TB/2006.361].

77. Yew WW, Chan CK, Chau CH, et al. Outcomes of patients with multidrug-resistant pulmonary tuberculosis treated with ofloxacin/levofloxacin containing regimens. Chest 2000; 117:744–751.

78. Veziris N, Truffot-Pernot C, Aubry A, et al. Fluoroquinolone-containing third-line regimen against Mycobacterium tuberculosis in vivo. Antimicrob Agents Chemother 2003; 47:3117–3122.

79. Andries K, Verhasselt P, Guillemont J, et al. A diarylquinoline drug active on the ATP synthase of Mycobacterium tuberculosis. Science 2005; 307:223–227.

80. Tyagi S, Nuermberger E, Yoshimatsu T, et al. Bactericidal activity of the nitroimidazopyran PA-824 in a murine model of tuberculosis. Antimicrob Agents Chemother 2005; 49:2289–2293.

81. Matsumoto M, Hashizume H, Tomishige T, et al. OPC-67683, a nitro-dihydro-imidazoox-azole derivative with promising action against tuberculosis in vitro and in mice. PLoS Med 2006; 3:e466.

82. Deidda D, Lampis G, Fioravanti R, et al. Bactericidal activities of the pyrrole derivative BM212 against multidrug-resistant and intramacrophagic M. tuberculosis strains. Antimicrob Agents Chemother 1998; 42:3035–3037.

83. Nikonenko BV, Protopopova M, Samala R, et al. Drug therapy of experimental tuberculosis (TB): improved outcome by combining SQ109, a new diamine antibiotic, with existing TB drugs. Antimicrob Agents Chemother 2007; 51:1563–1565.

84. Iseman MD, Madsen L, Goble M, et al. Surgical intervention in the treatment of pulmonary disease caused by drug-resistant Mycobacterium tuberculosis. Am Rev Respir Dis 1990; 141:623–625.

85. Pomerantz M, Brown JM. Surgery in the treatment of multidrug-resistant tuberculosis. Clin Chest Med 1997; 18:123–130.

86. Chan ED, Laurel V, Strand MJ, et al. Treatment and outcome analysis of 205 patients with multidrug-resistant tuberculosis. Am J Respir Crit Care Med 2004; 169:1103–1109.

87. Condos R, Rom WN, Schluger NW. Treatment of multidrug-resistant pulmonary tuberculosis with interferon-gamma via acrosol. Lancet 1997; 349:1513–1515.

88. Park SK, Cho S, Lee IH, et al. Subcutaneously administered interferon-gamma for the treatment of multidrug-resistant pulmonary tuberculosis. Int J Infect Dis 2007; 11:434–440.

89. Joloba ML, Johnson JL, Namale A, et al. Quantitative sputum bacillary load during rifampin-containing short course chemotherapy in human immunodeficiency virus-infected and non-infected adults with pulmonary tuberculosis. Int J Tuberc Lung Dis 2000; 4:528–536.

90. Jensen PA, Lambert LA, Iademarco MF, et al. Guidelines for preventing the transmission of *Mycobacterium tuberculosis* in health-care settings, 2005. MMWR Recomm Rep 2005; 54:1–141.

91. Rodrigues LC, Diwan VD, Wheeler JG. Protective effect of BCG against tuberculous meningitis and miliary tuberculosis: a meta analysis. Int J Epidemiol 1993; 22:1154–1158.

92. Colditz GA, Berkey CS, Mosteller F, et al. The efficacy of Bacille Calmette-Guerin vaccination of newborns and infants in the prevention of tuberculosis: meta-analysis of the published literature. Pediatrics 1995; 96:29–35.

93. Colditz GA, Brewer TF, Berkey CS, et al. Efficacy of BCG vaccine in the prevention of tuberculosis. JAMA 1994; 271:698–702.

94. Brewer TF. Preventing tuberculosis with bacillus Calmette-Guerin vaccine: a meta-analysis of the literature. Clin Infect Dis 2000; 31(suppl 3):S64—S67.

95. Leung CC, Tam CM, Chan SL, et al. Efficacy of BCG revaccination programme in a cohort given BCG vaccination at birth in Hong Kong. Int J Tuber Lung Dis 2001; 5:717–723.

96. Global Advisory Committee on Vaccine Safety. Revised BCG vaccination guidelines for infants at risk for HIV infection. Wkly Epidemiol Rec 2007; 82:193–196.

97. Cole ST, Brosch R, Parkhill J, et al. Deciphering the biology of Mycobacterium tuberculosis from the complete genome sequence. Nature 1998; 93:537–544.

98. Gupta UD, Katoch VM, McMurray DN. Current status of TB vaccines. Vaccine 2007; 25:3742–3751.

15

Nontuberculous Mycobacterial Respiratory Infections

BRENDAN J. CLARK
University of Colorado Health Sciences Center, Denver, Colorado, U.S.A.

CHARLES L. DALEY
National Jewish Health and University of Colorado Health Sciences Center,
Denver, Colorado, U.S.A.

I. Introduction

Shortly following the discovery of *Mycobacterium tuberculosis* by Koch in 1882, several other species of mycobacteria were described. However, it was not clear until the 1950s that some could cause disease in humans (1). The terms "mycobacteria other than tuberculosis" (TB), "environmental mycobacteria," "anonymous or atypical mycobacteria," and "nontuberculous mycobacteria" (NTM) have been used to describe these and refer to species other than those in the *M. tuberculosis* complex. Collectively, 130 species have been identified and many have been reported to cause pulmonary disease, lymphadenitis, soft tissue infections, bone and joint disease, genitourinary disease, eye infections, and disseminated disease. This chapter uses the term "NTM" and focuses on the pulmonary disease caused by these organisms.

II. Taxonomy

When Timpe and Runyon examined cultures of 88 human samples of NTM in 1954, they were able to divide them into three groups on the basis of phenotypic appearance (2). In 1959, Runyon further refined this classification system to divide the NTM into four groups on the basis of growth rate (rapid vs. slow) and pigmentation (pigmented vs. nonpigmented) (3). While this popular classification system is still commonly used today, molecular tools have replaced growth and biochemical tests to define new species of NTM. Species are now defined by analysis of two hypervariable regions in the highly conserved 16S ribosomal RNA (rRNA) sequence (4). Species differ by as little as 1% (3). The number of described species has nearly tripled from 50 in 1997 to 130 today as a result of these new techniques (5). A minority of these species is responsible for most of the pulmonary infections in humans. These most commonly include *M. avium* complex (MAC), *M. abscessus*, *M. kansasii*, *M. malmoense*, and *M. xenopi* (6).

III. Epidemiology

A. Incidence and Prevalence

Determining the incidence and prevalence of NTM disease is difficult because reporting is not mandatory in most parts of the world. The various study methods have difficulty discriminating between exposure and disease. Thus, the estimates between studies vary widely, even in the same location (7). Although not definitive, the existing data suggest that the incidence and prevalence of NTM are increasing.

Studies using a delayed type hypersensitivity reaction to subcutaneously injected mycobacterial antigens have estimated that 11% to 33.5% of the population in the United States has been exposed to NTM (7). The wide variation is partially explained by the different definitions used for exposure. Landmark skin testing studies done by Palmer (8) and Edwards (9) resulted in estimates of 33.5% and 29%, respectively. A recent study reported the results of skin testing with purified protein derivative-Battey (PPD-B) during two time periods in the National Health and Nutrition Examination Survey (NHANES) cohort. For the years 1971 to 1972 and 1999 to 2000, rates of a positive skin test were 11.2% and 16.6%, respectively (10). This markedly lower frequency of skin test reactivity to PPD-B compared with the study by Edwards is likely explained by a more strict definition of a positive test (5 mm induration and 3 mm greater than reaction to PPD-S). By assessing the same test in the same population separated by time, this study supports the observation that the prevalence of NTM infection is increasing.

Studies combining culture and clinical data may be more useful for estimating disease incidence and prevalence. A common theme of these studies is an increasing rate of NTM pulmonary infection or disease and a decreasing incidence of pulmonary TB. In Japan from 1971 to 1984, the incidence of pulmonary TB decreased from 133.1 to 46.3 per 100,000 while the incidence of NTM pulmonary disease increased from 0.89 to 2.15 (11). A similar report from Switzerland reported a decrease in the incidence of pulmonary TB from 16.2 to 13.2 per 100,000 over six years while the incidence of pulmonary NTM increased from 0.4 to 0.9 per 100,000 (12). Reports since the 1950s from Czechoslovakia (13), Wales (14), Ireland (15), Australia (16), and the United States (17) using different methods to assess incidence or prevalence have also reported increases. Marras and coworkers reported an increase in the number of pulmonary NTM isolates in Ontario from 9.1 per 100,000 in 1997 to 14.1 per 100,000 in 2003. One-third of the patients met diagnostic criteria for pulmonary disease (18). In contrast, a study from France prospectively evaluating the incidence of pulmonary NTM disease from 2001 to 2003 showed that the incidence did not change, remaining constant at 0.7 per 100,000 (19). Overall, however, the preponderance of evidence suggests that pulmonary disease due to NTM is increasing.

The reasons for the increase in incidence and prevalence have not been defined although several explanations have been proposed (7,16). The rise may not truly reflect an increase, but rather an increased awareness of the disease or improved diagnostic techniques. Alternatively, a true increase in incidence could be related to changes in the host such as an aging population, an increase in the number of immunocompromised individuals, or an increased prevalence of chronic lung disease. The consistent observation of a decreased incidence of pulmonary TB and an increased incidence of pulmonary NTM could be explained by cross-immunity between mycobacterial species.

Finally, an increase in the prevalence or virulence of organisms in the environment or changes in human behavior that would lead to increased exposure to organisms (e.g., showering) could be contributing.

B. Geographic Distribution

NTM have been reported to cause pulmonary disease in six continents. There is a marked variation in the prevalence of disease and predominant species both within and between countries. In the United States, the southeastern region seems to have the highest rate of infection (17,20,21). NTM have been recovered with higher frequency from water samples in the southeastern versus northern United States (22) and grow better at temperatures greater than 15.5°C (23), offering a possible explanation for this observation. The predominant species in North America have consistently been MAC, followed by *M. kansasii, M. abscessus, M. fortuitum, M. chelonae*, and *M. scrofulaceum* (16,17,20). MAC has also been reported as the predominant species in Central and South America, Europe, and Asia. *M. xenopi* is common in Europe and Canada (24), while *M. malmoense* is more common in northern Europe. Populations of miners in Czechoslovakia (13) and South Africa (25,26) have high rates of *M. kansasii*, likely reflecting different underlying risk factors.

IV. Pathogenesis, Risk Factors, and Specific Patient Populations

A. Pathogenesis and Risk Factors

NTM are ubiquitous in the environment and have been found in natural and drinking waters, biofilms, soil, aerosols, medical equipment, moldy buildings, and even cigarettes (27). Because human-to-human transmission has never been documented, the presumed source of infection is exposure to these environmental reservoirs. The mechanism by which an environmental exposure eventually leads to pulmonary infection is poorly understood. Because the pathologic response to TB and NTM are indistinguishable, it is presumed that the immune response is likely to be similar, eventually leading to granuloma formation (28). Important factors in granuloma formation include functional macrophages, T-cells, and cytokines [particularly interleukin (IL)-12, tumor necrosis factor (TNF)-α, and interferon (IFN)-γ]. Perturbations in each of these result in human hosts being predisposed to NTM pulmonary infection (6). Other proposed contributions to pathogenicity include the formation of biofilms and the ability to survive and escape immune surveillance in type II alveolar epithelial cells (29).

NTM are significantly less pathogenic than TB and likely require some degree of host impairment to establish infection (30). A number of risk factors for disease have been described. These can broadly be grouped into factors impairing host immunity, factors leading to impaired local (lung) immunity, and factors relating to patient demographics (Table 1). Increasing age has been consistently described as a risk factor for pulmonary NTM, both in patients with and without underlying lung disease (9,17,30,31). The most consistently reported risk factor is male gender, though there is also a population of elderly females who are at risk for nodular bronchiectatic lung disease (7,31). Smoking impairs pulmonary defenses against infection in a number of ways and has been described as a risk factor for other pulmonary infections, including TB (32).

Table 1 Risk Factors for NTM Respiratory Disease

Demographic factors	Immunodeficiency	Impaired local immunity
Age	IFN-γR mutations	Cystic fibrosis
Male—classic presentation	IL-12 p40/IL-12R mutations	Bronchiectasis
Female—nodular	HIV/AIDS	Pneumoconiosis
bronchiectasis	TNF-α antagonist therapy	α-1-Antitrypsin deficiency
Excessive alcohol	Diabetes	COPD
consumption	Chronic immunosuppressive	Prior TB
	therapy	Chronic aspiration
		Other causes of chronic lung disease

Abbreviations: NTM, nontuberculous mycobacteria; IFN, interferon; IL, interleukin; TNF, tumor necrosis factor; COPD, chronic obstructive pulmonary disease; TB, tuberculosis.

Perhaps the most important risk factor for the development of pulmonary NTM disease is underlying chronic lung disease. NTM disease has been described in association with COPD, cavitary lung disease, pneumoconiosis, bronchiectasis, prior TB, and pulmonary alveolar proteinosis (33). Factors including warmer climate and coastal location also seem to have an association.

B. Specific Patient Populations
Cystic Fibrosis
Mutations in the CFTR gene lead to viscous pulmonary secretions in patients with cystic fibrosis (CF). This predisposes them to a number of pulmonary infections and eventually leads to the development of bronchiectasis. Studies have documented a high prevalence of NTM from sputum cultures in patients with CF, with estimates ranging from 3% to 19.5% (34). A large prospective multicenter trial addressing this question estimated the prevalence to be 13% with MAC comprising 72% of these isolates (35). The diagnostic criteria for patients with CF do not differ from other patients. However, differentiating NTM infection from underlying CF can be difficult since CF shares many of the radiographic features of NTM infection (6). Additionally, bacterial overgrowth of sputum samples can hamper recovery of mycobacteria from sputum (36–38).

Bronchiectasis
Bronchiectasis can be both a cause and a consequence of NTM infection (39,40). Bronchiectasis seems to occur frequently in older women without underlying lung disease who are immunocompetent (31,41). The sensitivity of sputum culture in this population may be limited and alternative means of specimen collection such as sputum induction and bronchoscopy may be necessary to make a diagnosis (41). In contrast to patients with cavitary disease, patients with bronchiectasis are likely to be infected with two or more strains suggesting multiple or recurrent infections (42). In addition to antimicrobial therapy, chest physiotherapy to augment airway clearance is important although the optimal method is not known (43).

HIV and AIDS

NTM in AIDS most commonly causes disseminated disease presenting with nonspecific symptoms such as fever, night sweats, diarrhea, abdominal pain, and lymphadenopathy (44), with MAC being the most frequent isolate (45). Despite the fact that MAC is isolated from the sputum in up to 10% of patients with CD4 counts less than 50 cells/μL, pulmonary disease due to MAC is uncommon (46). Pulmonary disease been reported in 2.5% to 8% of patients with disseminated MAC (47) and has also rarely been reported in the absence of dissemination (47,48). Patients with pulmonary disease tend to have higher CD4 counts and focal alveolar infiltrates which rarely cavitate. Because it is much more common for MAC to colonize than to cause disease of the respiratory tract, other potential etiologies of respiratory infection in HIV infected patients should be excluded before considering MAC as a pathogen (6). *M. kansasii* is distinctly different from MAC in patients with HIV and AIDS. HIV imparted a 150-fold and AIDS a 900-fold risk for infection with *M. kansasii* in one study (49). In contrast to MAC, *M. kansasii* only rarely causes indolent disease and should almost always be treated as a pathogen (50).

Other Immunocompromised Patients

Pulmonary disease due to NTM has been described in several immunocompromised patient populations including transplant recipients. Rates may be as high as 6.5% following heart or lung transplant (51), 2.9% following bone marrow transplant (52), and are probably much lower in patients following liver or kidney transplant (53,54). Because of the susceptibility of this patient population to multiple opportunistic infections, patients with symptoms and nonresolving radiographic infiltrates should receive an aggressive diagnostic workup (53).

As discussed above, multiple cytokines are necessary for granuloma formation and eventual containment of mycobacterial infections. Principal among these are IFN-γ, IL-12, and TNF-α. Patient populations with defects in each of these are susceptible to infection with NTM. Mutations in IFN-γ receptor 1 (R1), IFN-γR2, IL-12 p40, and the IL-12 receptor have all been shown to lead to human disease (55). Dominant and recessive IFN-γR1 deficiencies have distinct clinical presentations (56). While there are no described mutations in TNF-α, large populations of patients with inflammatory bowel disease, rheumatoid arthritis, or psoriatic arthritis receive infusions of the TNF-α inhibitors infliximab, adalimumab, or etanercept. Although initially demonstrated to predispose to TB (57), recent reports have linked these therapies to NTM infections as well (58). Patients with mycobacterial infections should not receive these medications without proper antimycobacterial therapy.

V. Clinical Presentation and Radiographic Appearance

A. Fibrocavitary Lung Disease

The classical description of pulmonary infection with NTM is in middle-aged men who are smokers, consume alcohol, and have underlying chronic pulmonary disease, though patients may lack some or all of these risk factors. Presenting symptoms are difficult to differentiate from progression of underlying lung disease, often leading to a delay in diagnosis. They commonly include cough and dyspnea on exertion, while constitutional complaints such as fevers, night sweats, weight loss, and malaise are less common.

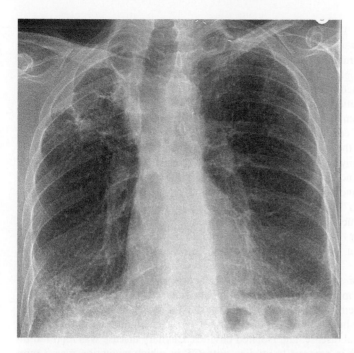

Figure 1 Chest radiograph of a 78-year-old man with underlying interstitial lung disease and *Mycobacterium intracellulare* lung disease. The chest radiograph demonstrates right upper lobe cavitary opacities with volume loss and pleural thickening. There are bibasilar lower lobe interstitial opacities related to his underlying interstitial lung disease.

There are no clinical features that reliably distinguish pulmonary NTM infection from other chronic pulmonary infections such as TB. MAC remains the most commonly isolated organism followed by *M. kansasii*, *M. abscessus*, and *M. fortuitum*. *M. xenopi* is more common in some areas such as Canada and Europe. Underlying lung disease is almost always present in *M. fortuitum*, in most cases of MAC and in half the cases of *M. kansasii* (1,17,59).

Radiographic findings in this form of disease will usually include apical linear opacities and nodules. Other findings include cavitation (44–88%), associated pleural thickening (37–56%), and bronchogenic spread (40–70%). Uncommon findings include adenopathy and pleural effusion (60). Fibrocavitary NTM lung disease can be radiographically indistinguishable from pulmonary TB (Fig. 1). However, larger thick-walled cavities and pleural calcification may be more suggestive of TB while diffuse bronchiectasis is more suggestive of infection with NTM (61,62).

B. Nodular Bronchiectasis

Although patients without predisposing risk factors were clearly present in prior studies (63), the study by Prince et al. in 1989 was the first to define this as a population of patients distinct from the classical presentation of pulmonary NTM (31). In this study, 21% of the 118 patients retrospectively reviewed were found to lack any of the traditional risk factors. These patients were predominantly women (81%), nonsmokers (62%), and in their seventh decade of life. Most presented with chronic cough, sometimes productive of purulent sputum, with symptoms persisting from about six months before diagnosis. Hemoptysis, fever, dyspnea on exertion, weight loss, night sweats, and malaise were all reported but were uncommon. In 1992, Reich and Johnson reported a similar series of six patients and suggested the term "Lady Windermere's syndrome" after the character from Oscar Wilde's Victorian-era play. His hypothesis was that habitual suppression of cough by older women leads to pooling of pulmonary secretions in dependent lobes of the lung and provided a favorable environment for NTM (64). Subsequent studies showing similar demographics and clinical characteristics have solidified this as a distinct presentation of NTM infection with MAC (41,65). Iseman et al. noted a markedly increased incidence of pectus excavatum and scoliosis in comparison to patients with TB and to the general population (66). He postulated this may lead to altered lung structure or impaired mucociliary function. Alternatively, this may be a phenotypic marker of a genetic predisposition that has not yet been described. The precise nature of what predisposes these women to infection with MAC remains unknown.

Initial reports of this disease only provided descriptions of chest radiograph findings. The most common pattern reported by Prince et al. was multiple discrete pulmonary nodules, seen in 71% of patients (31). Reich's report emphasized that nodules tended to be in the lingula and right middle lobe (64). Uncommon findings included consolidation, interstitial disease, and isolated cavities. Cavitary disease was reported in a total of 24%. This is in contrast to studies with CT in which cavitation was a rare finding, probably due to earlier detection of disease (67). With the more routine use of high-resolution CT, bronchiectasis was reported to almost universally accompany nodular infiltrates (Fig. 2) (67). Radiographic progression of the bronchiectasis argued

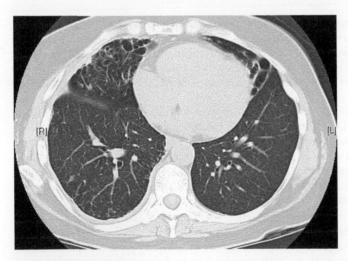

Figure 2 Chest CT in a 60-year-old woman with bronchiectasis and *Mycobacterium intracellulare* lung disease. The CT scan demonstrates right middle lobe and lingular bronchiectasis with scattered centrilobular nodules.

that MAC was the cause in at least some of the cases (68). When nodules accompany bronchiectasis, it is significantly more likely that MAC will be recovered from sputum cultures than when they do not (69).

C. Hypersensitivity-like Disease

A hypersensitivity-like disease has been described in patients who present with subacute dyspnea, cough, and fever and who have recently been exposed to indoor hot tubs. Disease has also been reported following exposure to metalworking fluids (70,71) and showers (72). High-resolution chest CT typically shows diffuse infiltrates with prominent nodularity throughout all lung fields, ground glass opacities, and a mosaic pattern (6). Biopsies show granulomas that are almost always well formed, rarely necrotic, and rarely stain positive for organisms (72). The diagnosis is made based on a combination of clinical, radiographic, microbiologic, and histopathologic findings. The finding of the same strains of MAC in both the hot tub and respiratory specimens from the patient is highly suggestive in the right clinical circumstances (6).

VI. Diagnosis
A. Diagnostic Criteria

Diagnosis of NTM pulmonary infection is based on the consensus opinion of experts and relies on the integration of clinical, radiographic, pathologic, and microbiologic data. Proposed criteria are summarized in Table 2. These guidelines were based on a large amount of experience with organisms such as MAC and *M. kansasii*. Given the fact that infections with the less common NTM organisms are generally indistinguishable, it is likely (but not proven) that the diagnostic criteria apply in these instances as well. Ultimately, the diagnosis must be confirmed by culture results, and empiric therapy other than that for TB is not recommended. Alternative diagnoses should be considered and excluded before making a diagnosis. A point of emphasis in the guidelines is continued follow-up and observation of patients when the diagnosis is in question;

Table 2 Diagnostic Criteria for NTM Pulmonary Infections

Clinical
  1. Pulmonary symptoms and radiographic evidence of disease
and
  2. Appropriate exclusion of other diagnoses
Microbiologic
  1. Positive culture results from at least two separate expectorated sputum samples. If nondiagnostic, consider repeat sputum acid-fast bacilli smears and cultures.
or
  2. Positive culture result from a bronchial wash or lavage
or
  3. Lung biopsy with histopathologic features consistent with mycobacterial infection and positive culture for NTM or a biopsy consistent with mycobacterial infection and a positive culture from a respiratory sample.

Abbreviation: NTM, nontuberculous mycobacteria.
Source: Modified from Ref. 6.

because of the indolent nature of NTM pulmonary infections, this is generally a safe approach (6).

B. Laboratory Diagnosis

The laboratory diagnosis of pulmonary disease due to NTM begins with the proper collection of a respiratory specimen. Three early morning specimens on different days should be collected and delivered to the laboratory without delay. Delays in processing of sputum samples can lead to bacterial overgrowth and decreased sensitivity of diagnostic techniques. If delays are anticipated, the specimen should be refrigerated at 4°C (73–75). Induction of sputum with hypertonic saline and bronchoscopy are alternatives for obtaining respiratory specimens in patients unable to produce sputum. These methods have never been prospectively evaluated in the diagnosis of NTM pulmonary disease, but have been demonstrated to have similar sensitivity in both immunocompetent (76) and immunocompromised (77) patients with pulmonary TB.

Once a respiratory specimen has been obtained, the goal of the microbiology laboratory is to provide timely species level identification of organisms (6). The armamentarium available to achieve this goal continues to expand rapidly. The laboratory evaluation begins with decontamination and microscopic examination for acid-fast bacilli (AFB). Although AFB smears are rapid and specific, they lack sensitivity (reports range from 22% to 65%), are unable to differentiate between TB and NTM, and are time consuming (74). Sensitivity may be enhanced by using fluorochrome staining and centrifugation (78,79). Culture on both liquid and solid media remains the gold standard and offers the ability to differentiate organisms on the basis of phenotype, to perform drug susceptibility testing, and to obtain sufficient numbers of organisms to perform further diagnostic testing. High-performance liquid chromatography (HPLC) and molecular methods are available for many of the commonly encountered NTM and help speed the identification of organisms from either respiratory specimens or culture. Analysis of the hypervariable regions in the 16S rRNA is often used to identify organisms to the species level (80). Susceptibility testing is performed using a broth-based method with either microdilution or macrodilution. The specific testing performed depends on the species. All MAC isolates should be tested for susceptibility to clarithromycin, *M. kansasii* for susceptibility to rifampin, and *M. abscessus* for susceptibility to multiple antibiotic agents such as clarithromycin, amikacin, cefoxitin, and linezolid (6).

VII. Treatment and Clinical Considerations in Specific Species

A. *Mycobacterium avium* Complex

M. avium complex comprises the species *M. avium* and *M. intracellulare*. Although there are differences in clinical presentation, with *M. intracellulare* being more important in pulmonary disease in the United States, there is no utility in identifying these organisms to the species level because this will not affect prognosis or treatment (6). As the most common NTM pulmonary pathogen worldwide, the treatment of MAC is the most extensively studied. A summary of the 18 trials examining the efficacy of regimens containing rifampin or ethambutol before 2001 was hampered by variations in trial design and clinical endpoints, but demonstrated an overall success rate of 39%. The longest follow up in these studies was 24 months (81). The first randomized controlled trial in pulmonary disease due to MAC, comparing rifampin and ethambutol with rifampin, ethambutol, and isoniazid demonstrated fewer failures of treatment with the three-drug regimen (16% vs. 41%) at two years (82). The results were even more disappointing when patients were followed out to five years when only 31% of the patients were alive and disease-free (83).

The introduction of the new macrolide, clarithromycin, and azalide, azithromycin, brought hope that their use would improve therapy of MAC infection. Both of these medications are present in high concentrations in lung tissue and phagocytes and showed much more substantial in vitro activity than the drugs discussed above (6). Many of the earlier trials with the newer macrolides were small, nonrandomized with limited follow-up, and with significant dropout rates. The success rates were reported to be between 26% and 71%, averaging 56% (81). In 2008, the largest randomized trial to date was published by the British Thoracic Society comparing 371 patients (170 with MAC) who received rifampicin and ethambutol plus either ciprofloxacin or clarithromycin. Patients were treated for two years and then monitored for another three years following completion of treatment. Only 31% in the clarithromycin and 34% in the ciprofloxacin group were alive and cured at five years (24). Because of the long duration of therapy and the potential dose-dependent side effects of the multiple medications in these regimens, the idea of thrice weekly macrolide-based therapy has also been investigated. Early noncomparative studies showed that this seemed to be as efficacious as daily therapy (84,85). However, a subsequent prospective study showed that this treatment strategy seemed to be less effective in patients with cavitary disease, with comorbidities such as COPD or bronchiectasis, who had failed a prior treatment course, or who had more severe disease (86).

The 2007 American Thoracic Society guidelines for NTM diseases provide treatment recommendations based on these and other studies as well as consensus expert opinion. The recommendations apply only to patients with macrolide-susceptible disease; patients with macrolide resistance should be referred for expert consultation. In vitro susceptibility testing to macrolides predicts clinical response (87–89), so all initial isolates should be tested against clarithromycin. Susceptibility testing to other antimycobacterial drugs is controversial. Thrice weekly regimens, including clarithromycin 1000 mg t.i.w. or azithromycin 500 to 600 mg t.i.w., rifampin 600 mg t.i.w., and ethambutol 25 mg/kg t.i.w. are recommended for initial therapy in patients with nodular/bronchiectatic disease. In patients with cavitary disease, extensive disease, and those who have been treated previously, a daily regimen of clarithromycin 500 to 1000 mg or azithromycin 250 to 300 mg, ethambutol 15 mg/kg, and rifampin 450 to 600 mg is recommended. Streptomycin or amikacin also should be considered in these patients. Patients should be monitored with monthly sputum cultures and treated until culture negative for 12 months (6). Surgery can be considered in patients such as those not responding to drug therapy, those with macrolide-resistant disease, or patients with complications from their infection and may be beneficial in other patient populations as well. Surgery may be associated with significant morbidity and should be performed by surgeons who have experience treating mycobacterial disease. Several retrospective studies indicate a high rate of culture negativity after resectional surgery (90–94).

Prolonged treatment with multiple medications often leads to significant side effects and requires close monitoring. Ethambutol can cause peripheral neuropathy and optic neuritis: Patients should be monitored symptomatically and with periodic assessment of visual acuity and red-green color discrimination. The rifamycins can cause nausea, vomiting, fever, rash, malaise, thrombocytopenia, hepatitis, renal failure, and can interact with numerous medications: Patients should have a complete blood count and serum chemistries monitored. The macrolides can cause nausea, vomiting, diarrhea, ototoxicity, and hepatitis: Patients may require periodic audiograms. Finally, streptomycin and amikacin can cause renal failure and ototoxicity so patients should be monitored based on their symptoms, physical examination, and audiograms. Amikacin levels should also be followed (6).

B. Mycobacterium kansasii

M. kansasii is the second most common cause of NTM pulmonary disease in the United States, though pockets in the United States and rest of the world exist where it is the most common (14,17,20,95). It is much more frequently pathogenic than MAC and there is controversy as to whether the diagnostic criteria apply, especially in high-risk populations (25,50,96). Although there are no randomized trials in the treatment of *M. kansasii*, it is clear that patients who receive rifampin as part of a multidrug regimen can achieve sputum culture negativity rates of nearly 100% with long-term rates of relapse as low as 0.8% (97–100). Rates of sputum conversion (from positive to negative culture) before the availability of rifampin were only 50% to 80% (98). The current recommendations for treatment of rifampin-susceptible disease are rifampin 10 mg/kg/day (maximum 600 mg), ethambutol 15 mg/kg/day, and isoniazid 5 mg/kg/day (maximum 300 mg) for 12 months once sputum cultures are negative. An alternative regimen with rifampin 600 mg/day, ethambutol 25 mg/kg/day, and clarithromycin 1000 mg/day was successful in all 56 patients treated with this regimen in Israel (101). Patients with rifampin-resistant disease should have therapy with three medications to which the organism is susceptible in vitro (102).

C. Rapidly Growing Mycobacteria

Rapidly growing mycobacteria (RGM) are distinguished by growth in subculture in less than seven days. *M. abscessus* is the third most common NTM infection in the United States and causes 80% of infections due to RGM while *M. fortuitum* is responsible for 15% of RGM cases. It is important to identify organisms within this group to the species level since this affects both treatment and prognosis (6,103). Most patients tend to present with nodular bronchiectasis; cavitation occurs only in about 15% (104). *M. abscessus* is typically resistant in vitro to most of the medications used to treat TB; the ideal medical treatment is unknown. Cure with medical therapy may be unrealistic for *M. abscessus* and the only chance for curative therapy may be with resection of local disease in addition to multidrug therapy. In contrast, *M. fortuitum* pulmonary infections can be treated with any combination of two drugs to which the isolate is susceptible until sputum cultures have been negative for 12 months.

VIII. Conclusion

Pulmonary infection with NTM is being recognized with increasing frequency in many parts of the world. A high index of suspicion is necessary as symptoms are nonspecific and may mimic underlying lung disease. Although the pathogenesis is poorly understood, several risk factors have been clearly defined and the disease has been well described in several distinct patient populations. The diagnosis is suspected based on clinical and radiographic data and ultimately confirmed by culture. The laboratory is able to use a multitude of techniques to identify organisms to the species level and guide the clinician in treatment. Treatment with multiple antimicrobial agents is typically prolonged with the potential for side effects and remains disappointing for most NTM. Further research regarding the treatment of pulmonary NTM and novel therapeutics that are more potent and have fewer side effects would ultimately improve the outcome in patients with pulmonary NTM.

IX. Case Scenarios
A. Case 1

A 67-year-old Caucasian woman presented to her local physician with a chronic cough associated with fatigue and weight loss. Over the past few years she has noted a increasingly frequent cough and exacerbations of her "bronchitis." Her cough would improve after treatment with oral antibiotics, only to return again a few weeks later. She was otherwise healthy and a lifelong nonsmoker. On exam she was thin, with pectus excavatum, and mitral valve prolapse. A chest radiograph was ordered that demonstrated opacities along the right and left heart borders. A subsequent chest CT scan demonstrated bronchiectasis in the right middle lobe and lingula with surrounding areas of centrilobular nodules in a tree-in-bud pattern. On the basis of these findings three sputum specimens were sent for mycobacterial culture and two were positive for MAC.

This case represents a classic example of a postmenopausal women presenting with right middle lobe and lingular bronchiectasis and underlying MAC infection. Isolation of MAC from respiratory specimens does not necessarily mean that the organisms are causing disease or that treatment is necessary. However, in this case, the patient meets the current American Thoracic Society and Infectious Diseases Society of America definition of disease with clinical and radiographic findings consistent with NTM infection plus at least two positive cultures.

B. Case 2

A 72-year-old man was evaluated for a chronic productive cough that had been present for nine months. He had a 50-pack-year smoking history and a history of ethanol abuse in the past. On exam he was thin with a low-grade fever and crackles in his posterior upper lung fields. Chest radiograph demonstrated bilateral upper lobe fibrocavitary abnormalities with multiple nodules. The patient was suspected of having pulmonary tuberculosis, so he was isolated and begun on a four-drug antituberculosis regimen. Three sputum specimens were obtained, one of which was smear positive. Eventually, the patient grew *M. kansasii* from two cultures. He was continued on isoniazid, rifampin, and ethambutol, but pyrazinamide was stopped. The patient was treated until he had 12 months of culture negativity.

M. kansasii can present like pulmonary tuberculosis with upper lobe cavitary disease. Typically, *M. kansasii* related cavities have thinner walls with less surrounding consolidation than is seen with tuberculosis. The physicians in this case appropriately suspected tuberculosis and ordered isolation and initiation of four-drug therapy. Once *M. kansasii* was identified, pyrazinamide was stopped because it has no activity against this organism. A three-drug regimen was continued for 14 months, or 12 months after he converted his cultures to negative. Unlike with many NTM pulmonary infections, the cure rate for pulmonary *M. kansasii* infection is high, averaging over 95%.

References

1. Wolinsky E. Nontuberculous mycobacteria and associated diseases. Am Rev Resp Dis 1979; 119(1):107–159.

2. Timpe A, Runyon EH. The relationship of "Atypical" acid-fast bacteria to human disease: a preliminary report. J Lab Clin Med 1954; 44:202–209.

3. Tortoli E. Impact of genotypic studies on mycobacterial taxonomy: the new mycobacteria of the 1990s. Clin Microbiol Rev 2003; 16(2):319–354.

4. Boddinghaus B, Rogall T, Flohr T, et al. Detection and identification of mycobacteria by amplification of rRNA. J Clin Microbiol 1990; 28(8):1751–1759.

5. Euzéby JP. List of prokaryotic names with standing in nomenclature: genus *Mycobacterium*. 2008. Available at: http://www.bacterio.cict.fr/m/mycobacterium.html. Accessed July 2008.

6. Griffith DE, Aksamit T, Brown-Elliott BA, et al. An official ATS/IDSA statement: diagnosis, treatment, and prevention of nontuberculous mycobacterial diseases. Am J Respir Crit Care Med 2007; 175(4):367–416.

7. Marras TK, Daley CL. Epidemiology of human pulmonary infection with nontuberculous mycobacteria. Clin Chest Med 2002; 23(3):553–567.

8. Palmer CE. Tuberculin sensitivity and contact with tuberculosis. Am Rev Tuberc 1953; 68(5):678–694.

9. Edwards FG. Disease caused by 'atypical' (opportunist) mycobacteria: a whole population review. Tubercle 1970; 51(3):285–295.

10. Khan K, Wang J, Marras TK. Nontuberculous mycobacterial sensitization in the United States: national trends over three decades. Am J Respir Crit Care Med 2007; 176(3):306–313.

11. Tsukamura M, Kita N, Shimoide H, et al. Studies on the epidemiology of nontuberculous mycobacteriosis in Japan. Am Rev Respir Dis 1988; 137(6):1280–1284.

12. Debrunner M, Salfinger M, Brandli O, et al. Epidemiology and clinical significance of nontuberculous mycobacteria in patients negative for human immunodeficiency virus in Switzerland. Clin Infect Dis 1992; 15(2):330–345.

13. Kubin M, Svandova E, Medek B, et al. *Mycobacterium kansasii* infection in an endemic area of Czechoslovakia. Tubercle 1980; 61(4):207–212.

14. Jenkins PA. The epidemiology of opportunist mycobacterial infections in Wales, 1952–1978. Rev Infect Dis 1981; 3(5):1021–1023.

15. Kennedy MP, O'Connor TM, Ryan C, et al. Nontuberculous mycobacteria: incidence in Southwest Ireland from 1987 to 2000. Respir Med 2003; 97(3):257–263.

16. O'Brien DP, Currie BJ, Krause VL. Nontuberculous mycobacterial disease in northern Australia: a case series and review of the literature. Clin Infect Dis 2000; 31(4):958–967.

17. O'Brien RJ, Geiter LJ, Snider DE Jr. The epidemiology of nontuberculous mycobacterial diseases in the United States. Results from a national survey. Am Rev Respir Dis 1987; 135(5):1007–1014.

18. Marras TK, Chedore P, Ying AM, et al. Isolation prevalence of pulmonary non-tuberculous mycobacteria in Ontario, 1997–2003. Thorax 2007; 62(8):661–666.

19. Dailloux M, Abalain ML, Laurain C, et al. Respiratory infections associated with nontuberculous mycobacteria in non-HIV patients. Eur Respir J 2006; 28(6):1211–1215.

20. Good RC. From the Center for Disease Control. Isolation of nontuberculous mycobacteria in the United States, 1979. J Infect Dis 1980; 142(5):779–783.

21. Good RC, Snider DE Jr. Isolation of nontuberculous mycobacteria in the United States, 1980. J Infect Dis 1982; 146(6):829–833.

22. Falkinham JO III, Parker BC, Gruft H. Epidemiology of infection by nontuberculous mycobacteria. I. Geographic distribution in the eastern United States. Am Rev Respir Dis 1980; 121(6):931–937.

23. George KL, Parker BC, Gruft H, et al. Epidemiology of infection by nontuberculous mycobacteria. II. Growth and survival in natural waters. Am Rev Respir Dis 1980; 122(1):89–94.
24. Jenkins PA, Campbell IA, Banks J, et al. Clarithromycin vs ciprofloxacin as adjuncts to rifampicin and ethambutol in treating opportunist mycobacterial lung diseases and an assessment of *Mycobacterium vaccae* immunotherapy. Thorax 2008; 63(7):627–634.
25. Corbett EL, Blumberg L, Churchyard GJ, et al. Nontuberculous mycobacteria: defining disease in a prospective cohort of South African miners. Am J Respir Crit Care Med 1999; 160(1):15–21.
26. Corbett EL, Churchyard GJ, Clayton T, et al. Risk factors for pulmonary mycobacterial disease in South African gold miners. A case-control study. Am J Respir Crit Care Med 1999; 159(1):94–99.
27. Falkinham JO III. Nontuberculous mycobacteria in the environment. Clin Chest Med 2002; 23(3):529–551.
28. Corpe RF, Stergus I. Is the histopathology of nonphotochromogenic mycobacterial infections distinguishable from that caused by *Mycobacterium tuberculosis*? Am Rev Respir Dis 1963; 87:289–291.
29. McGarvey J, Bermudez LE. Pathogenesis of nontuberculous mycobacteria infections. Clin Chest Med 2002; 23(3):569–583.
30. Robakiewicz M, Grzybowski S. Epidemiologic aspects of nontuberculous mycobacterial disease and of tuberculosis in British Columbia. Am Rev Respir Dis 1974; 109(6):613–620.
31. Prince DS, Peterson DD, Steiner RM, et al. Infection with Mycobacterium avium complex in patients without predisposing conditions. N Engl J Med 1989; 321(13):863–868.
32. Murin S, Bilello KS. Respiratory tract infections: another reason not to smoke. Cleve Clin J Med 2005; 72(10):916–920.
33. Field SK, Cowie RL. Lung disease due to the more common nontuberculous mycobacteria. Chest 2006; 129(6):1653–1672.
34. Kilby JM, Gilligan PH, Yankaskas JR, et al. Nontuberculous mycobacteria in adult patients with cystic fibrosis. Chest 1992; 102(1):70–75.
35. Olivier KN, Weber DJ, Wallace RJ, Jr., et al. Nontuberculous mycobacteria. I: multicenter prevalence study in cystic fibrosis. Am J Respir Crit Care Med 2003; 167(6):828–834.
36. Bange FC, Kirschner P, Bottger EC. Recovery of mycobacteria from patients with cystic fibrosis. J Clin Microbiol 1999; 37(11):3761–3763.
37. Whittier S, Hopfer RL, Knowles MR, et al. Improved recovery of mycobacteria from respiratory secretions of patients with cystic fibrosis. J Clin Microbiol 1993; 31(4):861–864.
38. Whittier S, Olivier K, Gilligan P, et al. Proficiency testing of clinical microbiology laboratories using modified decontamination procedures for detection of nontuberculous mycobacteria in sputum samples from cystic fibrosis patients. The Nontuberculous Mycobacteria in Cystic Fibrosis Study Group. J Clin Microbiol 1997; 35(10):2706–2708.
39. Barker AF. Bronchiectasis. N Engl J Med 2002; 346(18):1383–1393.
40. Fujita J, Ohtsuki Y, Shigeto E, et al. Pathological findings of bronchiectases caused by Mycobacterium avium intracellulare complex. Respir Med 2003; 97(8):933–938.
41. Huang JH, Kao PN, Adi V, et al. *Mycobacterium avium-intracellulare* pulmonary infection in HIV-negative patients without preexisting lung disease: diagnostic and management limitations. Chest 1999; 115(4):1033–1040.
42. Wallace RJ Jr., Zhang Y, Brown BA, et al. Polyclonal *Mycobacterium avium* complex infections in patients with nodular bronchiectasis. Am J Respir Crit Care Med 1998; 158(4):1235–1244.
43. Pryor JA. Physiotherapy for airway clearance in adults. Eur Respir J 1999; 14(6):1418–1424.

44. Jones D, Havlir DV. Nontuberculous mycobacteria in the HIV infected patient. Clin Chest Med 2002; 23(3):665–674.
45. Nightingale SD, Byrd LT, Southern PM, et al. Incidence of *Mycobacterium avium-intracellulare* complex bacteremia in human immunodeficiency virus-positive patients. J Infect Dis 1992; 165(6):1082–1085.
46. Chin DP, Hopewell PC, Yajko DM, et al. *Mycobacterium avium* complex in the respiratory or gastrointestinal tract and the risk of M. avium complex bacteremia in patients with human immunodeficiency virus infection. J Infect Dis 1994; 169(2):289–295.
47. Kalayjian RC, Toossi Z, Tomashefski JF Jr., et al. Pulmonary disease due to infection by Mycobacterium avium complex in patients with AIDS. Clin Infect Dis 1995; 20(5): 1186–1194.
48. Hocqueloux L, Lesprit P, Herrmann JL, et al. Pulmonary *Mycobacterium avium* complex disease without dissemination in HIV-infected patients. Chest 1998; 113(2):542–548.
49. Bloch KC, Zwerling L, Pletcher MJ, et al. Incidence and clinical implications of isolation of *Mycobacterium kansasii*: results of a 5-year, population-based study. Ann Intern Med 1998; 129(9):698–704.
50. Marras TK, Daley CL. A systematic review of the clinical significance of pulmonary *Mycobacterium kansasii* isolates in HIV infection. J Acquir Immune Defic Syndr 2004; 36(4):883–889.
51. Malouf MA, Glanville AR. The spectrum of mycobacterial infection after lung transplantation. Am J Respir Crit Care Med 1999; 160(5 pt 1):1611–1616.
52. Weinstock DM, Feinstein MB, Sepkowitz KA, et al. High rates of infection and colonization by nontuberculous mycobacteria after allogeneic hematopoietic stem cell transplantation. Bone Marrow Transplant 2003; 31(11):1015–1021.
53. Doucette K, Fishman JA. Nontuberculous mycobacterial infection in hematopoietic stem cell and solid organ transplant recipients. Clin Infect Dis 2004; 38(10):1428–1439.
54. Queipo JA, Broseta E, Santos M, et al. Mycobacterial infection in a series of 1261 renal transplant recipients. Clin Microbiol Infect 2003; 9(6):518–525.
55. Dorman SE, Holland SM. Interferon-gamma and interleukin-12 pathway defects and human disease. Cytokine Growth Factor Rev 2000; 11(4):321–333.
56. Dorman SE, Picard C, Lammas D, et al. Clinical features of dominant and recessive interferon gamma receptor 1 deficiencies. Lancet 2004; 364(9451):2113–2121.
57. Keane J, Gershon S, Wise RP, et al. Tuberculosis associated with infliximab, a tumor necrosis factor alpha-neutralizing agent. N Engl J Med 2001; 345(15):1098–1104.
58. Salvana EM, Cooper GS, Salata RA. Mycobacterium other than tuberculosis (MOTT) infection: an emerging disease in infliximab-treated patients. J Infect 2007; 55(6):484–487.
59. Aksamit TR. *Mycobacterium avium* complex pulmonary disease in patients with pre-existing lung disease. Clin Chest Med 2002; 23(3):643–653.
60. Miller WT, Jr. Spectrum of pulmonary nontuberculous mycobacterial infection. Radiology 1994; 191(2):343–350.
61. Christensen EE, Dietz GW, Ahn CH, et al. Initial roentgenographic manifestations of pulmonary *Mycobacterium tuberculosis*, *M kansasii*, and *M intracellularis* infections. Chest 1981; 80(2):132–136.
62. Levin DL. Radiology of pulmonary *Mycobacterium avium*-intracellulare complex. Clin Chest Med 2002; 23(3):603–612.
63. Rosenzweig DY. Pulmonary mycobacterial infections due to *Mycobacterium intracellulare-avium* complex. Clinical features and course in 100 consecutive cases. Chest 1979; 75(2): 115–119.
64. Reich JM, Johnson RE. *Mycobacterium avium* complex pulmonary disease presenting as an isolated lingular or middle lobe pattern. The Lady Windermere syndrome. Chest 1992; 101(6):1605–1609.

65. Kubo K, Yamazaki Y, Hachiya T, et al. Mycobacterium avium-intracellulare pulmonary infection in patients without known predisposing lung disease. Lung 1998; 176(6):381–391.
66. Iseman MD, Buschman DL, Ackerson LM. Pectus excavatum and scoliosis. Thoracic anomalies associated with pulmonary disease caused by Mycobacterium avium complex. Am Rev Respir Dis 1991; 144(4):914–916.
67. Hartman TE, Swensen SJ, Williams DE. *Mycobacterium avium-intracellulare* complex: evaluation with CT. Radiology 1993; 187(1):23–26.
68. Moore EH. Atypical mycobacterial infection in the lung: CT appearance. Radiology 1993; 187(3):777–782.
69. Swensen SJ, Hartman TE, Williams DE. Computed tomographic diagnosis of *Mycobacterium avium-intracellulare* complex in patients with bronchiectasis. Chest 1994; 105(1):49–52.
70. Biopsy-confirmed hypersensitivity pneumonitis in automobile production workers exposed to metalworking fluids—Michigan, 1994–1995. MMWR 1996; 45(28):606–610.
71. Respiratory illness in workers exposed to metalworking fluid contaminated with non-tuberculous mycobacteria—Ohio, 2001. MMWR 2002; 51(16):349–352.
72. Marras TK, Wallace RJ Jr., Koth LL, et al. Hypersensitivity pneumonitis reaction to *Mycobacterium avium* in household water. Chest 2005; 127(2):664–671.
73. Warren JR, Bhattacharya M, De Almeida KN, et al. A minimum 5.0 ml of sputum improves the sensitivity of acid-fast smear for *Mycobacterium tuberculosis*. Am J Respir Crit Care Med 2000; 161(5):1559–1562.
74. Somoskovi A, Mester J, Hale YM, et al. Laboratory diagnosis of nontuberculous mycobacteria. Clin Chest Med 2002; 23(3):585–597.
75. Hale YM, Pfyffer GE, Salfinger M. Laboratory diagnosis of mycobacterial infections: new tools and lessons learned. Clin Infect Dis 2001; 33(6):834–846.
76. Anderson C, Inhaber N, Menzies D. Comparison of sputum induction with fiber-optic bronchoscopy in the diagnosis of tuberculosis. Am J Respir Crit Care Med 1995; 152(5 pt 1):1570–1574.
77. Conde MB, Soares SL, Mello FC, et al. Comparison of sputum induction with fiberoptic bronchoscopy in the diagnosis of tuberculosis: experience at an acquired immune deficiency syndrome reference center in Rio de Janeiro, Brazil. Am J Respir Crit Care Med 2000; 162(6):2238–2240.
78. Somoskovi A, Hotaling JE, Fitzgerald M, et al. Lessons from a proficiency testing event for acid-fast microscopy. Chest 2001; 120(1):250–257.
79. Peterson EM, Nakasone A, Platon-DeLeon JM, et al. Comparison of direct and concentrated acid-fast smears to identify specimens culture positive for Mycobacterium spp. J Clin Microbiol 1999; 37(11):3564–3568.
80. Piersimoni C, Scarparo C. Pulmonary infections associated with non-tuberculous mycobacteria in immunocompetent patients. Lancet Infect Dis 2008; 8(5):323–334.
81. Field SK, Fisher D, Cowie RL. *Mycobacterium avium* complex pulmonary disease in patients without HIV infection. Chest 2004; 126(2):566–581.
82. First randomised trial of treatments for pulmonary disease caused by *M avium intracellulare*, *M malmoense*, and *M xenopi* in HIV negative patients: rifampicin, ethambutol and isoniazid versus rifampicin and ethambutol. Thorax 2001; 56(3):167–172.
83. Pulmonary disease caused by *Mycobacterium avium-intracellulare* in HIV-negative patients: five-year follow-up of patients receiving standardised treatment. Int J Tuberc Lung Dis 2002; 6(7):628–634.
84. Griffith DE, Brown BA, Cegielski P, et al. Early results (at 6 months) with intermittent clarithromycin-including regimens for lung disease due to *Mycobacterium avium* complex. Clin Infect Dis 2000; 30(2):288–292.

85. Griffith DE, Brown BA, Murphy DT, et al. Initial (6-month) results of three-times-weekly azithromycin in treatment regimens for *Mycobacterium avium* complex lung disease in human immunodeficiency virus-negative patients. J Infect Dis 1998; 178(1):121–126.

86. Lam PK, Griffith DE, Aksamit TR, et al. Factors related to response to intermittent treatment of *Mycobacterium avium* complex lung disease. Am J Respir Crit Care Med 2006; 173(11):1283–1289.

87. Wallace RJ Jr., Brown BA, Griffith DE, et al. Initial clarithromycin monotherapy for *Mycobacterium avium-intracellulare* complex lung disease. Am J Respir Crit Care Med 1994; 149(5):1335–1341.

88. Griffith DE, Brown-Elliott BA, Langsjoen B, et al. Clinical and molecular analysis of macrolide resistance in *Mycobacterium avium* complex lung disease. Am J Respir Crit Care Med 2006; 174(8):928–934.

89. Heifets L, Mor N, Vanderkolk J. Mycobacterium avium strains resistant to clarithromycin and azithromycin. Antimicrob Agents Chemother 1993; 37(11):2364–2370.

90. Pomerantz M, Denton JR, Huitt GA, et al. Resection of the right middle lobe and lingula for mycobacterial infection. Ann Thorac Surg 1996; 62(4):990–993.

91. Shiraishi Y, Fukushima K, Komatsu H, et al. Early pulmonary resection for localized *Mycobacterium avium* complex disease. Ann Thorac Surg 1998; 66(1):183–186.

92. Shiraishi Y, Nakajima Y, Katsuragi N, et al. Pneumonectomy for nontuberculous myco-bacterial infections. Ann Thorac Surg 2004; 78(2):399–403.

93. Shiraishi Y, Nakajima Y, Takasuna K, et al. Surgery for *Mycobacterium avium* complex lung disease in the clarithromycin era. Eur J Cardiothorac Surg 2002; 21(2):314–318.

94. Nelson KG, Griffith DE, Brown BA, et al. Results of operation in *Mycobacterium avium-intracellulare* lung disease. Ann Thorac Surg 1998; 66(2):325–330.

95. Ahn CH, Lowell JR, Onstad GD, et al. A demographic study of disease due to *Myco-bacterium kansasii* or *M intracellulare-avium* in Texas. Chest 1979; 75(2):120–125.

96. Marras TK, Morris A, Gonzalez LC, et al. Mortality prediction in pulmonary *Mycobacte-rium kansasii* infection and human immunodeficiency virus. Am J Respir Crit Care Med 2004; 170(7):793–798.

97. Griffith DE. Management of disease due to *Mycobacterium kansasii*. Clin Chest Med 2002; 23(3):613–621, vi.

98. Pezzia W, Raleigh JW, Bailey MC, et al. Treatment of pulmonary disease due to *Myco-bacterium kansasii*: recent experience with rifampin. Rev Infect Dis 1981; 3(5):1035–1039.

99. Ahn CH, Lowell JR, Ahn SS, et al. Chemotherapy for pulmonary disease due to *Myco-bacterium kansasii*: efficacies of some individual drugs. Rev Infect Dis 1981; 3(5): 1028–1034.

100. Ahn CH, Lowell JR, Ahn SS, et al. Short-course chemotherapy for pulmonary disease caused by *Mycobacterium kansasii*. Am Rev Respir Dis 1983; 128(6):1048–1050.

101. Shitrit D, Baum GL, Priess R, et al. Pulmonary *Mycobacterium kansasii* infection in Israel, 1999-2004: clinical features, drug susceptibility, and outcome. Chest 2006; 129(3): 771–776.

102. Wallace RJ, Jr., Dunbar D, Brown BA, et al. Rifampin-resistant *Mycobacterium kansasii*. Clin Infect Dis 1994; 18(5):736–743.

103. Daley CL, Griffith DE. Pulmonary disease caused by rapidly growing mycobacteria. Clin Chest Med 2002; 23(3):623–632, vii.

104. Griffith DE, Girard WM, Wallace RJ Jr. Clinical features of pulmonary disease caused by rapidly growing mycobacteria. An analysis of 154 patients. Am Rev Respir Dis 1993; 147(5):1271–1278.

16
Fungal Infections

TOM LIM, JOHN H. MACGREGOR, and CHRISTOPHER H. MODY
University of Calgary, Calgary, Alberta, Canada

I. Introduction

There are estimated to be 1.5 million species of fungi (1). Indeed, fungi represent an entire kingdom in the living world. Infections due to species within this kingdom are many and varied. However, for the purpose of this chapter, the focus will be on the pulmonary manifestations of fungal infections caused by the most common fungal species. The discussion is limited to the infections and only briefly mentions the allergic diseases such as allergic bronchopulmonary mycosis and allergic fungal sinusitis.

II. *Aspergillus* spp.

Aspergillus spp. comprise over 200 different species. The most common human pathogens are *Aspergillus fumigatus* ($\sim$56% of cases), *A. flavus* ($\sim$19% of cases), and *A. terreus* ($\sim$16% of cases). However, *A. niger* ($\sim$8% of cases), *A. clavatus*, *A. niveus*, and *A. nidulans* have also been consistently implicated in human infections (2).

A. Clinical Presentation

The spectrum of disease involving *Aspergillus* spp. is broad, ranging from invasive infection to chronic disease and even hypersensitivity reactions in which there is no active infection. Pulmonary involvement is the most frequent site of *Aspergillus* infection. However, disseminated infection and isolated extrapulmonary organ involvement, in particular, of the gastrointestinal tract, brain, kidneys, and liver has been documented. The pulmonary involvement can be divided into four main categories: invasive pulmonary aspergillosis (IPA), chronic necrotizing aspergillosis (CNA), aspergilloma, and allergic bronchopulmonary aspergillosis (ABPA), a hypersensitivity reaction. The common pathway for all types of pulmonary involvement begins with the inhalation of spores.

IPA is an acutely invasive form of pulmonary aspergillosis often involving angioinvasion and high fungal burden. The clinical picture of IPA often includes bronchopneumonia, fever, cough, sputum production, dyspnea, pleuritic chest pain, and small pulmonary infarcts (3). The mortality for IPA is as high as 50% for neutropenic patients and 90% for hematopoietic stem-cell transplantation patients (4).

In contrast, CNA is a locally invasive form of pulmonary aspergillosis seen in patients mildly immunocompromised or with chronic lung disease. It is chronic and a less frequent manifestation of the disease. The clinical presentation often has prominent constitutional features, with fever, weight loss, malaise, fatigue, and a chronic productive cough.

The third common presentation of aspergillosis is aspergilloma. An aspergilloma is a fungal ball consisting of fungal elements that often develops in a preexisting lung cavity or within a necrotic tumor. Clinically, aspergillomas may exist for years without causing symptoms, and consequently may present as an incidental finding on chest X ray. Cough or hemoptysis is the most common initial symptom and bleeding develops from local invasion or disruption of blood vessels lining the cavity wall (5).

Allergic bronchopulmonary aspergillosis is a hypersensitivity reaction to fungal elements and not a true invasion of fungi in the lungs. It is usually seen in poorly controlled asthmatic or cystic fibrosis patients. Often, patients present with uncontrolled asthma, wheezing, fever, brownish sputum, and pleuritic chest pain. The chronic nature of the symptoms often leads to mucus impaction and bronchiectasis (5).

B. Etiopathogenesis

Aspergillus spores are ubiquitous in the environment and cause no sequelae in normal healthy individuals who come in contact with the fungi. There is a wide spectrum of disease caused by *Aspergillus*, and the condition and severity is dependent on the individual characteristics of the host. Extrapulmonary infection often occurs after dissemination from invasive pulmonary involvement. However, disseminated and local infection can also occur through intravenous catheters, burns, and prolonged skin contact with adhesives (6).

Invasive aspergillosis is seen in immunocompromised hosts with defects in neutrophil function, prolonged neutropenia, corticosteroid therapy, organ transplantation, hematologic malignancy, cytotoxic therapy, neutrophil dysfunction, and the terminal stages of AIDS. Patients undergoing hematopoietic stem cell transplantation and lung transplants are at particularly high risk. IPA is a common precursor to extrapulmonary manifestations of *Aspergillus* infection. By contrast, CNA usually occurs in patients with chronic lung diseases and who are mildly immunocompromised. Unlike IPA, CNA does not usually disseminate to other organs as patients have a sufficient immunity to defend against such invasion. Aspergillomas often develop in patients with underlying structural lung disease such as preexisting cavities that are frequently the result of tuberculosis, sarcoidosis, bronchial cysts, bullae, and neoplasms.

The pathogenesis of the noninfectious form of aspergillosis, ABPA, is not well understood. It is usually on the background of hypersensitivity such as chronic asthma or altered mucous production such as in cystic fibrosis. It is felt to be a combination of: immunoglobulin (Ig)E-mediated direct hypersensitivity, immune complex–mediated hypersensitivity, and abnormal T-lymphocyte cellular immune responses (3).

C. Diagnosis

The gold standard for diagnosis of invasive aspergillosis involves histopathology. However, obtaining tissue is often difficult and early diagnosis is crucial because of the high mortality rates. Diagnostic tools include performing culture, microscopy, or a galactomannan assay for *Aspergillus* on bronchoalveolar lavage (BAL), sputum, or serum samples. Galactomannan is a constituent of hyphae released during growth, and a report indicates that serum levels have 71% sensitivity and 89% specificity for

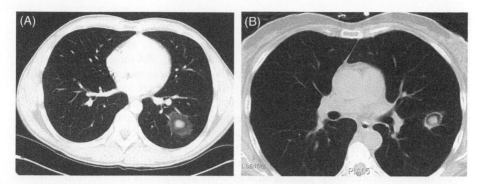

Figure 1 CT scan of the chest showing (**A**) halo sign and (**B**) air crescent sign.

Aspergillus infections (7). Moreover, BAL samples may be more effective with a sensitivity of 88% and a specificity of 87% in the galactomannan test (8). However, the galactomannan test is technically challenging to perform and not readily available in all centers. Microscopy and culture of BAL is useful (sensitivity up to 50% and specificity up to 97%), and in the presence of a new pulmonary infiltrate, a positive culture is considered diagnostic (3). Other tests, such as serum precipitant antibodies measured by immunodiffusion (or equivalent test), anti-*Aspergillus* IgE and IgG antibodies and skin reactivity to *Aspergillus* are useful in the diagnosis of ABPA.

Radiologic imaging is an important tool in the diagnosis of aspergillosis. CT scan is the modality of choice. IPA may present as ground glass changes, multiple nodules, cavitary lesions, consolidation, pulmonary hemorrhage and the halo and the air crescent signs (Fig. 1A and B) (5). Findings of CNA on CT are quite different and include upper lobe lesions, cavitations, and pleural thickening that gradually progress over months. CNA often manifests as an aspergilloma that becomes locally invasive. By contrast, aspergillomas present radiographically as an upper lobe intracavitary mass with a thick-walled cavity (9). Chronic ABPA is quite distinct and has features of bronchiectasis with dilated airways, the signet ring sign, tramlines, and mucoid impaction. A chest X ray is also helpful in the diagnosis of pulmonary aspergillosis but is not always useful in detecting early disease.

Overall the diagnosis of aspergillosis infection is difficult and the clinical history, the nature of impaired host defense, along with serologic tests, cultures, and radiographic imaging all play a role in making a diagnosis.

D. Treatment and Prevention

Treatment recommendations are based on the recently released Infectious Diseases Society of America (IDSA), and soon to be released American Thoracic Society (ATS) statements in the management of aspergillosis and fungal disease (10,11).

The management of aspergillosis depends on the severity of the infection and the nature of the underlying disease. For invasive aspergillosis, triazoles are the first line of therapy. Voriconazole 6 mg/kg b.i.d. IV for one day followed by 4 mg/kg b.i.d. is often the first choice. It may be possible to reduce the dose and switch to 200 mg b.i.d. PO when patients stabilize. Another triazole, itraconazole is reserved for more stable patients (400 mg PO daily). The echinocandin, caspofungin, is principally used as salvage therapy or in patients with refractory infections (10), and some data suggest that the combination of voriconazole plus caspofungin is superior to voriconazole alone (12). Liposomal amphotericin B can be used, but for the most part has been relegated to salvage therapy because of its high toxicity and increasing rates of resistance especially with *A. tereus* infections. The duration of treatment depends on the clinical context and severity of infection but often requires several months to more than a year.

Surgical management is generally reserved for severe necrosis, abscess drainage, or management of empyemas, invasion of bone, burn wounds, epidural abscesses, and vitreal disease. Unfortunately, patients with invasive aspergillosis often have significant comorbidities along with coagulopathies that may exempt them from major surgery.

Another clinical factor to consider in managing invasive aspergillosis is reversal of the immunodeficient state that permits *Aspergillus* proliferation. Reversal of neutropenia, if possible, is critical for recovery in patients receiving chemotherapy. Depending on the context this may involve granulocyte colony-stimulating factor (GCSF) treatment or decreasing the dose of immunosuppression.

Management of aspergillomas is reserved for symptomatic patients with hemoptysis. Although the mainstay of treatment is surgery with resection of cavity and fungus ball (13), many patients have sufficient debility that it precludes surgery. Medical therapy with voriconazole or itraconazole does not generally cure the infection, but has been used as suppressive treatment.

ABPA is generally managed with oral corticosteroids as the underlying disorder is a hypersensitivity reaction. Oral itraconazole has also been effective especially in cystic fibrosis, and can reduce the dose of steroid required (14).

E. Complications and Difficult Management Scenarios

There are many clinical challenges in aspergillosis. The high mortality rates make early diagnosis critical. However, diagnosis using traditional methods of fungal culture and histopathology are time consuming and insensitive. With the advent of galactomannan assays and polymerase chain reaction (PCR) based assays, diagnosis can be made earlier in high-risk populations. However, the availability of such tests and diagnostic accuracy in many centers are still barriers to management of patients.

Likewise the emergence of invasive *Aspergillus* infections in immunocompetent patient populations has made diagnosis more complex. The index of suspicion now has to be extended to patients in intensive care units (ICU) and patients on chronic corticosteroids. In studies of ICU patients, 60% of *Aspergillus* infections did not have the classical risk factors of leukemia, neutropenia or bone marrow transplant. These patients, however, had high rates of chronic obstructive pulmonary disease (COPD) and corticosteroid treatment (15). Thus, clinicians must be aware of the presentations of aspergillosis and maintain a high degree of suspicion in such patients. Finally, *A. tereus* is becoming increasingly resistant to amphotericin B, and *A. ustus* and *A. lentulus* are becoming increasingly more important pathogens. Consequently, clinicians must maintain a close working relationship with the clinical microbiology laboratory to promptly diagnose and treat these infections.

III. *Candida* spp.

Candidiasis is caused by the genus *Candida*, which contains approximately 200 species. The major pathogen is *Candida albicans* (~50% of cases), but other species include *C. tropicalis* (~15% of cases), *C. glabrata* (~15% of cases), *C. parapsilosis* (~15% of cases), *C. krusei* (~1% of cases), *C. lusitaniae* (~1% of cases) (16,17). The distinction between these species is important because of their differing susceptibilities to antifungal agents.

A. Clinical Presentation

There remains some controversy about the incidence of pulmonary candidiasis. Despite frequent microbial isolation from pulmonary secretions, many experts argue that pulmonary candidal infection only occurs in two scenarios. The first is in the context of disseminated candidiasis, and the second is following significant aspiration of organisms from an oropharyngeal source. Positive cultures obtained from throat swabs, sputum, or BAL, in the absence of disseminated disease or aspiration, probably represents colonization and should be managed as such.

B. Etiopathogenesis

There are a variety of risk factors for disseminated candidiasis, which include the presence of a central venous catheter, prolonged antibacterial therapy, hyperalimentation, surgery (especially if it transects the gut wall), prolonged ICU stay, renal failure, diabetes, cancer, other comorbidities, and colonization by *Candida* at multiple nonsterile sites (18). Although mucocutaneous candidiasis occurs in the setting of suppression of cell-mediated immunity such as AIDS, defects in neutrophil function predispose to disseminated *Candida* infections (19).

C. Diagnosis

Since mortality is proportional to the time it takes to institute therapy (20), rapid diagnosis is essential. Ideally, tissue is obtained, and invasive infection is confirmed by culture or histopathologic examination of the tissue. However, because of the urgency to initiate treatment, antifungal therapy is often started before this definitive evidence. Consequently, it is important to recognize the risk factors stated above. $(1\rightarrow3)$-β-D-glucan testing, if available, has been shown to be of value (21). However, treatment is often initiated on the basis of clinical judgment and prediction rules (22,23). Prediction rules take into account prior systemic antibiotic use, the presence of a central venous catheter, administration of total parenteral nutrition, corticosteroids, or other immunosuppressive agents, as well as renal dialysis, major surgery, or pancreatitis. The rules have high specificity but low sensitivity (23).

D. Treatment and Prevention

The mainstay of therapy for candidiasis is fluconazole. In nonneutropenic patients a loading dose of 800 mg/day, followed by 400 mg/day is often used. However, depending on the prevalence of *C. glabrata*, local fluconazole resistance, or recent use of azole antifungal agents, it may be necessary to select an echinocandin such as caspofungin as initial therapy. By contrast, when *C. parapsilosis* is isolated, fluconazole is often a superior agent. For most patients, amphotericin B has significant toxicity, while adding little to therapeutic efficacy.

E. Complications and Difficult Management Scenarios

The management of critically ill patients that have *Candida* isolated from cultures from external sites such as sputum, skin, urine, and wounds can be extremely challenging. The presence of multiple positive cultures in the setting of a central venous catheter, prolonged antibacterial therapy, hyperalimentation, visceral surgery, prolonged ICU stay, renal failure, diabetes, cancer, and other comorbidities will often prompt therapy, especially if the patient lacks physiologic reserve.

IV. *Blastomyces dermatitidis*

Blastomycosis is a multisystem disease caused by *Blastomyces dermatitidis*, a dimorphic fungus. Blastomycosis is endemic in southeastern and south central states bordering the Mississippi and Ohio River basins, the Midwestern states in the United States and Canadian provinces bordering the Great Lakes. Cases have also been encountered in Africa, Mexico, and Central and South America.

A. Clinical Presentation

The spectrum of pulmonary blastomycosis includes subclinical infection and acute or chronic respiratory disease. While less severe pulmonary presentations include lobar pneumonia, mass lesions, single or multiple nodules, and chronic fibronodular or fibrocavitary infiltrates, more severe infections can be manifest as disseminated infection with multiorgan system dysfunction and adult respiratory distress syndrome (ARDS) (24). Some patients will demonstrate extrapulmonary manifestations including verrucous or ulcerative skin disease, bone involvement, prostatitis, or epididymoorchitis.

B. Etiopathogenesis

Blastomyces is acquired by inhalation. In the United States most cases have been reported from Mississippi, Arkansas, Kentucky, Tennessee, and western Michigan and Wisconsin. In Canada, the disease occurs in Manitoba and western Ontario. Blastomyces grows in soil rich in organic debris or in rotting trees. Consequently, persons with blastomycosis are likely to have outdoor occupational or recreational exposure.

C. Diagnosis

B. dermatitidis appears as broad-based budding yeasts in BAL, sputum, or tissue biopsy. A test for *Blastomyces* urinary antigen has been shown to be useful, but does demonstrate cross-reactivity with *Histoplasma* urinary antigen. Culture provides a definitive diagnosis.

D. Treatment and Prevention Approach

Patients with mild-to-moderate pulmonary blastomycosis can be treated with itraconazole 200 mg orally twice daily for six months (the oral suspension is preferred). Current data suggest that response to fluconazole is inferior to itraconazole (65% vs. 95%) (25,26). Therapy should be extended to 12 months in patients with bone involvement, and therapeutic drug monitoring has been shown to be useful, aiming for trough levels greater than 1 µg/mL. Patients with severe pulmonary disease, central nervous system

(CNS) involvement, immunosuppression, or pregnancy are usually treated with amphotericin B. In particular, itraconazole is an inferior agent for meningeal infections because of high protein binding and poor CNS penetration. While there are data to support the use of voriconazole in savage therapy, there is little evidence to support its routine use as first-line therapy, and there are no current studies examining the clinical efficacy of posaconazole, which also has reduced CNS penetration (27–29).

E. Complications and Difficult Management Scenarios

The role of fluconazole in blastomycosis remains controversial. While *Blastomyces* is less susceptible to fluconazole in vitro than other azoles, fluconazole can be used in higher doses (800 mg/day) without significant toxicity, and its superior penetration into the CNS has some advantages. Consequently, fluconazole may play a role as adjuvant therapy with amphotericin B in CNS disease.

V. *Histoplasma capsulatum*

Histoplasmosis is a disease caused by the thermal dimorphic fungus *Histoplasma capsulatum* that preferentially grows in soil contaminated by bird or bat guano. Disease is contracted through inhalation of the spores from disturbance of the soil. Although *H. capsulatum* can be found anywhere in the world, it is endemic in states bordering the Ohio River valley and the lower Mississippi River in the United States.

A. Clinical Presentation

The most common manifestation of histoplasmosis is asymptomatic pulmonary nodules due to recent or remote exposure. The clinical presentations can vary from acute pulmonary manifestations with pneumonia, characterized by multifocal opacification to chronic pulmonary disease with progressive involvement. Chronic pulmonary disease, often with cavitary infiltrates, is more common in the setting of COPD. Disseminated disease can be particularly dangerous because it can progress to ARDS and multiorgan failure, including CNS disease. The pulmonary manifestations of histoplasmosis also include mediastinal lymphadenitis or granuloma, fibrosing mediastinitis, broncholithiasis, and pleural disease.

B. Etiopathogenesis

In nonimmunocompromised hosts, the severity of histoplasmosis is related to the size of the inoculum. By contrast, the nature of the immunodeficiency determines the likelihood of acquiring histoplasmosis in immunocompromised hosts. Persons at the extremes of age are predisposed, in addition to patients with AIDS, solid organ transplants, or patients receiving immunosuppressive monoclonal antibody therapy.

C. Diagnosis

Samples may be taken from lung (BAL, sputum, or tissue), blood, bone marrow, liver, skin lesions, or any site implicated in infection. *H. capsulatum* grows slowly, sometimes taking from four to six weeks before colonies emerge, and even then a DNA probe test is often required to confirm *Histoplasma* (30). Histopathology may reveal typical organisms that are 2 to 4 μm, oval, narrow-based budding yeasts, best seen on silver or periodic acid–Schiff staining.

An enzyme immunoassay is available to detect the galactomannan of *H capsulatum*. Urine provides superior results to serum and is positive in 95% of AIDS patients (31). However, because galactomannan is produced by other fungi, the test can be positive in other mycoses.

Serologic testing has been shown to be of value. The complement fixation (CF) test uses two separate antigens, yeast and mycelial (also called histoplasmin). A fourfold rise in CF antibody titer; or a single titer of greater than 1:32 is suggestive but not diagnostic of infection. Titers are often positive for years after fungal infection and therefore a low titer may be due to remote exposure. Furthermore, other fungal infections and even other granulomatous processes, including tuberculosis and sarcoidosis can lead to false-positive results (32,33).

Detection of M and H precipitin bands by immunodiffusion (ID) assay is more sensitive and specific than CF serology. The M band develops with acute infection and is often present for months to years after the infection. By contrast, the H band is less common and is usually accompanied by an M band. The H band is indicative of chronic or severe acute forms of histoplasmosis (32,34).

Other forms of the disease such as broncholithiasis or fibrosing mediastinitis may require bronchoscopic, pulmonary function or angiographic evaluation before proceeding to surgical consultation.

D. Treatment and Prevention

Treatment is usually offered for moderate to severe acute pulmonary disease. The earlier patients present following exposure and increased intensity of exposure should hasten a decision to treat. Progressive chronic pulmonary disease may also benefit from treatment. Itraconazole is more effective than fluconazole, and usual therapy is 200 mg b.i.d. for 6 to 12 weeks. Patients with moderate to severe disease, disseminated or CNS disease usually receive amphotericin B (0.7–1 mg/kg/day) may be withheld for healthy adults or in the setting in mild pulmonary disease as it is not clear if the risk of renal toxicity is low, or a lipid formulation of amphotericin B (3–5 mg/kg/day). By contrast, treatment may be withheld for healthy adults or in the setting in mild pulmonary disease as it is not clear if treatment speeds recovery in this setting.

E. Complications and Difficult Management Scenarios

Fibrosing mediastinitis is a particularly difficult problem. Unfortunately, fatal complications can arise. Some experts believe there is a role for a 12-week course of itraconazole, 200 mg twice daily (35), while others feel there is no role for antifungal therapy and early surgical consultation should be pursued.

VI. *Coccidioides immitis*

Coccidioidomycosis is an infection caused by a dimorphic fungus of the genus *Coccidioides*. *Coccidioides* species are endemic to semiarid regions of the western hemisphere, including the San Joaquin Valley of California, the south-central region of Arizona, and northwestern Mexico. They can also be found in parts of Central and South America.

A. Clinical Presentation

The most common manifestation of coccidioidomycosis is community-acquired pneumonia. Occasionally, patients will present with hilar adenopathy, peripheral blood eosinophilia, severe fatigue, night sweats, and the presence of erythema multiforme or erythema nodosum. Pulmonary manifestations include parapneumonic effusion, nodules, cavities that rupture or cause hemoptysis, chronic fibrocavitary disease, and even progression to ARDS and diffuse alveolar damage. Extrapulmonary manifestations include infections of the skin, arthritis, osteomyelitis, and meningitis.

B. Etiopathogenesis

The endemic areas for *Coccidioides immitis* are the arid regions of the southwestern Unities States including the San Joaquin Valley of California, the south-central region of Arizona, and northwestern Mexico. The organism resides in the soil, and when aerosols are generated, it is inhaled. Acquisition is common, and up to 60% of infections are asymptomatic, with the majority of symptomatic cases presenting as community acquired pneumonia (36). Patients with solid organ transplants, HIV infection or receiving TNF-α inhibitor therapy are especially at risk of coccidioidomycosis. African-American and Filipino-American men are also at increased risk for developing disseminated coccidioidomycosis (37).

C. Diagnosis

A variety of serologic tests have been employed for the diagnosis including anti-coccidioidal antibody in the serum measured by ELISA, immunodiffusion, or by tube precipitin and complement fixation assays. The diagnosis can also be made by identifying coccidioidal spherules in tissue or by culturing the fungus from tissue or respiratory secretions. The microbiology laboratory should be forewarned because special techniques need to be employed to isolate this pathogen.

D. Treatment and Prevention

In immunocompetent patients without identified risk factors, treatment is not required. However, when symptoms persist for more than six weeks, treatment should be offered. The approach to treatment in this setting is similar to the approach in immunosuppressed patients. Immunosuppressed patients such as those with solid organ transplants, HIV infection or other comorbidities such as chronic lung disease, chronic renal failure, or congestive heart failure are generally offered therapy. Antifungal therapy for chronic coccidioidomycosis generally requires 12 to 18 months of therapy and even longer in immunocompromised patients. Itraconazole 400 mg daily has been shown to be effective (38). Fluconazole has also been shown to be effective, although the response to itraconazole may be slightly superior, especially for bone and joint disease (38). Amphotericin B is reserved for patients with very severe disease. There are two recent trials examining the role of posaconazole. It has been shown to be effective as salvage therapy (39) in a phase II trial in which 85% of patients responded, but 33% relapsed (40).

Patients with diabetes mellitus are likely to develop chronic pulmonary coccidioidomycosis, particularly cavitary disease, and require close monitoring.

E. Complications and Difficult Management Scenarios

Surprisingly, one of the greatest challenges facing clinicians is the appropriate management of community-acquired pneumonia due to *C. immitis*. Despite the common nature of this disease, there is almost no data to guide our decisions. An abstract presented at the 2007 IDSA meeting by Ampel and colleagues presented the retrospective results of 104 patients that came to medical attention at the Tucson Veterans Affairs Hospital (41). The 51 patients that received no antifungal therapy had a somewhat lower symptom score than the 53 that were given treatment, but there was no significant difference in the duration of coccidioidal illness, anticoccidioidal complement fixation (CF) titer or chest radiograph abnormality. At the final visit, there was no difference in symptom score or CF titer in those initially treated or not treated, and no subject in either group developed disseminated disease at follow-up. This study outlines the desperate need for additional studies in this area.

VII. Cryptococcus spp.
Cryptococcus species consist of *Cryptococcus neoformans* var. *grubii* and *C. neoformans* var. *neoformans, C. gattii*, and other species such as *C. albidus, C. laurentii, and C. terreus*. Until recently, *C. gattii* was classified as serotype B and C of *C. neoformans*, but it is now clear that this represents a distinct species.

A. Clinical Presentation
Although meningitis is the most common and serious manifestation of cryptococcosis, pulmonary disease occurs in both immunocompetent and immunocompromised individuals. In immunocompetent patients, the pulmonary manifestations include asymptomatic colonization, often in patients with underlying structural lung disease (42,43). In symptomatic patients, the most common abnormalities are pulmonary nodules, masses, or interstitial pneumonitis (43–45). Pneumonia presents as patchy opacifications or ground glass opacities on the chest roentgenogram. However, pleural effusions, adenopathy, and even severe ARDS can occur with large fungal burdens (43,46).

B. Etiopathogenesis
Patients at risk of *C. neoformans* are those with severe T-cell immunodeficiencies, such as those with AIDS (CD4 T-cell count <100/µL). While therapy with cyclosporine and tacrolimus may reduce the risk of infection compared with other immunosuppressive regimens because of their direct antifungal activity (47,48), infections still occur in solid organ transplantation patients that receive these agents (49). Additionally, patients with hematologic malignancies and immunosuppression due to chemotherapeutic agents or monoclonal antibodies, patients receiving corticosteroids for solid organ transplantation or inflammatory diseases such as sarcoidosis, and patients with diabetes mellitus are also predisposed to cryptococcosis (50,51). Recently, treatment with novel immunosuppressive agents such as infliximab and alemtuzumab has also been identified as a risk factor for cryptococcosis (52–55).

By contrast, while sporadic cases of *C. gattii* appear around the world, there are two major endemic areas where nonimmunocompromised patients present. Traditionally, *C. gattii* has been endemic in northern Australia and Papua New Guinea (56). However, recently, cases have been identified on Vancouver Island in Canada, and the cases have very recently extended to the mainland of British Columbia and the adjacent Washington state (57,58).

C. Diagnosis

The diagnostic approach to cryptococcal infections includes a latex agglutination test for antigen and obtaining fluids or tissue for histopathologic examination of culture. The test for antigen has been shown to be of value in serum, CSF, and BAL (59). The organism is readily identified by mucicarmine or periodic acid–Schiff staining because of its polysaccharide capsule. Moreover, the organism grows readily on a variety of culture media, but prefers to grow at 30°C. Fortunately, *C. gattii* can readily be distinguished from *C. neoformans* by growth on selective media, and serologic identification need only be performed in difficult cases (60).

D. Treatment and Prevention

The approach to treatment is dictated by the severity of the illness and by the immune status of the patient. Immunocompetent patients that are simply colonized do not require therapy (61). Immunocompetent patients that are symptomatic can be treated with fluconazole. All patients should have serum cryptococcal antigen titers obtained. A lumbar puncture should be considered in all patients and should be performed if there is evidence of dissemination or CNS symptoms. Fluconazole 400 mg/day initially, tapering to 200 mg/day is often sufficient (43,61). Treatment should be given for six months and may have to be extended, particularly in patients with *C. gattii* infections (62). Patients with more severe disease should receive amphotericin B as described below.

For immunosuppressed patients, such as those with HIV, treatment is dictated by the high likelihood of dissemination and meningitis. The standard therapy for cryptococcosis in immunocompromised patients is amphotericin B (0.7 mg/kg/day) with or without flucytosine (100 mg/kg/day in four divided doses). If the CSF cultures are negative at two weeks, this therapy can be switched to fluconazole (400 mg/day) for an additional eight weeks.

E. Complications and Difficult Management Scenarios

Recently, *C. gattii* has emerged as an important pathogen on Vancouver Island, British Columbia, and the adjacent Washington state. The most common isolates are of the VGII molecular type, and clinicians should be aware of this disease, which is associated with a high mortality in patients that reside or have traveled to this region.

References

1. Hawksworth DL. Fungi: a neglected component of biodiversity crucial to ecosystem function and maintenance. Can Biodiversity 1992; 1:4–10.
2. Morgan J, Wannemuehler KA, Marr KA, et al. Incidence of invasive aspergillosis following hematopoietic stem cell and solid organ transplantation: interim results of a prospective multicenter surveillance program. Med Mycol 2005; 43(suppl 1):S49–S58.
3. Zmeili OS, Soubani AO. Pulmonary aspergillosis: a clinical update. QJM 2007; 100:317–334.
4. Yeghen T, Kibbler CC, Prentice HG, et al. Management of invasive pulmonary aspergillosis in hematology patients: a review of 87 consecutive cases at a single institution. Clin Infect Dis 2000; 31:859–868.
5. Soubani AO, Chandrasekar PH. The clinical spectrum of pulmonary aspergillosis. Chest 2002; 121:1988–1999.
6. Young RC, Bennett JE, Vogal CL, et al. Aspergillosis: the spectrum of disease in 98 patients. Medicine 1970; 49:147–173.

7. Pfeiffer CD, Fine JP, Safdar N. Diagnosis of invasive aspergillosis using a galactomannan assay: a meta-analysis. Clin Infect Dis 2006; 42:1417–1427.
8. Meersseman W, Lagrou K, Maertens J, et al. Galactomannan in bronchoalveolar lavage fluid: a tool for diagnosing aspergillosis in intensive care unit patients. Am J Respir Crit Care Med 2008; 177:27–34.
9. Tuncel E. Pulmonary air meniscus sign. Respiration 1984; 46:139–144.
10. Walsh TJ, Anaissie EJ, Denning DW, et al. Treatment of aspergillosis: clinical practice guidelines of the Infectious Diseases Society of America. Clin Infect Dis 2008; 46:327–360.
11. Limper AH, Knox KS, Sarosi GA, et al. American Thoracic Society statement on treatment of fungal infections in adult pulmonary and critical care patients. Am J Respir Crit Care Med 2009 (in press).
12. Marr KA, Boeckh M, Carter RA, et al. Combination antifungal therapy for invasive aspergillosis. Clin Infect Dis 2004; 39:797–802.
13. Chen JC, Chang YL, Luh SP, et al. Surgical treatment for pulmonary aspergilloma: a 28 year experience. Thorax 1997; 52:810–813.
14. Stevens DA, Schwartz HJ, Lee JY, et al. A randomized trial of itraconazole in allergic bronchopulmonary aspergillosis. N Engl J Med 2000; 342:756–762.
15. Vandewoude KH, Blot SI, Depuydt P, et al. Clinical relevance of *Aspergillus* isolation from respiratory tract samples in critically ill patients. Crit Care 2006; 10:R31.
16. Pappas PG, Rex JH, Lee J, et al. A prospective observational study of candidemia: epidemiology, therapy, and influences on mortality in hospitalized adult and pediatric patients. Clin Infect Dis 2003; 37:634–643.
17. Wisplinghoff H, Bischoff T, Tallent SM, et al. Nosocomial bloodstream infections in US hospitals: analysis of 24,179 cases from a prospective nationwide surveillance study. Clin Infect Dis 2004; 39:309–317.
18. Ostrosky-Zeichner L, Pappas PG. Invasive candidiasis in the intensive care unit. Crit Care Med 2006; 34:857–863.
19. Hachem R, Hanna H, Kontoyiannis D, et al. The changing epidemiology of invasive candidiasis: candida glabrata and *Candida krusei* as the leading causes of candidemia in hematologic malignancy. Cancer 2008; 112:2493–2499.
20. Morrell M, Fraser VJ, Kollef MH. Delaying the empiric treatment of candida bloodstream infection until positive blood culture results are obtained: a potential risk factor for hospital mortality. Antimicrob Agents Chemother 2005; 49:3640–3645.
21. Ostrosky-Zeichner L, Alexander BD, Kett DH, et al. Multicenter clinical evaluation of the $(1\rightarrow3)$ beta-D-glucan assay as an aid to diagnosis of fungal infections in humans. Clin Infect Dis 2005; 41:654–659.
22. Paphitou NI, Ostrosky-Zeichner L, Rex JH. Rules for identifying patients at increased risk for candidal infections in the surgical intensive care unit: approach to developing practical criteria for systematic use in antifungal prophylaxis trials. Med Mycol 2005; 43:235–243.
23. Ostrosky-Zeichner L, Sable C, Sobel J, et al. Multicenter retrospective development and validation of a clinical prediction rule for nosocomial invasive candidiasis in the intensive care setting. Eur J Clin Microbiol Infect Dis 2007; 26:271–276.
24. Lemos LB, Baliga M, Guo M. Acute respiratory distress syndrome and blastomycosis: presentation of nine cases and review of the literature. Ann Diagn Pathol 2001; 5:1–9.
25. Dismukes WE, Bradsher RW Jr., Cloud GC, et al. Itraconazole therapy for blastomycosis and histoplasmosis. NIAID Mycoses Study Group. Am J Med 1992; 93:489–497.
26. Pappas PG, Bradsher RW, Kauffman CA, et al. Treatment of blastomycosis with higher doses of fluconazole. The National Institute of Allergy and Infectious Diseases Mycoses Study Group. Clin Infect Dis 1997; 25:200–205.
27. Bakleh M, Aksamit AJ, Tleyjeh IM, et al. Successful treatment of cerebral blastomycosis with voriconazole. Clin Infect Dis 2005; 40:e69–e71.

28. Borgia SM, Fuller JD, Sarabia A, et al. Cerebral blastomycosis: a case series incorporating voriconazole in the treatment regimen. Med Mycol 2006; 44:659–664.
29. Gauthier GM, Safdar N, Klein BS, et al. Blastomycosis in solid organ transplant recipients. Transpl Infect Dis 2007; 9:310–317.
30. Stockman L, Clark KA, Hunt JM, et al. Evaluation of commercially available acridinium ester-labeled chemiluminescent DNA probes for culture identification of *Blastomyces dermatitidis*, *Coccidioides immitis*, *Cryptococcus neoformans*, and *Histoplasma capsulatum*. J Clin Microbiol 1993; 31:845–850.
31. Wheat LJ, Kauffman CA. Histoplasmosis. Infect Dis Clin North Am 2003; 17:1–19.
32. Picardi JL, Kauffman CA, Schwarz J, et al. Detection of precipitating antibodies to *Histoplasma capsulatum* by counterimmunoelectrophoresis. Am Rev Respir Dis 1976; 114:171–176.
33. Wheat J, French ML, Kamel S, et al. Evaluation of cross-reactions in Histoplasma capsulatum serologic tests. J Clin Microbiol 1986; 23:493–499.
34. Bauman DS, Smith CD. Comparison of immunodiffusion and complement fixation tests in the diagnosis of histoplasmosis. J Clin Microbiol 1975; 2:77–80.
35. Loyd JE, Tillman BF, Atkinson JB, et al. Mediastinal fibrosis complicating histoplasmosis. Medicine (Baltimore) 1988; 67:295–310.
36. Galgiani JN, Ampel NM, Blair JE, et al. Coccidioidomycosis. Clin Infect Dis 2005; 41: 1217–1223.
37. Gifford MA, Buss WC, Douds RJ. Data on coccidioides fungus infection, Kern County 1901–1936. Kern County Health Department Annual Report, 1937:39–54.
38. Galgiani JN, Catanzaro A, Cloud GA, et al. Comparison of oral fluconazole and itraconazole for progressive, nonmeningeal coccidioidomycosis. A randomized, double-blind trial. Mycoses Study Group. Ann Intern Med 2000; 133:676–686.
39. Stevens DA, Rendon A, Gaona-Flores V, et al. Posaconazole therapy for chronic refractory coccidioidomycosis. Chest 2007; 132:952–958.
40. Catanzaro A, Cloud GA, Stevens DA, et al. Safety, tolerance, and efficacy of posaconazole therapy in patients with nonmeningeal disseminated or chronic pulmonary coccidioidomycosis. Clin Infect Dis 2007; 45:562–568.
41. Ampel NM, Giblin A, Chavez S. Factors and outcomes associated with the decision to treat primary pulmonary coccidioidomycosis. Clin Infect Dis 2009; 48(2):172–178.
42. Rozenbaum R, Goncalves AJ. Clinical epidemiological study of 171 cases of cryptococcosis. Clin Infect Dis 1994; 18:369–380.
43. Aberg JA, Mundy LM, Powderly WG. Pulmonary cryptococcosis in patients without HIV infection. Chest 1999; 115:734–740.
44. Zlupko GM, Fochler FJ, Goldschmidt ZH. Pulmonary cryptococcosis presenting with multiple pulmonary nodules. Chest 1980; 77:575.
45. Khoury MB, Godwin JD, Ravin CE, et al. Thoracic cryptococcosis: immunologic competence and radiologic appearance. AJR Am J Roentgenol 1984; 142:893–896.
46. Penmetsa S, Rose TA, Crook ED. Rapid respiratory deterioration and sudden death due to disseminated cryptococcosis in a patient with the acquired immunodeficiency syndrome. South Med 1999; J 92:927–929.
47. Mody CH, Toews GB, Lipscomb MF. Cyclosporin A inhibits the growth of *Cryptococcus neoformans* in a murine model. Infect Immun 1988; 56:7–12.
48. Mody CH, Toews GB, Lipscomb MF. Treatment of murine cryptococcosis with cyclosporin-A in normal and athymic mice. Am Rev Respir Dis 1989; 139:8–13.
49. Blankenship JR, Singh N, Alexander BD, et al. *Cryptococcus neoformans* isolates from transplant recipients are not selected for resistance to calcineurin inhibitors by current immunosuppressive regimens. J Clin Microbiol 2005; 43:464–467.

50. Pappas PG, Perfect JR, Cloud GA, et al. Cryptococcosis in human immunodeficiency virus-negative patients in the era of effective azole therapy. Clin Infect Dis 2001; 33:690–699.
51. Vilchez RA, Irish W, Lacomis J, et al. The clinical epidemiology of pulmonary cryptococcosis in non-AIDS patients at a tertiary care medical center. Medicine (Baltimore) 2001; 80:308–312.
52. Hage CA, Wood KL, Winer-Muram HT, et al. Pulmonary cryptococcosis after initiation of anti-tumor necrosis factor-alpha therapy. Chest 2003; 124:2395–2397.
53. Shrestha RK, Stoller JK, Honari G, et al. Pneumonia due to *Cryptococcus neoformans* in a patient receiving infliximab: possible zoonotic transmission from a pet cockatiel. Respir Care 2004; 49:606–608.
54. Arend SM, Kuijper EJ, Allaart CF, et al. Cavitating pneumonia after treatment with infliximab and prednisone. Eur J Clin Microbiol Infect Dis 2004; 23:638–641.
55. Nath DS, Kandaswamy R, Gruessner R, et al. Fungal infections in transplant recipients receiving alemtuzumab. Transplant Proc 2005; 37:934–936.
56. Jenney A, Pandithage K, Fisher DA, et al. Cryptococcus infection in tropical Australia. J Clin Microbiol 2004; 42:3865–3868.
57. Hoang LM, Maguire JA, Doyle P, et al. *Cryptococcus neoformans* infections at Vancouver Hospital and Health Sciences Centre (1997–2002): epidemiology, microbiology and histopathology. J Med Microbiol 2004; 53:935–940.
58. MacDougall L, Kidd SE, Galanis E, et al. Spread of *Cryptococcus gattii* in British Columbia, Canada, and detection in the Pacific Northwest, USA. Emerg Infect Dis 2007; 13:42–50.
59. Baughman RP, Rhodes JC, Dohn MN, et al. Detection of cryptococcal antigen in bronchoalveolar lavage fluid: a prospective study of diagnostic utility. Am Rev Respir Dis 1992; 145:1226–1229.
60. Min KH, Kwon-Chung KJ. The biochemical basis for the distinction between the two *Cryptococcus neoformans* varieties with CGB medium. Zentralbl Bakteriol Mikrobiol Hyg [A] 1986; 261:471–480.
61. Nadrous HF, Antonios VS, Terrell CL, et al. Pulmonary cryptococcosis in non-immunocompromised patients. Chest 2003; 124:2143–2147.
62. Dromer F. Comparison of the efficacy of amphotericin B and fluconazole in the treatment of cryptococcosis in human immunodeficiency virus-negative patients: a retrospective analysis of 83 cases. Clin Infect Dis 1996; 22:S154–S160.

17
Emerging Infections: Influenza, Avian Influenza, and Pandemic Influenza

ALAN J. LESSE
Veterans Affairs Western New York Healthcare System and University at Buffalo,
State University of New York, Buffalo, New York, U.S.A.

Something old, something new, something borrowed, then something goes askew.

I. Introduction

It may be somewhat of a paradox to consider influenza as an emerging pathogen, with yearly epidemics and worldwide pandemics dating back at least a century. These "old" manifestations of influenza continue into the 21st century with continual adaptation by the influenza virus necessitating yearly changes in our vaccination strategies. However, avian influenza has recently emerged as a "new" threat, with concern that this avian virus may convert to the next great pandemic virus, similar to the devastating 1917 to 1918 "Spanish" influenza pandemic that resulted in over 50 million deaths. When the next new pandemic will occur, how severe it will be, and where it will originate from, depend, in part, on how the new pandemic strain "borrows" genetic elements from both zoonotic and human strains. How "askew" this goes, in large part, will be determined by several factors that cannot be predicted.

This chapter reviews the pathophysiology of influenza, both epidemic and pandemic strains. It will also discuss the development of avian influenza and the potential of this disease to spawn the next pandemic. Lastly, antiviral therapy of influenza is also reviewed, as are recent changes in antiviral recommendations.

II. Influenza

Influenza virus is a member of the Orthomyxoviridae family, a segmented, negative-strand, RNA virus (1,2). There are five members of the family of Orthomyxoviridae including influenza A, influenza B, influenza C, isavirus, and thogotovirus. Influenza A and B account for the majority of human disease, with only scattered reports of influenza C virus infection in humans. The only current member of the isavirus family is the *i*nfectious *s*almon *a*nemia virus that does not affect humans. The thogotovirus family, which includes the Thogoto, Batken, and Dhorhi viruses, does infect humans, but at the current time, infection is only seen in the immunocompromised host.

A. The Virus

The speciation of influenza virus into influenza A, B, or C, is based on the antigenic recognition of the nucleoprotein (NP) and the matrix (M) protein. If classified as an influenza A species, the virus is subtyped on the basis of the surface hemagglutinin (HA) and neuraminidase (NA) antigens. Influenza A virus has 16 different HA types and nine different NA types (1,2). Individual strains of viruses are named in accordance with the site of origin, the isolate number, and the year of isolation. For example, the 2008 to 2009 influenza virus vaccine for the northern hemisphere contained A/Brisbane/59/2007 (H1N1) that represents an H1N1 isolate (number 59) from Brisbane, Australia, recovered during the 2007 season. Influenza B isolates (and influenza C) are not subtyped, as HA and NA variation in these strains are not as large as influenza A.

B. Replication Cycle

The HA of the influenza virus binds to sialic acid residues on the cell surface of human, avian, and other animal cells (3–5). In humans, the sialic acid residues of the upper airway are linked via α-2,6 linkages, while avian cells contain predominantly α-2,3-linked sialic acid (6). This difference likely explains some, but not all, of the species specificity of strictly human and avian strains. Once the virus is bound to the cell, it is endocytosed in clathrin-coated pits. In the low pH of the endosome, the HA undergoes a shape change allowing the viral ribonucleic protein, in the form of eight segments, access to the host cell cytosol. The viral protein M2 is responsible for final acidification of the endosome and release into the cytoplasm. The adamantane drugs, amantadine and rimantadine (so-called M2 agents), block this acidification and inhibit influenza A replication (see sect. VI).

Trafficking in and out of the nucleus is unusual for viral infections; however, the influenza virus is dependent on the nucleus for viral RNA synthesis. "Naked" viral RNA does not exist in the cell, and viral RNA is always associated with one of four viral proteins [NP, basic polymerase 1 (PB1), PB2, and PA], with NP being the major protein and PA, PB1, and PB2 being part of a trimeric RNA-dependent, RNA-polymerase. The proteins and associated ribonucleic acid are then localized to the nucleus via nuclear localizing signals present in each of the four proteins. Once in the nucleus, viral negative-strand RNA produces both viral messenger RNA and viral RNA. After synthesis, the complexes are too large to leave the nucleus by passive diffusion and are transported out of the nucleus via the host cell CRM1/exportin-1 nuclear export protein. Once in the cytoplasm, the viral particles assemble at the apical surface and bud from the cell. At this point the activity of the NA is essential for replication, as the HA of the virus binds actively to the host cell after budding. NA is required to cleave the HA sialic acid bond to release the viral particles from the cell. In the absence of NA activity influenza replication and infectivity is inhibited.

C. Clinical Illness

Influenza is characterized by the sudden onset of fever, headache, and myalgia accompanied by cough and sore throat. Symptoms may range from mild to severe. Episodes of influenza may be particularly severe and accompanied by significant malaise and myalgia. The acute disease generally resolves over five to seven days, although cough may remain for several weeks.

D. Complications

Although uncommon, primary influenza pneumonia is a potentially lethal complication of influenza. Pregnant women and immunocompromised individuals are at increased risk of this complication. More commonly, severe pneumonia associated with influenza is often the result of secondary bacterial pneumonia. Common bacterial species are responsible for the pneumonia, including *Streptococcus pneumoniae* and *Haemophilus influenzae*. However, the incidence of *Staphylococcus aureus* pneumonia increases significantly after influenza infections, and recent reports show a marked increase in incidence, severity, and mortality of community-associated, methicillin-resistant *S. aureus* (CA-MRSA) strains in children following influenza outbreaks (7,8).

Myositis and rhabdomyolysis may be seen with influenza, and serum creatinine phosphokinase levels are frequently elevated in patients with influenza. Myocarditis, pericarditis, encephalitis, and other systemic complications are also described.

E. Outbreak Tracking

Tracking of the yearly influenza activity is done on a nationwide basis by the Centers for Disease Control and Prevention (CDC), as described on the CDC Web site (9):

> The Outpatient Influenza-like Illness Surveillance Network (ILINet) consists of about 2,400 healthcare providers in 50 states reporting approximately 16 million patient visits each year. Each week, approximately 1,300 outpatient care sites around the country report data to CDC on the total number of patients seen and the number of those patients with influenza-like illness (ILI) by age group.

Additional data are also gathered including virus isolation and identification of influenza virus at local and state health departments, hospital surveillance through the Emerging Infections Program, and monitoring of death certificates for increased mortality. The system represents a significant cooperation of the local, state, and federal facilities and provides a nationwide assessment of disease activity. The data are summarized weekly at the CDC Web site (9). This system is a key component in the worldwide effort to identify rapidly any new strain of influenza that may be the harbinger of the next global outbreak.

Perhaps as a reflection of the new information age and the impact of the Internet, nearly identical epidemiologic curves have been derived by Google using "Google Flu" (http://www.google.org/flutrends/). To generate the data, user queries to Google for flu-related symptoms are analyzed by Google, processed by a published algorithm, and posted on the Internet. Google Flu replicates the accuracy of the CDC with the additional benefit of being two weeks earlier than CDC data (10).

F. Antigenic Drift

Influenza occurs on a yearly basis, peaking in activity during the winter in each hemisphere. Yearly disease activity is the result of antigenic changes in the predominant strains of the virus circulating worldwide. Mutations in the HA and to a lesser degree, NA, result in antigenically different but related viruses that circulate on a yearly basis. This process represent *antigenic drift*, and is responsible for the yearly variation of infecting strains. Recent theories of influenza virus spread and evolution, based on whole genomic sequencing of over 1300 influenza A isolates, suggest that there is significant antigen pressure on selection of the HA antigen. The yearly or biyearly changes in virus isolation in the temperate climate are theorized to evolve from continual viral activity in the tropics, which serve as a "pool" for viral reassortment (11). Such antigenic drift is the basis for the need for yearly alteration of the influenza vaccine. Antigenic cross-reactivity provides some partial protection, and over time, the population maintains partial recognition of yearly antigenic drift. Although not sufficient to mitigate severe disease or epidemics, this antigenic cross-reactivity on a population basis is sufficient to slow any worldwide epidemic of strains selected by antigenic drift.

G. Antigenic Shift

A process called antigenic shift produces pandemic influenza with worldwide increases in both attack rates and severity. Because influenza virus is a segmented genome, infection of a cell with different strains of influenza virus can result in genetic reassortment between the strains and selection of a new strain with unique HA and NA types. Additionally, reassortment of the viral proteins may place a unique HA or NA in a background of highly efficient human-to-human transmission. Emergence of these strains leads to a rapid and widespread worldwide epidemic, or pandemic, of a new virus that is antigenically unrecognized by preexisting immunity in the population. These shifts can either result from entry of a zoonotic strain of influenza capable of significant human-to-human spread, or the genomic rearrangement of a zoonotic strain and a human strain.

Over the last century, there have been three pandemics: (*i*) 1918—Spanish influenza, (*ii*) 1957—"Asian" influenza, and (*iii*) 1968—"Hong Kong" influenza. The 1918 Spanish influenza was unmatched in the worldwide scope and mortality rate related to the pandemic. The sudden introduction of the Spanish H1N1 virus into the population, possibly from an avian influenza virus (see Section III, Spanish Influenza), resulted in an extraordinarily high rate of pneumonia and death. After this major antigenic shift, the H1N1 virus remained the predominant influenza virus over the next 40 years. In 1957, the sudden introduction of the H2N2 strain of Asian influenza represented the second antigenic shift of the 20th century and the second, although milder pandemic. Concomitant with the introduction of the H2N2 strain was the sudden and unexplained disappearance of the H1N1 strain. The H2N2 remained the predominant circulating virus until 1968, when the third antigenic shift of the century brought the Hong Kong strain of H3N2 virus (and disappearance of the H2N2 strain). The H3N2 strain has been present in yearly outbreaks since 1968. Interestingly, in 1977, the H1N1 strain from the 1950s reemerged by unknown mechanisms and has remained codominant with the H3N2 strains since that time.

Mechanisms for the antigenic shift and emergence of the Asian and Hong Kong strains of influenza A appear to be classic reassortment of avian and human strains of influenza. Sequence analysis of the 1957 pandemic strain shows striking sequence homology of the HA, NA, and basic polymerase 1(PB1) of the H2N2 Asian pandemic strain and avian viruses circulating at the time (12,13). The 1967 Hong Kong virus showed significant homology of the HA and PB1 segments of the H3N2 strain and circulating avian strains of that period (13,14). These reassortments suggest that antigenic shift occurs in the setting of coinfection of avian and human strains, which may not be as rare as originally expected. In addition, the availability of a third species that is readily infected by both avian and human strains may serve as an effective "mixing bowl" for viral reassortment. Pigs, in fact, are susceptible to both strains of influenza and have been shown to harbor avian-human reassortant viruses (15).

Although the last two major pandemics of influenza have been associated with marked increases in morbidity and mortality, they pale in comparison to the 1918 epidemic at the end of World War I. This global pandemic of Spanish influenza had astonishingly high death rates and had the unusual propensity to cause mortality in the otherwise healthy 25- to 40-year olds. The Spanish influenza virus is a stunning example of antigenic shift, but the mechanism was different that the Asian or Hong Kong pandemics.

III. Spanish Influenza

The great pandemic of 1918 to 1919 was unlike any other pandemic in recorded time (16). Over a third of the world's population was possibly infected and mortality is estimated at 50 million deaths, with some estimates ranging as high as 100 million. The exact etiology of this enhanced mortality is still unknown, but recent advances in our understanding have been made possible through amplification of viral RNA from pathology specimens preserved from the fall of 1918. This molecular analysis forms the basis for our current understanding of the pathophysiology of the 1918 to 1919 pandemic.

Sequence analysis from the 1918 Spanish influenza H1N1 virus began in 1995 when Taubenberger and colleagues isolated RNA from formalin-fixed, paraffin-embedded samples recovered from a victim of Spanish influenza who died in the fall of 1918 (17). The initial sequence analysis suggested introduction of a novel influenza virus, and subsequent analysis of the complete genome suggested to Taubenberger and others that the 1918 isolate was a human-adapted strain of avian influenza virus that was rapidly introduced into a naïve population with devastating effects (16–19). Other investigators, however, have recently questioned the phylogenetic analysis of the data and suggest the 1918 virus was also the result of a reassortant between avian and human influenza virus (20–22). Which interpretation is ultimately accurate can only be determined if human viral isolates before the 1918 strain are obtained. Some may conclude the disagreement is only of interest to academics, but the implications of the analysis are profound. The recently described avian influenza virus (H5N1) has been responsible for a number of human cases since 1997 and has shown marked biologic similarities to bioengineered H1N1 virus based on the 1918 strain (see below). If Taubenberger and colleagues are correct, then the emergence of this new avian strain causing human disease is a source of great concern.

Whatever the source of the 1918 pandemic strain, the virus was also introduced into the swine population at about the same time and serves as the origin of classic swine influenza. Fear of another pandemic of influenza surfaced in 1976 when one soldier died and 13 others were infected at the military training base at Fort Dix, New Jersey (23–26). Rapid analysis and concern that the virus was a promontory strain heralding the next pandemic resulted in a major government effort at mass immunization of the U.S. population for swine flu. The program was initiated, but no epidemic occurred. The National Influenza Immunization Program was marred by the subsequent development of vaccine-associated cases of Guillain-Barré syndrome and stopped in December 1976.

The epidemiology of the 1918 to 1919 pandemic is remarkable, not only in the introduction of the virus into a highly susceptible population, but also in the spread of the virus around the world. Unlike most outbreaks of influenza, the 1918 strain had a phenomenally high attack rate and had a unique, three-wave epidemic over an 18-month time frame from 1918 to 1919 (16). The initial wave was seen in the spring of 1918 with rapid spread across the United States, Europe, and Asia. The more devastating fall wave seen in October and November of 1918 was accompanied by an explosive attack rate and associated with a high rate of secondary pneumonia and death. Previous pandemics had high death rates with the second wave of infection, but the 1918 Spanish influenza also had a third wave of infection, with the three-wave time frame condensed into one 18-month period.

The epidemiologic pattern for influenza-associated death during the Spanish influenza pandemic was unlike anything seen before or after. While infection rates peaked in the 5- to 14-year age range, the mortality had a triphasic appearance with increased mortality in the very young, the elderly, and surprisingly, the 20- to 35-year age group (16,18). The mortality rate in this younger population was *not* associated with increased mortality in the elderly, as the epidemic only produced a small 0.6% increase in mortality in the greater than 65-year population when compared with prepandemic influenza-associated death rates from 1911 to 1917. This suggests that prior exposure of the older population to cross-reacting viruses from the 1880s may have provided protection against the pandemic virus. Much of the data suggest that a major cause of mortality in the epidemic was secondary bacterial pneumonia (27,28).

The enhanced mortality of the Spanish influenza virus has recently been studied by molecular "reconstruction" of the virus based on the sequencing of the 1918 pathologic material and reverse genetic engineering (29). This reconstructed Spanish strain appears to cause an aberrant and dysregulatory activation of the innate immune system, with ineffective viral clearance and high death rates in experimental models (30,31).

The pandemic caused millions of death worldwide, but the immune response in survivors was effective on a population basis and halted the epidemic. In fact, the immune response to this virus was particularly impressive, with survivors of the 1918 pandemic still possessing strong immunologic response more than 80 years later when measured using a bioengineered HA replicating the 1918 pandemic strain (32).

The H1N1 pandemic strain and the subsequent viral "drift" isolates remained the major influenza isolate until 1957. In that year, the sudden emergence of the Asian H2N2 influenza pandemic strain (a result of reassortment between H1N1 and an avian strain to produce H2N2) was accompanied by the unexplained disappearance of the H1N1 strain. The H1N1 virus reemerged in 1977 without a pandemic, and along with the H3N2 virus (introduced in the 1968 Hong Kong pandemic) serves as the major strains causing influenza worldwide since 1977.

Given the devastation of the 1918 to 1919 pandemic and the likelihood that the pandemic strains was an avian influenza isolate with efficient human-to-human transmission, the 1997 detection of H5N1 avian influenza raised the specter that H5N1 may represent a preview of the first great pandemic virus of the 21st century, the possibility of pandemic avian influenza.

IV. Avian Influenza

Although the number of NA and HA types affecting humans remains rather small, birds are the targets of many more strains of influenza. Sequence analyses of strains of avian influenza dating back to the turn of the last century suggest that that there is limited genetic pressure on the strains as compared with human strains. However, two HA combinations, namely the H5N1 and H7N1 strains, have been noted to cause highly pathogenic avian influenza (HPAI) epidemics in chicken and turkeys (33). The molecular basis of the enhanced virulence of these strains appears to be related to the insertion of basic amino acids between the HA1 and HA2 domains of the HA (33). In the native state, the HA must be cleaved between the two regions by tissue-specific proteases found only within the respiratory and gastrointestinal tract. Insertion of these basic amino acids renders the regions susceptible to proteases with a much wider tissue distribution. This wider distribution of protease activity is likely responsible for the disseminated disease seen with HPAI and the resulting high mortality.

In 1997, a strain of H5N1 HPAI was detected in Guangdong Province in China. Shortly thereafter, infected chickens were detected in Hong Kong. Eighteen human cases were reported with a 33% mortality. The Chinese government ordered the systematic culling (killing) of the entire 1.5 million chickens in poultry farms and markets of Hong Kong (33). This Draconian effort was successful in eliminating the virus from detection until February 2003, when the virus reappeared in Hong Kong. Two human cases were discovered in a father and son who had just returned from Fujian Province. A third case occurred in Beijing that was originally diagnosed as severe acute respiratory syndrome (SARS), but was later confirmed to be avian influenza. Cases began to appear in several countries of Southeast Asia. As of March 2009, there have been 409 human cases of avian influenza in humans with 256 deaths for a crude mortality rate of 63% (34). A map of the geographic distribution of the cases is shown in Figure 1.

Avian influenza in humans is a far different disease than classic influenza. Dissemination of the virus outside of the respiratory tract (see discussion on tissue protease distribution mentioned earlier in this section) is common, and associated viremia, a rare complication in human influenza, is seen in a majority of cases where blood was

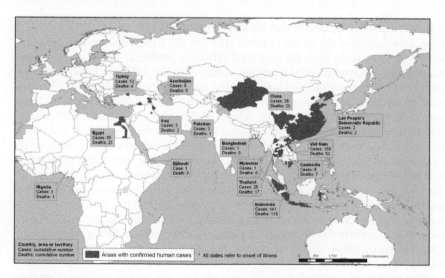

Figure 1   World Health Organization (WHO) tracking of human cases of avian influenza since 2003 as of 27 January, 2009. Reproduced with permission from the World Health Organization (WHO).

cultured for the virus. The H5N1 virus infects many organ systems, and pneumonia is quite common. Diarrhea is common as contrasted with classic human influenza, due, in part, to replication of the virus in the gastrointestinal tract (33).

Primary viral pneumonia occurs commonly in avian influenza with little evidence for secondary bacterial pneumonia commonly seen with human strains. This is probably related to the predilection of the NA of H5N1 and other avian strains for α-2,3-linked sialic acid. Although that linkage is rare in the upper respiratory tract in humans, it is present in the lower respiratory tract (6). Human strains of influenza have a predilection for α-2,6-linked sialic acid that is common in the upper airway of humans but not avian hosts. Infection with H5N1 virus in humans theoretically would require delivery of virus deeper into the respiratory tract of humans in order to gain access to α-2,3-linked sialic acid residues found in the distal pulmonary tree (6). This may explain the lower infectivity of these strains of HPAI for human (35). However, even genetically engineered strains of the 1918 influenza virus with HA that binds to both α-2,3 and α-2,6 linkages was not as effective as virus that bound solely to α-2, 6 linkages in the models, suggesting that a multitude of factors are involved with the species specificity and efficiency of transmission in these strains (36).

Infections with HPAI are quite severe in humans, as judged by the exceedingly high mortality (37). In addition, the majority of cases and death have been in the younger population, a feature seen in the 1918 to 1919 pandemic of H1N1 influenza in humans (33). In an interesting set of experiments, reverse-engineered H1N1 virus based on the Spanish influenza strain was highly pathogenic in mice without passage and capable of inducing a markedly enhanced but aberrant immune response and lymphocyte apoptosis (38,39). A similar accelerated immune response has been seen with HPAI, and the profound lymphopenia associated with the disease is thought to be mediated via apoptosis (40).

V.   Will HPAI Become the Next Pandemic Flu?

Since the identification of the strains of HPAI H5N1 in 1977, there has been concern that the strain will serve as the basis for next great influenza pandemic. At the current time, genetic pressure has resulted in at least four clades of avian influenza H5N1 infecting humans (33,41). There is confirmed human-to-human transmission of the virus (42), but the numbers are low. The factors that are responsible for the conversion of a strain from one species to another are just now being delineated. The current data are insufficient to predict exactly what genetic factors are required for this conversion, although additional insights continue to be learned (43). If Taubenberger and associates are correct and the great pandemic of Spanish influenza in1918 was the result of the introduction of a strain of avian origin into humans with effective human-to-human transmission, then H5N1 may be a precursor to the next pandemic. Much of the world has begun to plan for such a devastating conversion, with massive efforts going into vaccination, infection control, and antiviral therapy. Monitoring of avian and human cases of influenza may give us sufficient time to react to this introduction. However, if the introduction is anything like the 1918 epidemic, efforts aimed at control will likely only minimally mitigate the devastation of the virus.

Other models of conversion of this zoonosis into the human population predict that reassortment will be the key mechanism for selection of the next pandemic virus. As the incidence of human cases of avian influenza increase, the likelihood of simultaneous infection with H5N1 and either H3N2 or H1N1 in the same human rises. This increases the possibility of selection of a new reassorted virus with potentially effective human-to-human transmission. Similarly, coinfection could occur in the avian host, although this is reported to be much less common. More likely however is the possibility of reassortment in a host that is highly susceptible to both virus populations, such as swine. As with the introduction of H1N1 in 1918 to both human and swine populations, coinfection of swine with both avian and human strains of influenza have the great potential to produce a reassortant that is fully capable of efficient transmission in humans. Monitoring of nonavian animal populations for reassortant virus may give use our first look at the next pandemic strain. Even if the next pandemic is not of the caliber of the 50 million worldwide deaths of the 1918 outbreak, lethality in the four million or one million range, as seen with the Asian and Hong Kong pandemics, is clearly possible. Given the current world economic crisis in 2009, the introduction of highly lethal influenza pandemic may have an even greater consequence than originally predicted.

VI. Antiviral Therapy

Therapy of influenza, whether influenza or avian influenza is currently based on drugs which affect two stages in the replication cycle of the virus. Adamantanes (amantadine and rimantadine) work by inhibiting the ion channel of the M2 protein in influenza A. NA inhibitors (oseltamivir and zanamivir) work by inhibiting NA activity of the virus and prevent newly formed virus detachment from the infected cell. The adamantanes are only active against influenza A, but the NA inhibitors have activity against both influenza A and B.

A. Adamantanes

Amantadine was the first influenza antiviral medications developed for the prevention of influenza A (FDA approval in 1966). Amantadine was effective at preventing influenza A infection and was used as an adjunct to the primary prevention strategy of vaccination. The drug was primarily recommended during influenza outbreaks to prevent influenza A in closed communities (like nursing homes) where vaccination efficacy is often under 80% and a high-risk population may be exposed to virus. The major side effects of amantadine are confusion, lightheadedness, and other anticholinergic and CNS effects. In fact, the prominent CNS side effects are therapeutically useful for the treatment of early Parkinson's disease. In 1994 a highly related drug, rimantadine, was also approved for prevention and early treatment of influenza A infection. Rimantadine has fewer side effects than amantadine, especially with regard to the CNS effects.

B. Adamantane Resistance

It was quickly discovered that resistance to the adamantanes develops rapidly, and that patients treated with either agent may excrete resistant virus. For this reason, it is not recommended to use adamantanes for both treatment and prophylaxis in the same household, or closely confined population such as a nursing home. Resistance to the agents is easily conferred by single amino acid mutations in the M2 protein, most commonly a serine to asparagine change at amino acid 31. This change does not affect the infectivity or fitness of the virus. Adamantane-resistant virus can be shed in up to

30% of treated patients (44). Intrafamilial spread of adamantane-resistant strains is well documented.

Global resistance to the adamantanes increased slowly from their introduction through 2005, when the rapid global spread of an H3N2 Ser31Asn mutation resulted in over 90% resistance to the adamantanes (44). Some of the marked increase in resistance may have been traced to the SARS outbreak and heavy over-the-counter use of amantadine in China in 2003 (44). However, spontaneous antigenic drift in 1933 and 1934 produced amantadine-resistant H1N1 mutants 30 years before the introduction of the agents (45). In a large study on the development of adamantine resistance in H3N2 isolates, only 2% of U.S. adamantane-resistant isolates were obtained from patients on adamantanes, nursing home residents, or individuals in close contact with patients receiving adamantanes (45). This suggests that antigenic drift may be more important than drug selection pressure in the development of resistance to the agents.

Regardless of the exact molecular etiology of the resistance to adamantanes, the Centers for Disease Control and Prevention (CDC) in early 2005 advised against the use of the adamantanes for influenza infection as over 90% of the H3N2 virus tested was resistant to the agents (46,47). At the time, resistance to the newer NA inhibitors (see sect. VI.C) was quite low, and the adamantanes were removed from CDC recommendations and replaced with the NA inhibitors.

The use of the adamantanes for avian influenza at this time also appears to be limited. The original clade of avian influenza virus from Fujian Province is resistant to the adamantanes; however, a second clade of virus commonly seen in Indonesia, China, Russia, and Turkey maintains sensitivity to the adamantanes (46). However, because we cannot predict with any certainty whether M2 sensitive segments will be selected if a human-avian reassortant emerges, the next pandemic strain may be adamantane sensitive. During both the 1968 Hong Kong pandemic, and the accelerated transmissions associated with the 1977 Russian influenza outbreak, adamantanes remained effective agents (44).

C. NA Inhibitors

The most recent and powerful additions to the influenza antiviral compounds are two drugs that inhibit a key step in the replication of influenza virus in the host, NA. The two drugs, oseltamivir and zanamivir, inhibit the activity of influenza NAs. Inhibition of this viral enzyme results in massive virus accumulation at the site of infected cells and inability of the virus to spread, effectively interrupting the life cycle of the virus (48) (see life cycle above).

NA may also potentiate infectivity by directly cleaving mucin (49). Epithelial cell may be covered with thick layers of mucin, and the cleavage of mucin by NA allows the virus access to underlying sialic acid residues of respiratory tract epithelial cells, facilitating the infection of cells previously obscured by the mucin layer.

Unlike the adamantanes, the NA inhibitors are active against both influenza A and B. Although resistant virus has emerged on therapy (see below), the initial clinical trials with the NA inhibitors showed significantly lower rates of development of resistant virus that treatment with the adamantanes (48). These initial trials also found that NA inhibitor resistant viral isolates were less biologically fit (48). Spread of resistant virus from treated patients to intrahousehold contacts did not occur with any great frequency in the initial trials (48). Rates of resistance to oseltamivir in these initial trials were around 0.4% in adults and higher rates (4%) in children, probably owing to higher viral loads. Some of the resistance to oseltamivir in Japanese children was thought to be the result of lower dosing recommendations in Japan, but recent weight-based dosing trials have also shown selection of resistance among H1N1 strains to oseltamivir regardless of dosing (50).

Resistance to the NA inhibitors occurs via mutations in the NA protein. During the 2007 to 2008 influenza outbreak in Norway, oseltamivir resistance occurred in a remarkably high rate (67%) despite minimal use of oseltamivir in Norway and Western Europe (51). This clone has rapidly spread worldwide, so that nearly every U.S. H1N1 virus in the 2008 to 2009 influenza season is now oseltamivir resistant (52,53). This clearly demonstrates the biologic fitness of this oseltamivir-resistant mutant.

Resistance to the NA inhibitors is mediated through a histamine-to-tyrosine mutation at position 275 of the N1 NA (H275Y) of the H1N1 strains. This change alters the deformability of the active site of the NA (54). Molecular modeling of sialic acid, the natural ligand, and oseltamivir and zanamivir to the active site reveal that the structure of oseltamivir is bulkier than the structure of sialic acid and zanamivir (54). When the H275Y and/or other mutations are present (R2922K and N294S), the active site becomes more structurally rigid. Oseltamivir's structure requires flexibility of the active site in binding the bulkier oseltamivir. The H275Y mutation results in increased rigidity of the active site, excluding oseltamivir via steric hindrance as shown in the diagram below (55). The activity of zanamivir is maintained, however, as zanamivir more closely approximates the natural ligand, sialic acid, as shown in Figure 2.

High-level resistance to both zanamivir and oseltamivir has also be reported with key amino acid changes in the NA conferring resistance to all currently available NA inhibitors (56).

Unfortunately, the H275Y mutation occurs in the H5N1 strains of avian influenza. Further complicating the use of oseltamivir for avian influenza is the documented development of resistance during therapy and transmission of resistant virus to contacts (57). This will clearly have an impact on global pandemic plans, as oseltamivir is currently the sole NA stockpiled for pandemic preparation.

As of 2009, the CDC recommended that treatment for influenza is based on the likelihood of influenza A in the patient. Because of adamantane resistance in the H3N2 strains and oseltamivir resistance in H1N1 strains, the CDC recommends the use of BOTH rimantadine and oseltamivir OR zanamivir for treatment or prophylaxis. The H1N1 strains in circulation in 2009 have a high frequency of the H275Y mutation, are

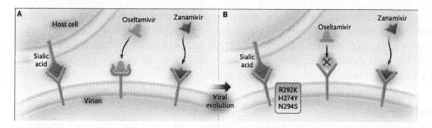

Figure 2 Schematic representation of neuraminidase binding of sialic acid and two neuraminidase inhibitors. (From Ref. 55, with permission from Massachusetts Medical Society, © 2005.)

oseltamivir resistant, but retain sensitivity to the adamantanes. The H3N2 have high rates of adamantane resistance but are oseltamivir sensitive. Therefore, the recommendation is for the use of rimantadine for possible H1N1 and oseltamivir for possible H3N2 virus. Zanamivir is also an acceptable single drug option as the NA mutation retains sensitivity to this agent, as detailed above. Use of zanamivir, however, is complicated by the fact that the drug must be given by inhalation and is not available for oral use. In addition, zanamivir can trigger bronchospasm in patients with chronic obstructive pulmonary disease (COPD), which limits its use. Known cases of influenza B can be treated with oseltamivir or zanamivir.

Treatment with either of the NA inhibitors must be given within the first 48 hours of symptoms to result in any benefit (48). A one-day reduction in symptoms is seen in patients treated within the first 48 hours, while a two- to three-day improvement was seen in patients treated within the first 12 hours. There are limited data on whether the agents prevent mortality related to influenza (58). Both agents are highly effective in preventing influenza in an outbreak.

Use of NA inhibitors in avian influenza is problematic. Development of resistant virus has been documented in patients treated with oseltamivir and infection with resistant virus has also been documented (42). Efficacy of the agent in avian influenza is uncertain based on the high mortality of the disease, limited number of cases, and the lack of any controlled trials. Should oseltamivir-resistant avian influenza evolve effective human-to-human transmission, the current stockpiles of oseltamivir will not protect the population from infection or treat those infected. The current worldwide spread of oseltamivir-resistant H1N1 further complicates the potential problem by providing a background strain for possible reassortment that already possess resistance to some of our most potent agents.

D. New Influenza Antivirals

One of the most pressing current needs is a parenteral formulation of a NA inhibitor. Both intravenous zanamivir and peramivir for intramuscular and intravenous injection are currently being studied (46,59). Other agents including long-acting NA inhibitors, HA inhibitors, siRNA, and polymerase inhibitors are also in various stages of development (46,59).

VII. The Future

On the basis of available data, a future global pandemic is nearly certain. The history of influenza, pandemic influenza, and most recently, avian influenza provide an opportunity to understand some of the biologic pressure on influenza virus. We must use this knowledge and continue to monitor influenza on a worldwide basis to predict the course of upcoming epidemics and the eventual pandemic that will arrive. When the virus goes askew and the next pandemic occurs, it will be important to act rapidly to control what will be a global threat of potentially historic proportions.

References
1. Dolin R. Influenza. In: Fauci AS, Braunwald E, Kasper DL, et al., eds. Harrison's Principles of Internal Medicine. 17th ed. McGraw-Hill, 2008:1127–1132.

2. Treanor JJ. Influenza. In: Mandell GL, Bennett JE, Dolin R, eds. Principles and Practice of Infectious Diseases. 6th ed. Philadelphia: Elsevier, 2005:2060–2085.
3. Vastrik I, D'Eustachio P, Schmidt E, et al. Reactome: a knowledge base of biologic pathways and processes. Genome Biol 2007; 8:R39.
4. Matthews L, Gopinath G, Gillespie M, et al. Reactome knowledgebase of human biological pathways and processes. Nucleic Acids Res 2009; 37:D619—D622.
5. Cros JF, Palese P. Trafficking of viral genomic RNA into and out of the nucleus: influenza, Thogoto and Borna disease viruses. Virus Res 2003; 95:3–12.
6. Shinya K, Ebina M, Yamada S, et al. Avian flu: influenza virus receptors in the human airway. Nature 2006; 440:435–436.
7. Unknown. Severe methicillin-resistant *Staphylococcus aureus* community-acquired pneumonia associated with influenza—Louisiana and Georgia, December 2006-January 2007. MMWR Morb Mortal Wkly Rep 2007; 56:325–329.
8. Bhat N, Wright JG, Broder KR, et al. Influenza-associated deaths among children in the United States, 2003-2004. N Engl J Med 2005; 353:2559–2567.
9. Centers for Disease Control and Prevention. Seasonal flu: flu activity & surveillance. Available at: http://www.cdc.gov/flu/weekly/fluactivity.htm
10. Ginsberg J, Mohebbi MH, Patel RS, et al. Detecting influenza epidemics using search engine query data. Nature 2009; 457:1012–1014.
11. Rambaut A, Pybus O, Nelson M, et al. The genomic and epidemiological dynamics of human influenza A virus. Nature 2008; 453:615–619.
12. Treanor J, Kawaoka Y, Miller R, et al. Nucleotide sequence of the avian influenza A/Mallard/ NY/6750/78 virus polymerase genes. Virus Res 1989; 14:257–269.
13. Kawaoka Y, Krauss S, Webster RG. Avian-to-human transmission of the PB1 gene of influenza A viruses in the 1957 and 1968 pandemics. J Virol 1989; 63:4603–4608.
14. Bean WJ, Schell M, Katz J, et al. Evolution of the H3 influenza virus hemagglutinin from human and nonhuman hosts. J Virol 1992; 66:1129–1138.
15. Castrucci MR, Donatelli I, Sidoli L, et al. Genetic reassortment between avian and human influenza A viruses in Italian pigs. Virology 1993; 193:503–506.
16. Taubenberger J, Morens DM. 1918 Influenza: the mother of all pandemics. Emerg Infect Dis 2006; 12:15–22.
17. Taubenberger JK, Reid AH, Krafft AE, et al. Initial genetic characterization of the 1918 "Spanish" influenza virus. Science 1997; 275:1793–1796.
18. Taubenberger J. The origin and virulence of the 1918 "Spanish"influenza virus. Proc Am Philos Soc 2006; 150:86–112.
19. Taubenberger J, Reid A, Lourens R, et al. Characterization of the 1918 influenza virus polymerase genes. Nature 2005; 437:889–893.
20. Antonovics J, Hood ME, Baker CH. Molecular virology: was the 1918 flu avian in origin? Nature 2006; 440:E9; discussion E-10.
21. Gibbs M, Gibbs A. Molecular virology: was the 1918 pandemic caused by a bird flu? Nature 2006; 440:E8; discussion E9–E10.
22. Vana G, Westover KM. Origin of the 1918 Spanish influenza virus: a comparative genomic analysis. Mole Phylogenet Evol 2008; 47:1100–1110.
23. Gaydos JC, Top FH Jr., Hodder RA, et al. Swine influenza a outbreak, Fort Dix, New Jersey, 1976. Emerg Infect Dis 2006; 12:23–28.
24. Sencer DJ, Millar JD. Reflections on the 1976 swine flu vaccination program. Emerg Infect Dis 2006; 12:29–33.
25. Dowdle WR. Influenza pandemic periodicity, virus recycling, and the art of risk assessment. Emerg Infect Dis 2006; 12:34–9.
26. Lessler J, Cummings DA, Fishman S, et al. Transmissibility of swine flu at Fort Dix, 1976. J R Soc Interface 2007; 4:755–762.

27. Brundage JF, Shanks GD. Deaths from bacterial pneumonia during 1918–1919 influenza pandemic. Emerg Infect Dis 2008; 14:1193–1199.

28. Gupta RK, George R, Nguyen-Van-Tam JS. Bacterial pneumonia and pandemic influenza planning. Emerg Infect Dis 2008; 14:1187–1192.

29. Tumpey TM, Basler CF, Aguilar PV, et al. Characterization of the reconstructed 1918 Spanish influenza pandemic virus. Science 2005; 310:77–80.

30. Kobasa D, Jones S, Shinya K, et al. Aberrant innate immune response in lethal infection of macaques with the 1918 influenza virus. Nature 2007; 445:319–323.

31. Kobasa D, Takada A, Shinya K, et al. Enhanced virulence of influenza A viruses with the haemagglutinin of the 1918 pandemic virus. Nature 2004; 431:703–707.

32. Yu X, Tsibane T, McGraw PA, et al. Neutralizing antibodies derived from the B cells of 1918 influenza pandemic survivors. Nature 2008; 455:532–536.

33. Peiris JS, de Jong MD, Guan Y. Avian influenza virus (H5N1): a threat to human health. Clin Microbiol Rev 2007; 20:243–267.

34. Matrosovich M, Matrosovich T, Uhlendorff J, et al. Avian-virus-like receptor specificity of the hemagglutinin impedes influenza virus replication in cultures of human airway epithelium. Virology 2007; 361:384–390.

35. World Health Organization. Confirmed Human Cases of Avian Influenza A (H5N1). Available at: http://www.who.int/csr/disease/avian_influenza/country/en/

36. Tumpey TM, Maines TR, Van Hoeven N, et al. A two-amino acid change in the hemagglutinin of the 1918 influenza virus abolishes transmission. Science 2007; 315:655–659.

37. Thanh TT, van Doorn HR, de Jong MD. Human H5N1 influenza: current insight into pathogenesis. Int J Biochem Cell Biol 2008; 40:2671–2674.

38. Kash JC, Basler CF, Garcia-Sastre A, et al. Global host immune response: pathogenesis and transcriptional profiling of type A influenza viruses expressing the hemagglutinin and neuraminidase genes from the 1918 pandemic virus. J Virol 2004; 78:9499–9511.

39. Kash J, Tumpey T, Proll S, et al. Genomic analysis of increased host immune and cell death responses induced by 1918 influenza virus. Nature 2006; 443:578–581.

40. de Jong MD, Hien TT. Avian influenza A (H5N1). J Clin Virol 2006; 35:2–13.

41. Abdel-Ghafar AN, Chotpitayasunondh T, Gao Z, et al. Update on avian influenza A (H5N1) virus infection in humans. N Engl J Med 2008; 358:261–273.

42. Wang H, Feng Z, Shu Y, et al. Probable limited person-to-person transmission of highly pathogenic avian influenza A (H5N1) virus in China. Lancet 2008; 371:1427–1434.

43. Van Hoeven N, Pappas C, Belser JA, et al. Human HA and polymerase subunit PB2 proteins confer transmission of an avian influenza virus through the air. Proc Natl Acad Sci U S A 2009; 106:3366–3371.

44. Hayden FG. Antiviral resistance in influenza viruses–implications for management and pandemic response. N Engl J Med 2006; 354:785–788.

45. Bright RA, Medina MJ, Xu X, et al. Incidence of adamantane resistance among influenza A (H3N2) viruses isolated worldwide from 1994 to 2005: a cause for concern. Lancet 2005; 366:1175–1181.

46. Hayden F. Developing new antiviral agents for influenza treatment: what does the future hold? Clin Infect Dis 2009; 48(suppl 1):S3–S13.

47. Bright RA, Shay DK, Shu B, et al. Adamantane resistance among influenza A viruses isolated early during the 2005–2006 influenza season in the United States. JAMA 2006; 295:891–894.

48. Moscona A. Neuraminidase inhibitors for influenza. N Engl J Med 2005; 353:1363–1373.

49. Matrosovich MN, Matrosovich TY, Gray T, et al. Neuraminidase is important for the initiation of influenza virus infection in human airway epithelium. J Virol 2004; 78:12665–12667.

50. Stephenson I, Democratis J, Lackenby A, et al. Neuraminidase inhibitor resistance after oseltamivir treatment of acute influenza A and B in children. Clin Infect Dis 2009; 48:389–396.

51. Hauge SH, Dudman S, Borgen K, et al. Oseltamivir-resistant influenza viruses A (H1N1), Norway, 2007–2008. Emerg Infect Dis 2009; 15:155–162.
52. Dharan NJ, Gubareva LV, Meyer JJ, et al. Infections with oseltamivir-resistant influenza A (H1N1) virus in the United States. JAMA 2009; 301:1034–1041.
53. Gooskens J, Jonges M, Claas EC, et al. Morbidity and mortality associated with nosocomial transmission of oseltamivir-resistant influenza A (H1N1) virus. JAMA 2009; 301:1042–1046.
54. Collins P, Haire L, Lin Y, et al. Crystal structures of oseltamivir-resistant influenza virus neuraminidase mutants. Nature 2008; 453:1258–1261.
55. Moscona A. Oseltamivir resistance: disabling our influenza defenses. N Engl J Med 2005; 353:2633–2636.
56. Sheu TG, Deyde VM, Okomo-Adhiambo M, et al. Surveillance for neuraminidase inhibitor resistance among human influenza A and B viruses circulating worldwide from 2004 to 2008. Antimicrob Agents Chemother 2008; 52:3284–3292.
57. de Jong MD, Tran TT, Truong HK, et al. Oseltamivir resistance during treatment of influenza A (H5N1) infection. N Engl J Med 2005; 353:2667–2672.
58. Bowles SK, Lee W, Simor AE, et al. Use of oseltamivir during influenza outbreaks in Ontario nursing homes, 1999–2000. J Am Geriatr Soc 2002; 50:608–616.
59. Moscona A. Global transmission of oseltamivir-resistant influenza. N Engl J Med 2009; 360:953–956.

18
Emerging Modalities for Diagnosis (Including Biomarkers)

DAVID R. MURDOCH
University of Otago and Canterbury Health Laboratories, Christchurch, New Zealand

I. Introduction

The clinical diagnosis of many respiratory infections can be made relatively easily using clinical and radiographic tools, but determining the etiological diagnosis can be much more challenging. This difficulty is largely due to the limitations of conventional diagnostic tests that, despite many advances, are still suboptimal. For example, even in the most rigorous prospective studies an etiological diagnosis is not made in up to half of the patients. In the real world the diagnostic rate is much less. For some respiratory infections, such as ventilator-associated pneumonia, making a syndromic diagnosis can also be difficult. In these situations, clinicians often look for other laboratory markers to supplement clinical decision-making.

This chapter reviews the current state of laboratory diagnostics for respiratory infections, focusing on new and emerging technologies.

II. Conventional Diagnostic Tests
A. Microscopy and Culture

Microscopy and culture of sputum or other respiratory tract samples are the main diagnostic tools for identifying the microbial cause of respiratory infections. The identification of respiratory pathogens in good-quality samples collected directly from the site of infection provides good evidence of likely causative microorganisms. This is especially so for microorganisms that do not normally colonize the human upper respiratory tract, such as *Legionella* spp. The rapid detection of *Pneumocystis jiroveci* infection still relies a lot on microscopy of respiratory tract samples using special stains, and direct immunofluorescence assays have long been used to reliably detect respiratory viruses in respiratory tract samples. For other microorganisms that can colonize the upper airways, such as *Streptococcus pneumoniae*, the challenge is to distinguish colonization from infection. This requires that respiratory samples be checked for quality before processing, confirming that they have been obtained from the lower respiratory tract (1,2). A major limitation of microscopy and culture is the inability to obtain lower respiratory tract samples from many people. Many patients with pneumonia do not produce sputum, and invasive procedures such as bronchoscopy are infrequently performed. Another limiting factor of culture is the inability of some respiratory pathogens (e.g., *Mycoplasma pneumoniae*) to be readily isolated in diagnostic laboratories.

Blood cultures are an important diagnostic tool for pneumonia, but only a small minority of patients with pneumonia have documented bloodstream infections.

B. Antigen Detection

Antigen detection assays have been used to detect respiratory pathogens for almost 100 years (3) and play an important role in contemporary diagnostics. Depending on the infecting microorganism, antigens can be detected in respiratory or nonrespiratory samples. Among bacterial respiratory pathogens, assays for *Legionella pneumophila* and *S. pneumoniae* are the most developed. Detection of soluble *Legionella* antigen in urine is an established and valuable tool for the diagnosis of Legionnaires' disease, although current commercial assays can only reliably detect infection caused by *L. pneumophila* serogroup 1 (4). Detection of pneumococcal antigen in urine is also useful for diagnosing pneumococcal pneumonia in adults, especially using new-generation immunochromatographic tests that detect the C-polysaccharide cell wall antigen (5). Unfortunately, the latter test cannot be used reliably in children as it detects pneumo-coccal carriage in this age group (6).

Antigen detection is also an important tool for the diagnosis of viral respiratory tract infections. Many commercial rapid tests are now available (particularly for influenza and respiratory syncytial viruses) using immunochromatographic, ELISA, or other formats. The ease of performance of these kits has been responsible for their widespread use, despite their not being as sensitive as direct immunofluorescence (7).

C. Antibody Detection

Antibody detection assays exist for most respiratory tract pathogens and have provided useful epidemiological data. However, because of the need in most cases to test both acute and convalescent sera collected several weeks apart to document a fourfold or greater rise in reciprocal antibody titers, these assays have limited impact on clinical decision making. Measurement of antibody titers in only acute serum samples is rarely sufficient for diagnostic purposes. Furthermore, most serological assays for respiratory pathogens have suboptimal sensitivity and specificity. For a small number of respiratory infections, such as *M. pneumoniae* infection, antibody detection remains an important diagnostic tool while improved alternative methods are being developed.

III. Emerging Diagnostic Tools for Determining the Microbial Etiology of Respiratory Tract Infections
A. Nucleic Acid Amplification Tests

Nucleic acid amplification tests (NAATs) such as polymerase chain reaction (PCR) are in use for about 20 years. Although NAATs have been widely applied to the diagnosis of respiratory tract infections, they can still be regarded as emerging, given that a relatively small proportion of diagnostic laboratories have employed them in routine use. The situation is changing rapidly with the increased availability of commercial diagnostic NAATs for all common respiratory pathogens. NAATs have particularly contributed to understanding the role of respiratory viruses, *Legionella* spp. and *Chlamydophila pneumoniae* in acute respiratory infections (8) (Table 1).

NAATs have many features that make them attractive tools for diagnosing the etiology of respiratory tract infections (9). They can detect very low levels of nucleic

Table 1 Current and Emerging Diagnostic Modalities for Pneumonia Pathogens

	Diagnostic modalities	
Pneumonia pathogen	Current	Emerging
Streptococcus pneumoniae	• Microscopy/culture of respiratory tract samples • Blood cultures • Urinary antigen detection	• Improved antigen detection methods • Quantitative NAATs
Haemophilus influenzae, *Moraxella catarrhalis,* *Staphylococcus aureus*	• Microscopy/culture of respiratory tract samples • Blood cultures	
Mycoplasma pneumoniae	• Antibody detection	• NAATs
Legionella spp.	• Culture of respiratory tract samples • Urinary antigen detection • Antibody detection • NAATs	• Improved NAATs • Improved antigen detection methods
Chamydophila pneumoniae	• Antibody detection • NAATs	• Improved NAATs
Respiratory viruses	• Antigen detection in respiratory tract samples • Culture of respiratory tract samples • Antibody detection • NAATs	• Multiplex NAATs
Bordetella pertussis	• Culture of respiratory tract samples • Antibody detection • NAATs	• Improved NAATs
Pneumocystis jiroveci	• Microscopy of respiratory tract samples	• NAATs
Mycobacteria	• Microscopy/culture of respiratory tract samples	• NAATs • Breath analysis

Abbreviation: NAATs, nucleic acid amplification tests.

acid from potentially all respiratory pathogens, do not depend on the viability of the target microbe, can provide results within a clinically relevant time frame, are probably less affected by prior antibiotic administration than culture-based methods, and have the potential to provide supplementary information such as the presence of antibiotic resistance genes. NAATs have been particularly useful for diagnosing infections that are difficult or impossible to rapidly diagnose by other methods.

The development of NAATs for respiratory tract pathogens has followed a similar pattern of evolution as for other infections. PCR is the NAAT that has been most widely evaluated, with greater use over time of real-time, commercial, and multiplex assays (8,10). To date, few comparative studies between different assays have been reported and limited efforts have been made to produce standardized methods. The accurate calculation of clinical specificity for NAATs is hindered by the lack of suitable comparator standards, an inherent problem with NAATs that are likely to be more sensitive than most comparator culture-based methods.

The further development of NAATs needs to focus on clarifying the clinical usefulness of these assays, creating standardized methods, producing even more user-friendly platforms, and exploring the role of quantitative assays.

Common Bacterial Pneumonia Pathogens
Streptococcus pneumoniae

The use of NAATs to diagnose pneumococcal pneumonia has been evaluated in both adults and children. For pneumonia, PCR has a sensitivity for detecting *S. pneumoniae* in blood samples ranging from 29% to 100% (9), although there is a tendency for the performance to be better in children than adults. The generally poor performance of PCR in blood samples may be due to the rapid clearance of the *S. pneumoniae* from the blood stream and sampling errors resulting from the small sample volumes used in PCR reactions. In addition, positive pneumococcal PCR results have also been recorded from asymptomatic control subjects (11–13), and these findings are not readily explained.

When testing sputum samples, reported PCR positivity rates have ranged from 68% to 100% from patients with pneumonia (9), although it is unclear how often this reflects colonization of the upper respiratory tract rather than infection (14). This is a particular concern given the presence of the pneumolysin gene, a common pneumococcal PCR target, in some nonpneumococcal viridans streptococci (15). Further refinement of PCR assays, including the use of multiple targets, has increased the specificity (16), with *lytA* assays potentially offering advantages over other assays (17). Some investigators have suggested that quantitative PCR may help distinguish colonization from infection, with a higher bacterial burden in pneumococcal disease than in a carrier state. Although this has not been systematically evaluated, initial data suggest that this might be worth exploring further (18). A recent study from Malawi showed that high pneumococcal DNA loads in blood and cerebrospinal fluid were associated with fatal outcome in children with invasive pneumococcal disease (19).

PCR has also been successfully applied to other invasive samples, such as pleural fluid (20,21) and lung aspirates (22).

Mycoplasma pneumoniae

As culture of *M. pneumoniae* is difficult, the diagnosis of mycoplasma pneumonia has traditionally relied on antibody detection that has suboptimal sensitivity and specificity. Recently, NAATs have shown to be sensitive and specific and are considered by many to be the methods of choice for direct pathogen detection (23).

Numerous studies have evaluated the use of NAATs for the detection of *M. pneumoniae* in clinical samples (9). Despite differences in assays, sample type, and study populations, there has generally been good correlation between NAAT and serological test results, although most studies have reported a significant number of samples positive by only one of these two methods. An extensive evaluation of 13 antibody detection assays using PCR as the comparator standard concluded that few commercial serological assays for detection of *M. pneumoniae* performed with sufficient sensitivity and specificity and highlighted the increasing importance of NAATs (24). There have been few direct comparisons between different NAATs. Most have shown good concordance between different assays (25,26), although a recent comparison of real-time simplex and multiplex nucleic acid sequence-based amplification (NASBA) and PCR indicated that simplex real-time NASBA was more sensitive for detecting *M. pneumoniae* (27).

Both upper and lower respiratory tract samples are suitable for testing for *M. pneumoniae* by NAATs. Throat swabs and nasopharyngeal samples may be the preferred sample types because of both high sensitivity and specificity and convenience. One study found that throat swabs were less affected by PCR inhibitors than nasopharyngeal aspirates (28), although it is unclear whether this is still an issue with modern nucleic acid extraction techniques. During the investigation of a large outbreak of *M. pneumoniae* infection in a closed community, 15% of patients continued to have *M. pneumoniae* DNA detected in their throats two to six weeks after initiation of antibiotics (29). *M. pneumoniae* has also been detected by PCR in transthoracic needle aspirate samples, although this approach may be less sensitive than testing upper respiratory samples (30).

In practice, PCR has been successfully used to rapidly diagnose mycoplasma pneumonia during outbreaks, and was particularly useful in young children, immunocompromised patients, and in early stage disease (31,32).

Legionella spp.

NAATs are a useful adjunct to culture and antigen detection for the diagnosis of Legionnaires' disease (4). When testing lower respiratory tract samples, PCR has repeatedly been shown to have sensitivity equal to or greater than culture (33–39). The main disadvantage with this approach is that less than half of patients with Legionnaires' disease produce sputum (4). Bronchoalveolar lavage fluid is an alternative sample type (34–37) when it is important to make an etiological diagnosis.

Nonrespiratory samples have also been evaluated. *Legionella* DNA can be detected by PCR in urine samples from patients with legionellosis with sensitivities ranging from 30% to 86% (40–44). The sensitivity of testing acute serum samples by PCR had a similar range although tended to be less than for testing urine when both samples types were directly compared in the same population (43,45–47). The sensitivity of testing serum may be higher in patients with more severe disease (48). Animal and human studies have also indicated that peripheral leukocyte and whole blood samples may also be useful for testing (49–51).

An interesting complication in the development of NAAT assays for detecting *Legionella* spp. has been the recognition that some commercial DNA extraction kits and reagents have been intermittently contaminated with *Legionella* DNA (52–54). This contamination presumably occurred during the manufacturing process and is a potential cause of false-positive results.

Chlamydophila pneumoniae

PCR is a promising tool for the rapid diagnosis of *C. pneumoniae* infection and has been extensively evaluated using a variety of assays (55). A standardized approach to *C. pneumoniae* diagnostic testing was published in 2001 by the U.S. Centers for Disease Control and Prevention and the Canadian Laboratory Centre for Disease Control (56). However, there are still few evaluations that have extensively used clinical samples, and the great variety in the methods used makes it difficult to make firm conclusions about performance. To further complicate matters, significant interlaboratory discordance of detection rates have been recorded for given assays, which may be partly related to contamination (57,58).

Pertussis

NAATs have revolutionized the laboratory diagnosis of pertussis, which has traditionally relied on slow and variably sensitive culture methods. The diagnostic yield from PCR is consistently greater than for culture when testing nasopharyngeal samples (9). Positive PCR results have been recorded in people without symptoms of *Bordetella pertussis* infection (59), and this may represent asymptomatic infection or colonization. PCR remains positive for a longer period after the onset of symptoms and, thus, is useful for individuals who present late in their illness (60). In the investigation of a pertussis outbreak, the combination of PCR and culture for samples obtained less than or equal to two weeks after illness onset and PCR alone for samples obtained more than two weeks after illness onset proved to be the most diagnostically useful (61). Of the 149 cases in this outbreak, 138 had positive PCR results and 79 had positive culture results for *B. pertussis* (11 had negative PCR results and positive culture results).

Respiratory Viruses

NAATs have revolutionized the diagnosis of respiratory viruses and have contributed greatly to understanding the epidemiology and importance of respiratory virus infections in humans of all ages. NAATs have a much faster turnaround time than culture-based methods and are able to detect many viral pathogens that are unable to be readily detected by direct immunofluorescence and culture. Recent outbreaks of severe acute respiratory syndrome (SARS) (62) and human cases of H5N1 influenza infection (63) have focused attention on severe viral pneumonias, and NAATs are an essential diagnostic tool in the investigation and management of these infections.

Various NAAT assays are available for all respiratory pathogens and have been evaluated in a variety of populations (8,64) and, like tests for other pathogens, there is a general lack of standardization. In general, when compared with conventional methods NAATs have a higher positivity rate than culture and direct immunofluorescence, presumably reflecting greater sensitivity (64). Perhaps more so than for other respiratory pathogens, considerable effort has been directed toward the development of multiplex assays to enable the simultaneous detection of multiple viral pathogens. Given the increasingly large number of respiratory viruses, this can be a challenging task.

Pneumocystis jiroveci

PCR has greater sensitivity than cytological methods for the detection of *P. jiroveci*, although it has been difficult to interpret the common finding of PCR-positive samples that are negative by standard methods (9). The latter may reflect *P. jiroveci* colonization of uncertain clinical significance. The performance of PCR has been shown to vary with different assays (65).

Mycobacteria

The desperate need for improved diagnostic methods for tuberculosis has focused attention on the potential role of NAATs. Despite some advances and the release of several commercial assays, NAATs for mycobacteria have yet to provide greater sensitivity than culture-based methods. The relatively high false-negative rate with NAATs for *Mycobacterium tuberculosis* probably reflects a combination of the paucibacillary nature of samples, presence of inhibitors in samples, and suboptimal DNA extraction methods. For direct detection of *M. tuberculosis* in respiratory samples, all commercial assays have high specificity (>98%), but variable sensitivities: 90% to 100% for smear-positive samples and 33% to 100% for smear-negative samples (9). Consequently, it is recommended that use of these tests is restricted to smear-positive samples only. Interestingly, initial evaluations of PCR for the diagnosis of tuberculosis in populations with high prevalence of both tuberculosis and HIV infection have been promising (66,67). Among 1396 patients with suspected tuberculosis in Nairobi, Kenya, PCR had a sensitivity and specificity of 93% and 84%, respectively, compared with culture (67). The use of NAATs for the diagnosis of tuberculosis in patients with smear-positive sputum samples was recently evaluated in a population with a low prevalence of tuberculosis (Liverpool, U.K.) (68). In this study, the NAAT result had a significant clinical impact in 39% of tested patients, particularly due to the rapid availability of results.

B. Antigen Detection

There are ongoing efforts to develop improved rapid antigen detection assays for respiratory pathogens. Investigation of alternative pneumococcal antigens for diagnostic purposes has shown promising results, although no candidate antigen has been demonstrated to perform better than existing commercial C-polysaccharide antigen assays. Detection of a pneumococcal virulence factor in clinical samples might theoretically help distinguish colonization from infection. Pneumolysin, in particular, has been investigated as a potential diagnostic target. Pneumolysin antigen detection applied to urine (69–71) specimens has shown promising results, but has yet to be demonstrated as superior to the cell wall C-polysaccharide (NOW) assay (69). It is possible that the combination of the pneumolysin-specific antigen detection, ELISA, and the NOW test is likely to result in a better diagnostic yield due to the higher specificity of the pneumolysin detection ELISA (70). Other candidate antigens are currently undergoing evaluation.

Although the development of urinary antigen detection assays has been a major advance in diagnostics for Legionnaires' disease, existing commercial tests are limited by their ability to only reliably detect *L. pneumophila* serogroup 1 (4). Some assays have been intended to detect other legionellae (72), although the performance is not as good as for *L. pneumophila* serogroup 1.

IV. Biomarkers

Laboratory testing for respiratory infections has largely focused on identifying a causative microbe, but there is also considerable interest in the detection of compounds in blood or other samples that help guide antibiotic therapy and provide diagnostic and prognostic information. Inflammatory markers, such as the peripheral white cell count and C-reactive protein (CRP), have been widely used for this purpose over a long period of time. More recently, numerous other potential biomarkers have been promoted, although few have been introduced into routine use. Many of these are still in the early stages of development. For other promising biomarkers, the time has come for rigorous evaluation in intervention studies.

A. Breath Analysis

Breath analysis has enormous diagnostic potential, but has not yet been extensively evaluated for the diagnosis or monitoring of respiratory tract infections (73–75). Alveolar breath contains many biomarkers derived from the blood by passive diffusion across the alveolar membrane (73), and also direct markers of lung injury (76–78). Furthermore, breath testing is noninvasive, easily repeatable and requires minimal sample work-up. Various testing methodologies and sample types have been used in breath research, usually involving the measurement of exhaled permanent gases, detection of volatile organic compounds, or analysis of exhaled breath condensate. To date most breath analysis research on lung diseases has focused on the recognition, severity assessment, and response to treatment of asthma and chronic obstructive pulmonary disease (COPD) using biomarkers such as nitric oxide (73,79).

The use of breath analysis for the investigation of respiratory infections is still in its infancy. Detection of molecules or patterns of molecules in breath may aid in the diagnosis of pneumonia per se. Electronic nose devices detect volatile molecules as they interact with chemical sensor assays (80–82). On the basis of the reactivity of multiple sensors to the volatile molecules, an electronic signature is generated. Different signatures can be grouped as "like" or "not like," using statistical models and pattern recognition algorithms. Testing of exhaled breath by a portable electronic nose has been used to diagnose pneumonia in mechanically ventilated patients (83–85) and bacterial sinusitis (86). In each study, electronic nose results correlated well with clinical scores and/or radiographic findings. The clinical impact of this device needs further evaluation, but it could be used as a trigger for further diagnostic studies in pneumonia such as bronchoscopy.

Bacteria produce volatile metabolites that may be used as biomarkers (87). Detection of these biomarkers in breath samples by gas chromatography/mass spectroscopy (GC/MS) or similar methods may provide an etiological diagnosis of pneumonia. For this to occur, specific biomarkers are needed, and it may be difficult to identify unique markers for each pathogen produced in sufficient quantities to enable detection. Potential biomarkers have been reported for some respiratory pathogens, such as *Aspergillus fumigatus* (88) and *M. tuberculosis* (89), but it is still uncertain whether they will prove to be useful as clinical diagnostic tools.

Analysis of exhaled breath condensate (EBC), collected by cooling or freezing exhaled air, is a promising technique in the assessment of airways inflammation. Assays have been developed to assess cytokine levels (78) and oxidant production (76,77) in the lower airways. Levels of hepatocyte growth factor in EBC may reflect local production of hepatocyte growth factor and may be useful for the monitoring of recovery process after pneumonia (90). Again, the potential of EBC analysis has yet to be fully realized.

B. C-Reactive Protein

CRP is an acute phase protein synthesized by hepatocytes (91). Production of CRP is stimulated by cytokines, particularly interleukin (IL)-6, IL-1, and tumor necrosis factor (TNF), in response to infection or tissue inflammation. CRP levels in healthy individuals are normally less than 10 mg/L, but increase within six to eight hours in disease states to peak levels more than 300 mg/L (91). CRP levels rapidly decline upon resolution of inflammation or tissue destruction.

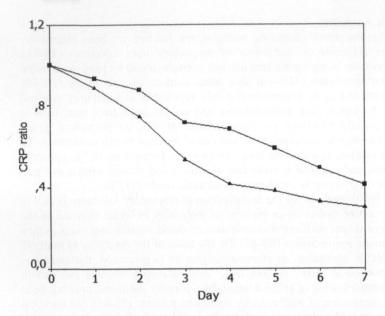

Figure 1 Time-dependent analysis of the C-reactive protein ratio during antibiotic therapy, showing a significant difference between survivors (▲) and nonsurvivors (■), $p = 0.039$ *Source*: From Ref. 93.

In lower respiratory tract infections, CRP has been proposed as a tool to help distinguish pneumonia from bronchitis, to distinguish bacterial from viral infections, and to monitor response to therapy. The findings of studies that have evaluated CRP as a rapid tool to identify bacterial infection and guide antibiotic prescription have been inconsistent. A recent systematic review concluded that testing for CRP is neither sufficiently sensitive nor specific to detect radiographically proved pneumonia or to distinguish between bacterial and viral infections (92). However, CRP may be useful for monitoring therapy in pneumonia (93) (Fig. 1), with persistently high levels suggestive of antibiotic treatment failure or the development of complications (94–96). CRP may also be an independent predictor of severity in community-acquired pneumonia. In one study of adults hospitalized with pneumonia, admission CRP less than 100 mg/L were associated with reduced 30-day mortality (OR, 0.18), reduced need for mechanical ventilation and/or inotropic support (OR, 0.21), and a reduction in complicated pneumonia (OR 0.05) (97). Furthermore, failure of CRP to fall by ≥50% within 4 days of admission was associated with increased 30-day mortality (OR, 24.5), need for mechanical ventilation and/or inotropic support (OR, 7.1), and complicated pneumonia (OR, 15.4).

C. Procalcitonin

PCT is the polypeptide precursor of the calcium regulatory hormone calcitonin (98). Production of PCT is normally confined to the thyroid C-cells, although it can be produced in extrathyroidal tissue in response to inflammation. PCT concentrations rise within hours of onset of disease states, with levels peaking at about six hours. The highest concentrations of PCT are seen in systemic bacterial infections, but also occur in multiorgan dysfunction following trauma (99).

An algorithm has been developed at the University Hospital Basel that classifies patients with lower respiratory tract infections according to the probability of bacterial infection on the basis of PCT levels (100). This algorithm has been evaluated in several intervention trials comparing PCT-guided antibiotic therapy with standard therapy. In 243 patients admitted with suspected lower respiratory tract infections (36% with pneumonia, 25% with exacerbation of COPD, 24% with acute bronchitis), PCT-guidance reduced antibiotic use by about 50% without compromising outcome (101). When used outside a trial setting in routine practice, the magnitude of this effect may be less (102). In a subsequent trial of 302 adults with community-acquired pneumonia, PCT-guidance reduced antibiotic prescriptions on admission (85% vs. 99%) and antibiotic treatment duration (median 5 vs. 12 days), with similar outcomes in both groups (103). Using a similar intervention for exacerbations of COPD, PCT guidance reduced antibiotic prescriptions over a six-month follow-up period (40% vs. 72%) (104). As a tool for predicting radiographic pneumonia and bacterial infection in adults with lower respiratory tract infection in primary care, PCT measurement had a positive predictive value that was judged as too low for use in clinical practice (105). The role of PCT measurement in the diagnosis of ventilator-associated pneumonia is still unclear (100). PCT levels, with other markers, may also be useful to monitor treatment failure in pneumonia (96).

As a prognostic tool for the assessment of lower respiratory tract infections, PCT levels correlate reasonably well with other markers and, in general, without offering any major advantage over other prognostic tools. Among 1651 patients seen in U.S. emergency departments with community-acquired pneumonia, PCT levels added little prognostic information beyond the pneumonia severity index and CURB-65 (106). PCT levels on admission predicted the severity and outcome of community-acquired pneumonia in 1671 adults in Germany with a similar prognostic accuracy as the CRB-65 score and a higher accuracy compared with CRP and leukocyte count (107). Other investigators have concluded that PCT levels are a useful adjunct to other clinical and laboratory parameters in the severity assessment of community-acquired pneumonia (108–110), but not necessarily as a stand-alone tool.

D. Other Biomarkers

The triggering receptor expressed on myeloid cells-1 (TREM-1) is expressed on neutrophils and mature monocytes when activated by bacteria and fungi, and mediates the acute inflammatory response to microbial products (111). When measured in bronchoalveolar lavage fluid from patients receiving mechanical ventilation, TREM-1 level was a better predictor of pneumonia than clinical or other laboratory measurements (112). In a separate study, alveolar (but not plasma) levels of TREM-1 were higher in patients with culture-positive pulmonary aspiration syndrome compared with those with culture-negative disease (113). An alveolar diagnostic cut-off of 250 pg/mL had a sensitivity of 66% and specificity of 92% for predicting culture-positive pulmonary aspiration syndrome. Other investigators have found that serum levels of TREM-1 greater than 50 pg/mL were an independent predictor of mortality (relative risk 7.0) in adults admitted with community-acquired pneumonia (114). The latter study also evaluated the prognostic value of serum cytokine levels and found that IL-6 levels greater than 80 pg/mL were associated with a nearly threefold increased risk of death. Serum TREM-1 levels are also increased in patients with stable COPD (115), thus limiting its usefulness in this group.

Other potential biomarkers include pro-adrenomedullin, which has been associated with severity and outcome in community-acquired pneumonia (116), and copeptin, which has been linked to prognosis in patients hospitalized with acute exacerbation of COPD (117), with ventilator-associated pneumonia (118), and with community-acquired pneumonia (119).

V. Future prospects

NAATs have now been developed to a stage whereby multiplex assays that detect all common respiratory pathogens are commercially available in user friendly platforms, and further improvements in design and performance are expected. The emphasis should now be placed on developing standardized methods and assessing the clinical impact of these assays in intervention trials. It is unclear whether NAATs will eventually make culture obsolete, although this is unlikely in the near future. Antigen detection assays in immunochromatographic or similar formats are fast and simple to perform. In many ways these methods are among the most attractive diagnostic tools, but further development is reliant on the discovery of suitable antigens that can be reliably detected in readily obtained samples. Breath analysis is an exciting new area with enormous potential. However, its application to the diagnosis of respiratory infections is still in the early stages of evaluation and it is uncertain whether the potential will be fully realized. Biomarkers can make important contributions to the diagnosis of respiratory infections when used in conjunction with clinical information and pathogen detection tests. Further emphasis should be place on clarifying the situations when biomarkers can be useful and assessing their impact in intervention trials.

References

1. Murray PR, Washington JAI. Microscopic and bacteriologic analysis of expectorated sputum. Mayo Clin Proc 1975; 50:339–344.
2. Musher DM, Montoya R, Wanahita A. Diagnostic value of microscopic examination of gram-stained sputum and sputum cultures in patients with bacteremic pneumococcal pneumonia. Clin Infect Dis 2004; 39:165–169.
3. Dochez AR, Avery OT. The elaboration of specific soluble substance by pneumococcus during growth. J Exp Med 1917; 26:477–493.
4. Murdoch DR. Diagnosis of Legionella infection. Clin Infect Dis 2003; 36:64–69.
5. Werno AM, Murdoch DR. Laboratory diagnosis of invasive pneumococcal disease. Clin Infect Dis 2008; 46:926–932.
6. Dowell SF, Garman RL, Liu G, et al. Evaluation of Binax NOW, an assay for the detection of pneumococcal antigen in urine samples, performed among pediatric patients. Clin Infect Dis 2001; 32:824–825.
7. Smit M, Beynon KA, Murdoch DR, et al. Comparison of the NOW Influenza A & B, NOW Flu A, NOW Flu B, and Directigen Flu A+B assays, and immunofluorescence with viral culture for the detection of influenza A and B viruses. Diagn Microbiol Infect Dis 2007; 57:67–70.

8. Ieven M. Currently used nucleic acid amplification tests for the detection of viruses and atypicals in acute respiratory infections. J Clin Virol 2007; 40:259–276.
9. Murdoch DR. Molecular genetic methods in the diagnosis of lower respiratory tract infections. APMIS 2004; 112:713–727.
10. Barken KB, Haagensen JAJ, Tolker-Nielsen T. Advances in nucleic acid-based diagnostics of bacterial infections. Clin Chim Acta 2007; 384:1–11.
11. Dagan R, Shriker O, Hazan I, et al. Prospective study to determine clinical relevance of detection of pneumococcal DNA in sera of children by PCR. J Clin Microbiol 1998; 36:669–673.
12. Rudolph KM, Parkinson AJ, Black CM, et al. Evaluation of polymerase chain reaction for diagnosis of pneumococcal pneumonia. J Clin Microbiol 1993; 31:2662–2666.
13. Salo P, Ortqvist A, Leinonen M. Diagnosis of bacteremic pneumococcal pneumonia by amplification of pneumolysin gene fragment in serum. J Infect Dis 1995; 171:479–482.
14. Murdoch DR, Anderson TP, Beynon KA, et al. Evaluation of a PCR assay for detection of *Streptococcus pneumoniae* in respiratory and nonrespiratory samples from adults with community-acquired pneumonia. J Clin Microbiol 2003; 41:63–66.
15. Keith ER, Podmore RG, Anderson TP, et al. Characteristics of *Streptococcus pseudopneumoniae* isolated from purulent sputum samples. J Clin Microbiol 2006; 44:923–927.
16. Sheppard CL, Harrison TG, Morris R, et al. Autolysin-targeting LightCycler assay including internal process control for detection of *Streptococcus pneumoniae* DNA in clinical samples. J Med Microbiol 2004; 53:189–195.
17. Carvalho MDS, Tondella ML, McCaustland K, et al. Evaluation and improvement of real-time PCR assays targeting *lytA*, *ply*, and *psaA* genes for detection of pneumococcal DNA. J Clin Microbiol 2007; 45:2460–2466.
18. Kais M, Spindler C, Kalin M, et al. Quantitative detection of *Streptococcus pneumoniae*, *Haemophilus influenzae*, and *Moraxella catarrhalis* in lower respiratory tract samples by real-time PCR. Diagn Microbiol Infect Dis 2006; 55:169–178.
19. Carrol ED, Guiver M, Nkhoma S, et al. High pneumococcal DNA loads are associated with mortality in Malawian children with invasive pneumococcal disease. Pediatr Infect Dis J 2007; 26:416–422.
20. Falguera M, López A, Nogués A, et al. Evaluation of the polymerase chain reaction method for detection of *Streptococcus pneumoniae* DNA in pleural fluid samples. Chest 2002; 122:2212–2216.
21. Lahti E, Mertsola J, Kontiokari T, et al. Pneumolysin polymerase chain reaction for diagnosis of pneumococcal pneumonia and empyema in children. Eur J Clin Microbiol Infect Dis 2006; 25:783–789.
22. Scott JAG, Marston EL, Hall AJ, et al. Diagnosis of pneumococcal pneumonia by *psaA* PCR analysis of lung aspirates from adult patients in Kenya. J Clin Microbiol 2003; 41:2554–2559.
23. Daxboeck F, Krause R, Wenisch C. Laboratory diagnosis of *Mycoplasma pneumoniae* infection. Clin Microbiol Infect 2003; 9:263–273.
24. Beersma MFC, Dirven K, van Dam AP, et al. Evaluation of 12 commercial tests and the complement fixation test for *Mycoplasma pneumoniae*-specific immunoglobulin G (IgG) and IgM antibodies, with PCR use as the "gold standard". J Clin Microbiol 2005; 43: 2277–2285.
25. Templeton KE, Scheltinga SA, Graffelman AW, et al. Comparison and evaluation of real-time PCR, real-time nucleic acid sequence-based amplification, conventional PCR, and serology for diagnosis of *Mycoplasma pneumoniae*. J Clin Microbiol 2003; 41:4366–4371.
26. Ursi D, Dirven K, Loens K, et al. Detection of *Mycoplasma pneumoniae* in respiratory samples by real-time PCR using an inhibition control. J Microbiol Methods 2003; 55: 149–153.

27. Loens K, Beck T, Ursi D, et al. Evaluation of different nucleic acid amplification techniques for the detection of *M. pneumoniae*, *C. pneumoniae* and *Legionella* spp. in respiratory specimens from patients with community-acquired pneumonia. J Microbiol Methods 2008; 73:257–262.

28. Reznikov M, Blackmore TK, Finlay-Jones JJ, et al. Comparison of nasopharyngeal aspirates and throat swab specimens in a polymerase chain reaction based test for *Mycoplasma pneumoniae*. Eur J Clin Microbiol Infect Dis 1995; 14:58–61.

29. Waring AL, Halse TA, Csiza CK, et al. Development of a genomics-based PCR assay for detection of *Mycoplasma pneumoniae* in a large outbreak in New York state. J Clin Microbiol 2001; 39:1385–1390.

30. Falguera M, Nogues A, RuizGonzalez A, et al. Detection of Mycoplasma pneumoniae by polymerase chain reaction in lung aspirates from patients with community-acquired pneumonia. Chest 1996; 110:972–976.

31. Kim NH, Lee JA, Eun BW, et al. Comparison of polymerase chain reaction and the indirect particle agglutination antibody test for the diagnosis of *Mycoplasma pneumoniae* pneumonia in children during two outbreaks. Pediatr Infect Dis J 2007; 26:897–903.

32. Liu F-C, Chen P-Y, Huang F-L, et al. Rapid diagnosis of *Mycoplasma pneumoniae* infection in children by polymerase chain reaction. J Microbiol Immunol Infect 2007; 40:507–512.

33. Cloud JL, Carroll KC, Pixton P, et al. Detection of *Legionella* species in respiratory specimens using PCR with sequencing confirmation. J Clin Microbiol 2000; 38:1709–1712.

34. Jaulhac B, Nowicki M, Bornstein N, et al. Detection of *Legionella* spp. in bronchoalveolar lavage fluids by DNA amplification. J Clin Microbiol 1992; 30:920–924.

35. Jonas D, Rosenbaum A, Weyrich S, et al. Enzyme-linked immunoassay for detection of PCR-amplified DNA of legionellae in bronchoalveolar fluid. J Clin Microbiol 1995; 33:1247–1252.

36. Kessler HH, Reinthaler FF, Pschaid A, et al. Rapid detection of *Legionella* species in bronchoalveolar lavage fluids with the EnviroAmp *Legionella* PCR amplification and detection kit. J Clin Microbiol 1993; 31:3325–3328.

37. Lisby G, Dessau R. Construction of a DNA amplification assay for detection of *Legionella* species in clinical samples. Eur J Clin Microbiol Infect Dis 1994; 13:225–231.

38. Matsiota-Bernard P, Pitsouni E, Legakis N, et al. Evaluation of commercial amplification kit for detection of *Legionella pneumophila* in clinical specimens. J Clin Microbiol 1994; 32:1503–1505.

39. Weir SC, Fischer SH, Stock F, et al. Detection of *Legionella* by PCR in respiratory specimens using a commercially available kit. Am J Clin Pathol 1998; 110:295–300.

40. Helbig JH, Engelstädter T, Maiwald M, et al. Diagnostic relevance of the detection of *Legionella* DNA in urine samples by the polymerase chain reaction. Eur J Clin Microbiol Infect Dis 1999; 18:716–722.

41. Maiwald M, Schill M, Stockinger C, et al. Detection of *Legionella* DNA in human and guinea pig urine samples by the polymerase chain reaction. Eur J Clin Microbiol Infect Dis 1995; 14:25–33.

42. Matsiota-Bernard P, Waser S, Vrioni G. Detection of *Legionella pneumophila* DNA in urine and serum samples from patients with pneumonia. Clin Microbiol Infect 2000; 6:223–225.

43. Murdoch DR, Walford EJ, Jennings LC, et al. Use of the polymerase chain reaction to detect Legionella DNA in urine and serum samples from patients with pneumonia. Clin Infect Dis 1996; 23:475–480.

44. Socan M, Kese D, Marinic-Fiser N. Polymerase chain reaction for detection of legionellae DNA in urine samples from patients with community-acquired pneumonia. Folia Microbiol 2000; 45:469–472.

45. Lindsay DS, Abraham WH, Fallon RJ. Detection of mip gene by PCR for diagnosis of Legionnaires' disease. J Clin Microbiol 1994; 32:3068–3069.
46. Lindsay DSJ, Abraham WH, Findlay W, et al. Laboratory diagnosis of legionnaires' disease due to *Legionella pneumophila* serogroup 1: comparison of phenotypic and genotypic methods. J Med Microbiol 2004; 53:183–187.
47. Matsiota-Bernard P, Vrioni G, Nauciel C. Use of the polymerase chain reaction for the detection of *Legionella pneumophila* DNA in serum samples. Clin Infect Dis 1997; 25:939.
48. Diederen BMW, De Jong CMA, Marmouk F, et al. Evaluation of real-time PCR for the early detection of *Legionella pneumophila* DNA in serum samples. J Med Microbiol 2007; 56:94–101.
49. Aoki S, Hirakata Y, Miyazaki Y, et al. Detection of *Legionella* DNA by PCR of whole-blood samples in a mouse model. J Med Microbiol 2003; 52:325–329.
50. Murdoch DR, Chambers ST. Detection of Legionella DNA in peripheral leukocytes, serum, and urine from a patient with pneumonia caused by *Legionella dumoffii*. Clin Infect Dis 2000; 30:382–383.
51. Murdoch DR, Jennings LC, Light GJ, et al. Detection of *Legionella* DNA in guinea pig peripheral leukocytes, urine and plasma by the polymerase chain reaction. Eur J Clin Microbiol Infect Dis 1999; 18:445–447.
52. Evans GE, Murdoch DR, Anderson TP, et al. Contamination of Qiagen DNA extraction kits with *Legionella* DNA. J Clin Microbiol 2003; 41:3452–3453.
53. van der Zee A, Peeters M, de Jong C, et al. Qiagen DNA extraction kits for sample preparation for *Legionella* PCR are not suitable for diagnostic purposes. J Clin Microbiol 2002; 40:1126.
54. Shen H, Rogelj S, Kieft TL. Sensitive, real-time PCR detects low-levels of contamination by *Legionella pneumophila* in commercial reagents. Mol Cell Probes 2006; 20:147–153.
55. Kumar S, Hammerschlag MR. Acute respiratory infection due to *Chlamydia pneumoniae*: current status of diagnostic methods. Clin Infect Dis 2007; 44:568–576.
56. Dowell SF, Peeling RW, Boman J, et al. Standardizing *Chlamydia pneumoniae* assays: recommendations from the Centers for Diseases Control and Prevention (USA) and the Laboratory Centre for Disease Control (Canada). Clin Infect Dis 2001; 33:492–503.
57. Apfalter P, Assadian O, Blasi F, et al. Reliability of nested PCR for detection of *Chlamydia pneumoniae* DNA in atheromas: results from a multicenter study applying standardized protocols. J Clin Microbiol 2002; 40:4428–4434.
58. Apfalter P, Blasi F, Boman J, et al. Multicenter comparison trial of DNA extraction methods and PCR assays for detection of *Chlamydia pneumoniae* in endarterectomy specimens. J Clin Microbiol 2001; 39:519–524.
59. Lind-Brandberg L, Welinder-Olsson C, Lagergard T, et al. Evaluation of PCR for diagnosis of *Bordetella pertussis* and *Bordetella parapertussis* infections. J Clin Microbiol 1998; 36:679–683.
60. Muller FM, Hoppe JE, Wirsing von Konig CH. Laboratory diagnosis of pertussis: state of the art in 1997. J Clin Microbiol 1997; 35:2435–2443.
61. Sotir MJ, Cappozzo DL, Warshauer DM, et al. Evaluation of polymerase chain reaction and culture for diagnosis of pertussis in the control of a county-wide outbreak focused among adolescents and adults. Clin Infect Dis 2007; 44:1216–1219.
62. Peiris JSM, Yuen KY, Osterhaus A, et al. Current concepts: The severe acute respiratory syndrome. N Engl J Med 2003; 349:2431–2441.
63. The Writing Committee of the World Health Organization Consultation on Human Influenza. Avian Influenza A (H5N1) infection in humans. N Engl J Med 2005; 353:1374–1385.
64. Fox JD. Nucleic acid amplification tests for detection or respiratory viruses. J Clin Virol 2007; 40(suppl 1):S15–S23.

65. Robberts FJL, Liebowitz LD, Chalkley LJ. Polymerase chain reaction detection of *Pneumocystis jiroveci*: evaluation of 9 assays. Diagn Microbiol Infect Dis 2007; 58: 3850–392.

66. Kibiki GS, Mulder B, van der Ven AJAM, et al. Laboratory diagnosis of pulmonary tuberculosis in TB and HIV endemic settings and the contribution of real time PCR for *M. tuberculosis* in bronchoalveolar lavage fluid. Trop Med Int Health 2007; 12:1210–1217.

67. Kivihya-Ndugga L, van Cleeff M, Juma E, et al. Comparison of PCR with the routine procedure for diagnosis of tuberculosis in a population with high prevalences of tuberculosis and human immunodeficiency virus. J Clin Microbiol 2004; 42:1012–1015.

68. Taegtmeyer M, Beeching NJ, Scott J, et al. The clinical impact of nucleic acid amplification tests on the diagnosis and management of tuberculosis in a British hospital. Thorax 2008; 63:317–321.

69. Cima-Cabal MD, Méndez FJ, Vázquez F, et al. Immunodetection of pneumolysin in human urine by ELISA. J Microbiol Methods 2003; 54:47–55.

70. García-Suárez MDM, Cima-Cabal MD, Villaverde R, et al. Performance of a pneumolysin ELISA assay for the diagnosis of pneumococcal infections. J Clin Microbiol 2007; 45:3549–3554.

71. Rajalakshmi B, Kanungo R, Srinivasan S, et al. Pneumolysin in urine: a rapid antigen detection method to diagnose pneumococcal pneumonia in children. Ind J Med Microbiol 2002; 20:183–186.

72. Harrison T, Uldum S, Alexiou-Daniel S, et al. A multicenter evaluation of the Biotest legionella urinary antigen EIA. Clin Microbiol Infect 1998; 4:359–365.

73. Cao W, Duan Y. Breath analysis: potential for clinical diagnosis and exposure assessment. Clin Chem 2006; 52:800–811.

74. Corradi M, Mutti A. Exhaled breath analysis: from occupational to respiratory medicine. Acta Biomed 2005; 76(suppl 2):20–29.

75. Risby TH, Solga SF. Current status of clinical breath analysis. Appl Physics B 2006; 85:421–426.

76. Majewska E, Kasielski M, Luczynski R, et al. Elevated exhalation of hydrogen peroxide and thiobarbituric acid reactive substances in patients with community acquired pneumonia. Respir Med 2004; 98:669–676.

77. Romero PV, Rodríguez B, Martínez S, et al. Analysis of oxidative stress in exhaled breath condensate from patients with severe pulmonary infections. Arch Bronconeumol 2006; 42:113–119.

78. Sack U, Scheibe R, Wötzel M, et al. Multiplex analysis of cytokines in exhaled breath condensate. Cytometry Part A 2006; 69A:169–172.

79. Kharitonov SA, Barnes PJ. Exhaled biomarkers. Chest 2006; 130:1541–1546.

80. Nagle HT, Schiffman SS, Gutierrez-Osuna R. The how and why of electronic noses. IEEE Spectr 1998; 35:22–34.

81. Pearce TC. Computational parallels between the biological olfactory pathway and its analogue 'The Electronic Nose': Part I. Biological olfaction. BioSystems 1997; 41:43–67.

82. Thaler ER, Hanson CW. Medical applications of electronic nose technology. Exp Rev Med Dev 2005; 2:559–566.

83. Hanson CW, Thaler ER. Electronic nose prediction of a clinical pneumonia score: biosensors and microbes. Anesthesiology 2005; 102:63–68.

84. Hockstein NG, Thaler ER, Lin Y, et al. Correlation of pneumonia score with electronic nose signature: a prospective study. Ann Otol Rhinol Laryngol 2005; 114:504–508.

85. Hockstein NG, Thaler ER, Torigian D, et al. Diagnosis of pneumonia with an electronic nose: correlation of vapor signature with chest computed tomography scan findings. Laryngoscope 2004; 114:1701–1705.

86. Thaler ER, Hanson CW. Use of an electronic nose to diagnose bacterial sinusitis. J Rhinol 2006; 20:170–172.

87. Allardyce RA, Langford VS, Hill AL, et al. Detection of volatile metabolites produced by bacterial growth in blood culture media by selected ion flow tube mass spectrometry (SIFT-MS). J Microbiol Methods 2006; 65:361–365.

88. Syhre M, Scotter JM, Chambers ST. Investigation into the production of 2-Pentylfuran by *Aspergillus fumigatus* and other respiratory pathogens *in vitro* and human breath samples. Med Mycol 2008; 46:209–215.

89. Syhre M, Chambers ST. The scent of *Mycobacterium tuberculosis*. Tuberculosis 2008; 88:317–323.

90. Nayeri F, Millinger E, Nilsson I, et al. Exhaled breath condensate and serum levels of hepatocyte growth factor in pneumonia. Respir Med 2002; 96:115–119.

91. Clyne B, Olshaker O. The C-reactive protein. J Emerg Med 1999; 17:1019–1025.

92. van der Meer V, Knuistingh Neven A, van den Broek PJ, et al. Diagnostic value of C reactive protein in infections of the lower respiratory tract: systematic review. BMJ 2005; 331:26–31.

93. Coelho L, Póvoa P, Almeida E, et al. Usefulness of C-reactive protein in monitoring the severe community-acquired pneumonia clinical course. Critical Care 2007; 11:R92.

94. Smith RP, Lipworth BJ. C-reactive protein in simple community-acquired pneumonia. Chest 1995; 107:1028–1031.

95. Smith RP, Lipworth BJ, Cree IA, et al. C-reactive protein. A clinical marker in community-acquired pneumonia. Chest 1995; 108:1288–1291.

96. Menéndez R, Cavalcanti M, Reyes S, et al. Markers of treatment failure in hospitalized community-acquired pneumonia. Thorax 2008; 63:447–452.

97. Chalmers JD, Singanayagam A, Hill AT. C-reactive protein is an independent predictor of severity in community-acquired pneumonia. Am J Med 2008; 121:219–225.

98. Schneider H-G, Lam QT. Procalcitonin for the clinical laboratory: a review. Pathology 2007; 39:383–390.

99. Wanner GA, Keel M, Steckholzer U, et al. Relationship between procalcitonin plasma levels and severity of injury, sepsis, organ failure, and mortality in injured patients. Crit Care Med 2000; 28:950–957.

100. Christ-Crain M, Müller B. Biomarkers in respiratory tract infections: diagnostic guides to antibiotic prescription, prognostic markers and mediators. Eur Respir J 2007; 30:556–573.

101. Christ-Crain M, Jaccard-Stolz D, Bingisser R, et al. Effect of procalcitonin-guided treatment on antibiotic use and outcome in lower respiratory tract infections: cluster-randomised, single-blinded intervention trial. Lancet 2004; 363:600–607.

102. Bignardi GE, Dhar R, Heycock R, et al. Can procalcitonin testing reduce antibiotic prescribing for respiratory infections? Age Ageing 2006; 35:625–626.

103. Christ-Crain M, Stolz D, Bingisser R, et al. Procalcitonin guidance of antibiotic therapy in community-acquired pneumonia. A randomized trial. Am J Respir Crit Care Med 2006; 174:84–93.

104. Stolz D, Christ-Crain M, Bingisser R, et al. Antibiotic treatment of exacerbations of COPD. A randomized, controlled trial comparing procalcitonin-guidance with standard therapy. Chest 2007; 131:9–19.

105. Holm A, Pedersen SS, Nexoe J, et al. Procalcitonin versus C-reactive protein for predicting pneumonia in adults with lower respiratory tract infection in primary care. Br J Gen Pract 2007; 57:555–560.

106. Huang DT, Weissfeld LA, Kellum JA, et al. Risk prediction with procalcitonin and clinical rules in community-acquired pneumonia. Ann Emerg Med 2008; 52:48–58.

107. Krüger S, Ewig S, Marre R, et al. Procalcitonin predicts patients at low risk of death from community-acquired pneumonia across all CRB-65 classes. Eur Respir J 2008; 31:349–355.

108. Don M, Valent F, Korppi M, et al. Efficacy of serum procalcitonin in evaluating severity of community-acquired pneumonia in childhood. Scand J Infect Dis 2007; 39:129–137.
109. Hirakata Y, Yanagihara K, Kurihara S, et al. Comparison of usefulness of plasma procalcitonin and C-reactive protein measurements for estimation of severity in adults with community-acquired pneumonia. Diagn Microbiol Infect Dis 2008; 61:170–174.
110. Müller B, Harbarth S, Stolz D, et al. Diagnostic and prognostic accuracy of clinical and laboratory parameters in community-acquired pneumonia. BMC Infect Dis 2007; 7:10.
111. Bouchon A, Facchetti F, Weigand MA, et al. TREM-1 amplifies inflammation and is a crucial mediator of septic shock. Nature 2001; 410:1103–1107.
112. Gibot S, Cravoisy A, Levy B, et al. Soluble triggering receptor expressed on myeloid cells and the diagnosis of pneumonia. N Engl J Med 2004; 350:451–458.
113. El Solh AA, Akinnusi ME, Peter M, et al. Triggering receptors expressed on myeloiod cells in pulmonary aspiration syndromes. Intensive Care Med 2008; 34:1012–1019.
114. Tejera A, Santolaria F, Diez M-L, et al. Prognosis of community acquired pneumonia (CAP): value of triggering receptor expressed on myeloid cells-1 (TREM-1) and other mediators of the inflammatory response. Cytokine 2007; 38:117–123.
115. Radsak MP, Taube C, Haselmayer P, et al. Soluble triggering receptor expressed on myeloid cells 1 is released in patients with stable chronic obstructive pulmonary disease. Clin Dev Immunol 2007; 2007:52040.
116. Christ-Crain M, Morgenthaler NG, Stolz D, et al. Pro-adrenomedullin to predict severity and outcome in community-acquired pneumonia [ISRCTN04176397]. Crit Care 2006; 10: R96.
117. Stolz D, Christ-Crain M, Morgenthaler NG, et al. Copeptin, C-reactive protein, and procalcitonin as prognostic biomarkers in acute exacerbation of COPD. Chest 2007; 131:1058–1067.
118. Seligman R, Papassotiriou J, Morgenthaler NG, et al. Copeptin, a novel prognostic biomarker in ventilator-associated pneumonia. Crit Care 2008; 12:R11.
119. Müller B, Morgenthaler N, Stolz D, et al. Circulating levels of copeptin, a novel biomarker, in lower respiratory tract infections. Eur J Clin Invest 2007; 37:145–152.

19
New Management Modalities

THOMAS M. FILE, JR.
Northeastern Ohio Universities College of Medicine, Rootstown; and Summa Health System, Akron, Ohio, U.S.A.

I. Introduction

Community-acquired pneumonia (CAP), Hospital-acquired (or nosocomial) pneumonia (HAP), ventilator-associated pneumonia (VAP), and health care–associated pneumonia (HCAP) are important causes of morbidity and mortality despite improvements in supportive care and prevention. Optimal outcomes of these infections rely on timely and appropriate management strategies. However, despite advances in general knowledge, mortality for many of these infections remains high. It is appropriate therefore that new approaches to management of pneumonia be explored with the hopes that such strategies will lead to better outcomes in the future. This chapter considers newer approaches to management and prevention that include new antimicrobials, novel methods of administration of antimicrobials, and new approaches to modification of the host response and prevention.

II. New Antimicrobials

Multidrug-resistant (MDR) respiratory pathogens are being isolated with increasing frequency in microbiology laboratories worldwide. The efficacy of empiric therapy is threatened today by the emergence these pathogens. It is therefore vital that new agents be developed to address the issue of resistance to our presently available antimicrobials. Despite a general decline in new anti-infective development, there are some new drugs on the market as well as drugs currently in development that will assist in the fight against resistant pathogens in the future.

There are two main approaches to dealing with the problem of MDR isolates. The first is the implementation of control measures for appropriate antibiotic use, including improved prescriber education, formulary restriction, and approval policies using infectious disease specialists and support teams, antimicrobial cycling, and/or program termination. These measures can reduce antibiotic use and treatment cost and have been shown to have variable results in controlling resistance. Nevertheless, it is paramount that appropriate infection control and antimicrobial prescribing practices be followed to reduce untoward emergence of resistance.

The second approach to dealing with multidrug resistance is the development and use of new antimicrobial agents. Research and development into new antimicrobial agents has reduced dramatically in recent years (1). Current drugs must be used wisely and judiciously to sustain their activity and to avoid the development of resistance for as long as possible. The drugs that have come onto the market since 2000 are few in number but important additions to the clinical armamentarium. New antimicrobial agents and those currently in development are listed in Table 1.

Among the antimicrobial agents currently in development, many are relatively narrow-spectrum agents that focus on gram-positive organisms; this is likely due to recent increases in the prevalence of methicillin-resistant *Staphylococcus aureus* (MRSA) and vancomycin-resistant *Enterococci* (VRE). Thus, in the near future, there are more likely to be several options of therapy for resistant gram-positive organisms, but with continued shortage of agents suitable for the treatment of such problematic gram-negative pathogens as *Pseudomonas*, *Acinetobacter*, *Enterobacter*, and *Klebsiella*.

A. Problem Pathogens

Resistance to commonly used antibiotics for CAP presents a major consideration in choosing empirical therapy. Resistance patterns clearly vary by geography. Local antibiotic prescribing patterns are a likely explanation. However, clonal spread of resistant strains is well documented. Therefore, antibiotic recommendations must be modified on the basis of local susceptibility patterns. The most significant etiological pathogen of CAP is *Streptococcus pneumoniae*, and the emergence of drug-resistant *S. pneumoniae* (DRSP) isolates is well documented (2).

The incidence of resistance appears to have stabilized somewhat in the last few years. Resistance to penicillin and cephalosporins may even be falling, while macrolide resistance continues to increase (2). However, the clinical relevance of DRSP for pneumonia is uncertain and few well-controlled studies have examined the impact of in vitro resistance on clinical outcomes of CAP. Current levels of β-lactam resistance do not generally result in CAP treatment failures when appropriate agents (i.e., amoxicillin, ceftriaxone, or cefotaxime) and doses are used, even in the presence of bacteremia. The available data suggest that the clinically relevant level of penicillin resistance is a minimal inhibitory concentration (MIC) value of at least 4 mg/L (2). Data exist suggesting that resistance to macrolides and older fluoroquinolones (ciprofloxacin and levofloxacin) results in clinical failure (2). To date, no failures have been reported for the newer fluoroquinolones (moxifloxacin and gemifloxacin).

Recently, serotype A19 *S. pneumoniae*, which is not contained in the conjugate vaccine, has emerged as a cause of clinical infection (3). This strain may be resistant to clindamycin and the more potent β-lactams such as ceftriaxone, but does retain susceptibility to the ketolides (e.g., telithromycin and cethromycin), faropenem, and respiratory fluoroquinolones.

An increasing incidence of pneumonia due to community-associated methicillin-resistant *S. aureus* (CA-MRSA) has been observed over the past decade. Most contain the gene for Panton–Valentine leukocidin (PVL), a toxin associated with clinical features of necrotizing pneumonia, shock, and respiratory failure, as well as formation of abscesses and empyemas (4). CA-MRSA pneumonia has been reported often associated with preceding influenza. This strain should also be suspected in patients who present with cavitary infiltrates without risk factors for anaerobic aspiration pneumonia (gingivitis and a risk for loss of consciousness, such as seizures or alcohol abuse, or esophogeal motility disorders). Diagnosis is usually straightforward with high yields from sputum and blood cultures in this characteristic clinical scenario. CA-MRSA CAP remains rare in most communities but is expected to be an emerging problem in CAP treatment.

Table 1 Recently Approved Antimicrobials and Antimicrobials Under Clinical Development for Therapy of Lower Respiratory Tract Infections

Antimicrobial	Class/target	Spectrum	IV/PO	Comments
Recently approved agents				
Linezolid	Oxazolidinone (ribosome)	Gram positive	IV, PO	Half-life bioavailability, as a protein inhibitor, reduces toxin
Tigecycline	Tetracycline (ribosome)	Gram-positive, gram-negative, anaerobes	IV	Active against MRSA and many MDR gram-negative bacilli, *not* active against *P aeruginosa*
Daptomycin	Lipoglycopeptide (cell wall)	Gram positive	IV	*Not* effective for pneumonia, inactivated by surfactant
Agents under development				
Dalbavancin	Lipoglycopeptide (cell wall)	Gram positive	IV	Long half-life allowing once weekly dose
Doripenem	Carbapenem (cell wall)	Gram-positive, gram-negative, anaerobes	IV	More active in vitro against *P. aeruginosa*
Oritavancin	Glycopeptide (cell wall)	Gram positive	IV	Long half-life
Telavancin	Lipoglycopeptide (cell wall, membrane)	Gram positive	IV	
Iclaprim	Dihydrofolate reductase inhibitor	Primarily gram positive	IV (PO in development)	
Rib-X-1741	Oxazolidinones (ribosome)	Gram positive	PO	
EDP-420	Bicylic macrolide (ribosome)	Community respiratory pathogens	PO	
PZ-601	Carbapenem (cell wall)	Gram-positive, gram-negative, anaerobes	IV	Active against MRSA, less active against *P. aeruginosa*
Ceftobiprole	Cephalosporin (cell wall)	Gram positive (including MRSA), gram negative	IV	Active against MRSA
Ceftaroline	Cephalosporin (cell wall)	Gram positive (including MRSA), gram negative	IV	Active against MRSA
Faropenem	Penem (cell wall)	Community respiratory pathogens	PO	Not active against atypicals
BC-3205	Pleuromutilin (protein synthesis)	Community respiratory pathogens	PO	Active against DRSP and atypicals

Abbreviations: MDR, multidrug resistant; MRSA, methicillin-resistant *Staphylococcus aureus*; DRSP, drug-resistant *S. pneumoniae*.

While methicillin-resistant strains of *S. aureus* are still the minority, the excess mortality of inappropriate antibiotic therapy would suggest that empirical coverage should be considered when CA-MRSA is a concern. The most effective therapy is yet to be defined. Presently vancomycin or linezolid is recommended (4). However, vancomycin has never been specifically studied for CAP, while linezolid has been found to be better than ceftriaxone for bacteremic *S. pneumoniae* in a nonblinded study and superior to vancomycin in retrospective analysis of studies involving nosocomial MRSA pneumonia (5,6). One concern with vancomycin is the increasing MICs of MRSA that have emerged over the past decade that may reduce the efficacy of vancomycin in pulmonary infection. An additional concern with CA-MRSA is necrotizing pneumonia associated with PVL and other toxin production. Vancomycin does not decrease toxin production while linezolid has been shown to affect toxin production in a laboratory setting (7). Newer agents for MRSA have recently become available and others are anticipated. Of the presently available agents, daptomycin should not be used for CAP.

Important bacterial pathogens as causes of HAP or VAP include the gram-negative pathogens, *Pseudomonas* and *Acinetobacter*, and MRSA *Pseudomonas* and *Acinetobacter* are often resistant to many of the commonly used antimicrobial agents in intensive care units both in North America and in Europe. In some cases, an older agent, colistin, is the only active antimicrobial, and as such colistin has reemerged as a useful agent.

B. Recently Approved Antimicrobials
Linezolid
Linezolid is an oxazolidinone antibiotic that is active against a vast array of gram-positive species. It has been shown to be useful in treating patients with serious infections caused by vancomycin-resistant or vancomycin-intermediate organisms, although it is not specifically approved for the latter. Linezolid has documented efficacy in both CAP and VAP (4). As indicated above linezolid has a potential advantage over vancomycin since it has been shown to reduce toxin production in laboratory studies. Prospective, randomized controlled studies are pending to confirm whether or not this agent is superior to vancomycin for MRSA.

Daptomycin
Daptomycin is the first agent in a new class, the cyclic lipopeptides (8). It has activity against a broad range of gram-positive organisms. Daptomycin can inhibit many organisms that are resistant to oxacillin, vancomycin, or linezolid. However, it is not indicated for pneumonia. In a randomized, controlled trial in CAP, it was found to be inferior to ceftriaxone. Subsequent studies found that it is inactivated by surfactant (9).

Tigecycline
Tigecycline is a broad-spectrum antimicrobial of the glycylcycline class. It is a first-in-class agent designed to avoid bacterial resistance to tetracyclines by efflux and ribosomal protection. It has broad-spectrum activity including DRSP, MRSA, VRE, extended spectrum β-lactamase (ESBL) producing Enterobacteriaceae and *Acinetobacter* (10). However, it has little activity against *Pseudomonas*, *Proteus*, and *Providencia* spp.

Tigecycline was compared with levofloxacin in two randomized controlled trials in patients requiring hospitalization for CAP (11). Both studies showed comparable results of tigecycline and levofloxacin. However in a HAP/VAP trial, tigecycline (±ceftazidime and amikacin) was non-inferior to imipenem (±amikacin and vancomycin) for the modified intent to treat population but not for the clinically evaluable population, driven by results in VAP patients. Further exploration of these results is pending at this time (12).

Telithromycin

Telithromycin is a ketolide related to the macrolides. Because it targets additional domains of the ribosome as compared with the macrolides, it is usually active against macrolide-resistant *S. pneumoniae* (13). It has been used for the treatment of mild-to-moderate CAP, including multidrug-resistant strains of *S. pneumoniae*, and its effectiveness in CAP has been demonstrated in randomized trials. However, concern with use has occurred because of rare cases of severe hepatotoxicity and visual disturbances. Serious exacerbations of myasthenia gravis and loss of consciousness have also been reported. Telithromycin is most appropriately considered as an option for therapy if the prevalence of "high-level" macrolide resistance is common in the community (i.e., >25% of strains with MIC >16 µg/mL) or the patient has risk factors for macrolide-resistant pneumococci. The risk-benefit ratio should be carefully weighed by each prescriber, and telithromycin should not be prescribed in patients with known liver disease.

Doripenem

Doripenem is the newest carbapenem approved by the FDA in 2007 for treatment of complicated urinary tract and intra-abdominal infections (14). It has a similar spectrum of activity as meropenem, although it appears to have more potent in vitro activity against *Pseudomonas aeruginosa* than meropenem. At this time, it is not approved for pneumonia; however, it has been compared with piperacillin/tazobactam in a study of HAP and with imipenem in a VAP trial (see a description of the VAP study in sect. II.D) (15).

C. Investigational Antimicrobials Under Development

Dalbavancin

Dalbavancin is a glycopeptide antimicrobial that, like vancomycin, inhibits bacterial wall synthesis (16). It is active against resistant gram-positive organisms including MRSA. It is typically bactericidal and a half-life of 170 to 210 hours, making once-weekly dosing possible. To date there are no published clinical trials for the treatment of pneumonia.

Telavancin

Telavancin is a rapidly acting bactericidal lipoglycopeptide (17). It acts in two ways: It inhibits transglycosylation, thus inhibiting cell wall synthesis, and it also causes bacterial cell membrane depolarization leading to changes in cell permeability. Telavancin has activity against resistant gram-positive organisms, including MRSA. Telavancin has been evaluated in the treatment of HAP but the results have not yet been published.

Oritavancin

Oritavancin is a semisynthetic glycopeptide that has a very long plasma terminal half-life (360 hours), making once-daily to once-weekly administration feasible (18). It is active against vancomycin-intermediate and resistant organisms. There have been no published trials of this agent in pneumonia.

Ceftobiprole

Ceftobiprole is an extended-spectrum β-lactam that binds tightly to and inhibits PBP2a, a protein that is responsible for staphylococcal resistance to β-lactams (19). Ceftobiprole is delivered as a prodrug that is hydrolyzed to the active molecule in vivo. It is active against MSSA and MRSA as well as most gram-negative bacilli. Studies of CAP and HAP/VAP have been performed but not published as yet.

Ceftaroline

Ceftaroline is a broad-spectrum cephalosporin, administered as a prodrug that has a similar antimicrobial spectrum as ceftibiprole. Studies in CAP are underway.

Iclaprim

Iclaprim is a potent inhibitor of bacterial dihydrofolate reductase (DHFR) and is highly selective for bacterial over human DHFR (20). Compared with trimethoprim, it has better binding to DHFR, possibly due to lipophilic interactions. Iclaprim is active in vitro against trimethoprim-resistant *S. aureus*. The MIC for both MSSA and MRSA is approximately 0.06 µg/mL. To date there are no published trials in pneumonia.

Cethromycin

Cethromycin is a ketolide antimicrobial that has shown higher in vitro potency and a broader range of activity than macrolides against gram-positive bacteria associated with respiratory tract infections, and, again in in vitro tests, it appears to be effective against penicillin- and macrolide-resistant bacteria (21). In preclinical studies, there have been minimal safety concerns. The drug has been evaluated for CAP in randomized controlled trials. The phase III CAP pivotal development program was comprised of two double-blind, randomized, well-controlled, multicenter, multinational, comparator trials designed to assess the safety and effectiveness of cethromycin in CAP patients compared with clarithromycin (22).

Faropenem

Faropenem medoxomil represents a novel antimicrobial subclass within the β-lactams, the penems, which maintains an intrinsic stability against the majority of β-lactamases that render many structurally related β-lactam antibiotics ineffective. Faropenem medoxomil is an orally available, broad-spectrum antibacterial agent with proven efficacy against a wide variety of bacterial pathogens, including those etiological agents responsible for community respiratory tract infections (including DRSP) (23). Faropenem has been shown to be comparable to commonly use agents in mild community respiratory infections; however, the FDA issued a nonapprovable letter in October 2006 requesting additional information and possible superiority trials pending reconsideration of an evaluation of trial designs for mild respiratory infections.

BC-3205

BC-3205 (Nabriva Pharmaceuticals, Vienna, Austria) is a new class of antimicrobial of the pleuromutilins. BC-3205 is an oral agent with activity against gram positive and gram-negative bacteria and atypical organisms. BC-3205 is currently in a multi-dose phase I trial. Pleuromutilin antibiotics are a novel clinically validated class of antibiotics that specifically inhibit bacterial protein synthesis. Their antibacterial profile covers resistant pathogens, including MRSA, that cause diseases such as respiratory tract and skin infections.

PZ-601

PZ-601 (also known as SMP-601 and SM-216601) is a novel investigational broad-spectrum injectable carbapenem antibiotic being developed by Protez Pharmaceuticals, Malvem, Pennslyvania, U.S. A key feature of PZ-601 is its potent activity versus multiresistant gram-positive organisms including MRSA and VRE, in addition to activity versus the Enterobacteriaceae (including extended-spectrum beta lactamase producers) and anaerobes. Currently clinical studies are underway.

RX-1741

RX-1741 (Rib-X Pharmaceuticals, Greater New York, New York, U.S.) is an oxazoli-dinone antibiotic that exhibits activity against MRSA and other gram-positive organisms (such as *S. pneumoniae*), and has demonstrated both greater spectrum and potency of activity than linezolid. It has in vitro activity against the atypical pathogens and is currently undergoing studies in CAP.

EDP-420

EDP-420 (Enanta Pharmaceuticals, Inc., Greater Boston Area, Massachusetts, U.S.) is a bicyclic macrolide antibiotic with improved activity profile relative to currently marketed macrolides and ketolides, including DRSP. There are no published trials in pneumonia at this time.

D. Pharmacodynamic Principles in Therapy of Pneumonia

Advances in the science of antimicrobial pharmacodynamics have provided insight into the link between drug exposures and clinical efficacy (24). Pharmcodynamic properties of antimicrobials have become particularly important for the potential to improve outcome of respiratory tract infections in the face of increasing drug resistance. Knowing which pharmacodynamic measure is representative of the antimicrobial activity of an antimicrobial allows the potential to optimize a dosing strategy. As an example, because the area under the curve/minimal inhibitory concentration (AUC/MIC) ratio best describes activity of the fluoroquinolone class, a large, once-daily dose can be utilized. By increasing the dose of levofloxacin to 750 mg once daily for the treatment of CAP, Dunbar et al. demonstrated a faster resolution of clinical illness as compared with 500 mg once daily (25). β-Lactams exhibit time-dependent killing and recent strategies have evolved to provide for continuous infusion or prolonged intermittent infusion. In an effort to improve clinical outcomes of the treatment of *P. aeruginosa* infections in critically ill patients, Lodise et al. compared in a cohort-control study, intermittent infusions of piperacillin-tazobactam (3.375 g IV for 30 minutes every 4 or 6 hours) to extended infusions of piperacillin-tazobactam (3.375 g IV for 4 hours every 8 hours) (26). Of a total of 194 patients, 102 received extended infusions and 92 received intermittent infusions of piperacillin-tazobactam. No differences in baseline clinical characteristics were noted between the two patient groups. Among patients with Acute Physiological and Chronic Health Evaluation–II (APACHE-II) scores greater than 17, 14-day mortality rate was significantly lower with extended-infusion therapy than with intermittent-infusion therapy (12.2% vs. 31.6%, respectively; $p = 0.04$), and the median duration of hospital stay after collection of samples for culture was also significantly shorter (21 days vs. 38 days; $p = 0.02$). On the basis of a Monte Carlo Simulation of probability of attainment of the pharmacodynamic target, the prolonged infusion group attained the target for 100% of isolates with an MIC of 16 µg/mL whereas the 30-minute infusion group attained the target for only 27% of the isolates with the same MIC. These results strongly suggest that improved outcomes may be realized by extended-infusion piperacillin-tazobactam therapy and indicate that is a suitable alternative to intermittent-infusion piperacillin-tazobactam therapy.

More recently, Chastre et al. compared prolonged infusion of doripenem with standard dosing of imipenem in the treatment of VAP (27). Patients were randomly assigned to doripenem 500 mg every eight hours via a four-hour infusion or imipenem 500 mg every six hours or 1000 mg every eight hours via 30- or 60-minute infusion for 7 to 14 days. Vancomycin and/or amikacin were added at the discretion of the investigator. Clinical cure rates were 68.3% and 64.2% in the doripenem and imipenem groups respectively. Although sample sizes were small, clinical cure was 80% for doripenem and 42.9% for imipenem in patients with *P. aeruginosa* infection. Only 18% (5 of 28) of *P. aeruginosa* isolates had MICs greater than equal to 8 µg/mL at baseline or following therapy in the doripenem arm compared with 64% (16 of 25) in the imipenem treatment group ($p = 0.001$). Doripenem has greater stability in saline compared with the other carbapenems and is therefore suitable for use in an extended infusion, an important factor in optimizing the pharmacodynamic profile of the drug against less susceptible pathogens.

III. Aerosolized Antimicrobials

For antimicrobials to be effective they must reach the site of infection, remain there for an adequate length of time, and affect some target site to disrupt the microbe. One method to potentially improve the response of an antimicrobial for pneumonia is to directly deliver the drug to the lower respiratory tract via nebulization. Drug concentrations in the lower bronchi following inhalation of aerosolized drug are often significantly higher than the concentrations following intravenous administration; this may allow treatment of pathogens with higher MICs. Additional potential benefits are reduced systemic exposure and a reduction in systemic side effects.

Although aerosolized antimicrobials are widely recognized therapy for patients with cystic fibrosis, there remains a paucity of clinical data to support this approach for pneumonia and few anitmicrobials have been developed for administration by this route. Prevention and treatment of ventilator-associated pneumonia with nebulized agents have been examined. Wood and Boucher compared the use of aerosolized ceftazidime, 250 mg every 12 hours by nebulization ($n = 20$) to placebo ($n = 20$) for up to seven days. Although there was no difference in the incidence of pneumonia, aerosolized ceftazidime did result in a reduction in the number of cases of pneumonia at ICU day 14 (28). Interestingly, concentrations of tumor necrosis factor α (TNF-α) and interleukin-8 (IL-8) were significantly attenuated in the treated group and this correlated with less development of pneumonia.

Selection of an appropriate nebulizer is also a critical consideration when administering drug via inhalation. Recently Niederman et al. reported the results of a double-blind, placebo-controlled, feasibility study of nebulized amikacin in patients with gram-negative VAP using a Pulmonary Drug Delivery System (PDDS™) (29). In bench models, the PDDS Clinical has high efficiency for aerosol delivery with lower respiratory tract delivery of 50% to 70%. Patients were randomized to receive aerosol containing 400 mg amikacin once daily with placebo (saline) 12 hours later; 400 mg amikacin twice a day or placebo twice a day. Intravenous antibiotics (agent and duration) were determined by the treating physician, but chosen in accordance to current guidelines. Mean number of intravenous antibiotics at the end of study (mean 7 days), were two times greater with placebo than twice-daily amikacin ($p < 0.02$). For once and twice-daily amikacin, peak serum drug levels were 1.3 and 1.8 µg/mL, respectively, on day 1, and 2.3 and 3.2 µg/mL on day 3. Mean trough levels were 0.87 and 1.49 µg/mL. Tracheal aspirate levels (mean) on day 3 were 6.9 mg/mL and 16.2 mg/mL, respectively. The nebulized amikacin was well tolerated; and further efficacy studies are planned.

Mohr et al. reviewed retrospectively the medical records of 22 patients who received aerosolized aminoglycosides in conjunction with parenteral antibiotics for VAP in the surgical ICU. Sixteen patients received inhaled tobramycin, and six received inhaled amikacin (30). The average duration of mechanical ventilation was 31 ± 12 days, the mean ICU length of stay (LOS) was 41 ± 13 days, and the mean hospital LOS was 71 ± 25 days. The average duration of mechanical ventilation after initiation of aerosolized antibiotics was 4.3 days. Seven patients (40%) developed recurrent pneumonia with the same pathogen, but only one had a change in antibiotic susceptibility pattern. There were no renal or pulmonary complications of aminoglycoside treatment. The authors concluded that aerosolized aminoglycosides are potentially valuable adjuncts in select patients with minimal risk of antibiotic resistance.

An uncontrolled, prospective study evaluated 60 critically ill patients with VAP who were treated with aerosolized colistin for the treatment of MDR pathogens (*Acinetobacter* in 37; *Pseudomonas* in 12; *Klebsiella* in 11) (31) Half of the pathogens isolated were susceptible only to colistin. Virtually all patients received concomitant intravenous therapy with colistin or other antimicrobial agents. Therapy was considered beneficial (bacteriological and clinical response) in 50 (83%) patients and no significant adverse effects were noted. Controlled trials are needed to establish the safety and efficacy of adjunctive aerosolized antibiotics.

In a meta-analysis of five randomized controlled trials, Ioannidou et al. determined the effects of administration of antimicrobials administered via the respiratory tract (either inhaled or endotracheally instilled) in the treatment of nosocomial pneumonia (32). Administration directly into the respiratory tract was associated with better treatment success in intent to treat and clinically evaluable patient populations; however, there were no statistically significant differences for all-cause mortality or microbiological eradication or without concurrent usage of systemic antibiotics.

Aerosolized antibiotics may also be useful to treat microorganisms that, on the basis of high MIC values, are "resistant" to systemic therapy. Anecdotal reports have appeared of patients with VAP due to MDR *P. aeruginosa* that is unresponsive to systemic antibiotics, but who have improved with the addition of aerosolized amino-glycosides or polymyxin B. Concerns about aerosolized antibiotics leading to an increased risk of pneumonia due to resistant microorganisms were raised when these agents were used as prophylaxis, not as therapy. One side effect of aerosolized anti-biotics has been bronchospasm, which can be induced by the antibiotic or the associated diluents present in certain preparations. Further investigation into the use of aerosolized antibiotics is warranted.

IV. Host Factors

One of the most significant factors that influence the outcome of pneumonia is the inflammatory response of the host. A balance between the inflammatory response to infection and the concomitant anti-inflammatory response is critical for an appropriate response (33). Therefore managing inflammation is an attractive adjunctive to anti-microbial therapy. This may be more important than the specific microorganism causing the infection or the type of antibiotic administered. Various strategies have been eval-uated to improve outcomes of severe pneumonia by modifying the host response.

A. Immunomodulating Effects of Macrolides

In addition to direct antibacterial effects, the macrolides have some immunomodulating properties. Such properties may be beneficial to the host response during respiratory infections and may in part explain the results of studies showing that the outcome of patients with pneumococcal bacteremia improves if a macrolide is included as part of combination therapy (usually with a cephalosporin).

Some studies have shown that clarithromycin and erythromycin enhance attrac-tion of neutrophils to the site of infection (chemotaxis) and the avidity with which they engulf bacteria (phagocytosis) (34). The drugs likewise enhance neutrophil production of the reactive oxygen species that they use to kill engulfed bacteria. All of these actions, which would not be reflected in in vitro antimicrobial susceptibility tests, would be expected to enhance the body's natural ability to resist infection and thus supplement the drugs direct antibacterial activity.

At the same time that macrolides enhance the immune system's antibacterial activity, they also modify the body's inflammatory response (35). Indeed, not only has erythromycin been found helpful for treating bronchial asthma, but macrolides are now the standard treatment for diffuse panbronchiolitis, a chronic inflammation of the bronchioles. This anti-inflammatory activity, which has been confirmed in animal studies, apparently results from macrolides' ability to reduce monocyte synthesis of inflammatory cytokines. Although a reduction in the inflammatory response may not directly contribute to bacterial cure, it would be expected to promote more rapid symptom resolution.

Macrolides reduce bacterial infectivity in other ways as well, without invoking either the immune system or antibiotic mechanisms. Specifically they reduce the ability of pathogens to adhere to mucosal surfaces and they interfere with expression of viru-lence factors. In addition, clarithromycin has been shown to reduce sputum production and sputum elasticity, as well as decreasing mucus production in purulent rhinitis. Neurally induced contraction of airway smooth muscles is likewise attenuated. All these effects tend to reduce the severity of respiratory symptoms, and the reductions in sputum and mucus production may render the environment less hospitable to bacterial growth.

Macrolides may also have benefit in nosocomial pneumonia. A randomized trial of 200 patients with sepsis and VAP showed that those who received clarithromycin (in addition to standard treatment including antibiotics) had significantly faster resolution of VAP (10 versus 15.5 days) and weaning from mechanical ventilation (16 versus 22.5 days) compared to those who received placebo (36). Among those who died of sepsis, time to death was significantly prolonged in those who received clarithromycin.

Further studies are needed to identify factors associated with the beneficial effects of macrolide therapy as an immunomodifier and to clarify appropriate dosing regimens.

B. Drotrecogin Alfa Activated

Drotrecogin alfa activated is the first immunomodulatory therapy approved for severe sepsis. In the United States, the FDA recommended the use of drotrecogin alfa activated for patients at high risk of death. The high-risk criterion suggested by the FDA is an APACHE II score greater than or equal to 25 (4). Among patients who benefit the best from this therapy are those with sepsis due to severe CAP. The greatest reduction in the mortality rate was for *S. pneumoniae* infection. The benefit appears to be greatest when the treatment is given as early in the hospital admission as possible.

Although the benefit of drotrecogin alfa activated is clearly greatest for patients with CAP who have high APACHE II scores, this criterion alone may not be adequate to select appropriate patients. Further studies are needed to optimize selection of patients for therapy.

C. Glucocorticoids

In a longitudinal translational study involving patients with sepsis-induced ARDS (most with pneumonia), Meduri and collaborators demonstrated that tissue associated glucocorticoid resistance is a central pathogenetic mechanism in sepsis-associated dysregulated systemic inflammation, and that prolonged low-dose glucocorticoid administration can restore cellular sensitivity to glucocorticoids and their anti-inflammatory action (37). The relevance of these findings was tested prospectively in two randomized trials.

Confalonieri et al. prospectively tested the hypothesis that a seven-day low-dose glucocorticoid infusion (hydrocortisone 240 mg/day) attenuates systemic inflammation in severe CAP and leads to earlier resolution of pneumonia and a reduction in systemic inflammation-associated complications (38). Twenty-three patients receive hydrocortisone (200 mg IV loading dose followed by 10 mg/hr for 7 days) and 23 received placebo in addition to standard of care. These results indicate that modulation of systemic inflammation with early use of glucocorticoids may improve resolution of CAP.

Meduri and collaborators investigated in a randomized trial prolonged methylprednisolone infusion (1 mg/kg/day) in 91 patients with early ARDS, 43% caused by severe CAP (39). The primary endpoint was a one-point reduction in lung injury score (LIS) by study day 7. In intention-to-treat analysis, the response of the two groups (63 treated and 28 control) clearly diverged by day 7, with twice the proportion of treated patients achieving a one-point reduction in LIS (69.8% vs. 35.7%; $p = 0.002$) and breathing without assistance (53.9% vs. 25.0%; $p = 0.01$). By day 7, treated patients had a significant reduction in C-reactive protein levels (2.9 ± 4.1 vs. 13.1 ± 6.8; $p < 0.001$)

and lung injury score (2.14 ± 0.12 vs. 2.68 ± 0.14; $p < 0.001$) and multiorgan dysfunction score (MODS) score (0.90 ± 1.1. vs. 1.9 ± 1.4; $p = 0.002$). Treatment was associated with a reduction in the duration of mechanical ventilation (5 vs. 9.5 days; $p = 0.002$), ICU stay (7 vs. 14.5 days; $p = 0.007$), and ICU mortality (57.4% vs. 79.4%; $p = 0.03$). Among those with severe CAP, methylprednisolone-treated patients had by day 7 a higher rate of extubation (61% vs. 14%; $p = 0.07$) and lower C-reactive protein (2.5 ± 1.8 vs. 12.1 ± 8.1; $p = 0.06$). Treatment was associated with a reduction in median duration of mechanical ventilation (5 vs. 10 days; $p = 0.13$) and hospital mortality (16.5% vs. 42.5%; $p = 0.3$).

Before widespread use of glucocorticoids in patients with severe pneumonia can be recommended, the encouraging results of the studies need to be confirmed by larger studies. Studies regarding the particular glucocorticoids to be used and treatment timing, dosage, duration, and tapering strategies are needed to identify the best and safest manner for administration.

D. Genetic Variability

Increasingly, data suggests that the host response to infection and organ failure may be determined by the genetic predisposition of the patient rather than characteristics of the infection or its treatment (40). Organ dysfunction or failure in CAP can therefore be conceived of as different pathways of response initiated by pneumonia but determined by genetic predisposition. An extremely large number of polymorphisms have now been described within the pro- and anticoagulant hemostatic pathways, many of which have been suggested to influence coagulation. The value of genetic studies in CAP and other severe infections will be when the management of an individual patient can be optimized by therapy based on individual genotype for factors important in outcome. Development of new therapeutic agents based on gene variants or even gene therapy may play a role in management but not in the near future.

The real hope is improving use the pharmaceutical agents already available or developed in the future are genetic profiles that will be accurate markers and therefore more appropriate to identify patients for drotrecogin alfa therapy or other future immunomodulatory agents. Once clinically important gene variants have been identified, clinical trials with patients entered or at least stratified by genotype to confirm the benefit of the particular agent in that specific genotype would need to follow.

V. Prevention

Presently the best approach is to reduce the burden of disease due to lower respiratory tract infections is by prevention by immunization and smoking cessation, as well as reducing comorbidities to the extent possible, for example, better control of diabetes, congestive heart failure (CHF) and chronic obstructive pulmonary disease (COPD); and reducing malnutrition and risks for aspiration.

Vaccination is the mainstay for prevention of CAP. Pneumococcal polysaccharide and inactivated influenza vaccines are recommended for all older adults and for younger persons with medical conditions that place them at high risk for pneumonia and its complications. The new live, attenuated influenza vaccine is recommended for healthy persons (without comorbid illness that places them at higher risk of pneumonia) 2 to 49 years of age. The efficacy of the pneumococcal polysaccharide vaccine has been documented for prevention of invasive infection (e.g., bacteremia) among the elderly and younger adults with certain chronic medical conditions. The vaccine reduces invasive pneumococcal disease among persons 65 years or older by a relative 44% to 75% (41). Efficacy decreases with advancing age, and although one randomized clinical trial suggested some protection against pneumococcal pneumonia among high-risk elderly persons, other trials did not demonstrate efficacy against lower respiratory tract infection without bacteremia (42,43). The 7-valent pneumococcal conjugate vaccine is currently only licensed for use in children aged 2 to 59 months, but has reduced disease in adults by decreasing transmission from children.

The effect of influenza vaccine seems to have additional benefits besides simply protecting against direct infection. A large observational study of adults 65 years or older found that vaccination against influenza was associated with a relative reduction in the risk of hospitalization for cardiac disease (19% reduction), cerebrovascular disease (16–23% reduction), and pneumonia or influenza (29–32% reduction) and a relative reduction in the risk of death from all causes (48–50% reduction) (44).

New strategies for preventive vaccines are necessary. The development of more potent vaccines could potentially further reduce complications in the elderly. At the time of this writing, a 13-valent pneumococcal conjugate vaccine is being evaluated for adults. In addition, it will be important to determine whether new recommendations for influenza vaccination of children will have a similar effect of reducing the disease burden in older adults as has been observed with the use of the conjugate pneumococcal vaccine for invasive pneumococcal disease. One study in Japan showed that the mortality in elderly individuals significantly decreased as more school children were vaccinated for influenza (45). The role of vaccines for other respiratory viruses (e.g., respiratory syncytial virus, parainfluenza, adenovirus, and metapneumovirus) needs to be explored.

In addition to immunization, another consideration to potentially lessen the burden of CAP in the elderly may be directed at reducing the impact of comorbid conditions. Risk factors associated with CAP in elderly patients include COPD, chronic heart failure, diabetes, malnutrition, and swallowing disorders, which increase the risk of aspiration (46). In addition to predisposing to CAP, these conditions significantly worsen the outcome of CAP in elderly patients. While the effect of comorbid conditions on CAP is well established, whether optimally controlling these conditions will reduce the burden of CAP in elderly persons is unclear. Will interventions such as more intensive treatment of diabetes, COPD, and CHF; supplementation of nutritional deficiencies; or evaluation of risk factors for aspiration reduce the predisposition or severity of pneumonia? Previous studies have shown that hyperglycemia at the time of admission adversely affects patients with a wide variety of clinical illnesses, including CAP (47). However, no prospectively controlled trials have assessed the effect of more rigorous control of blood glucose levels, or other comorbidities, on the incidence and outcome of CAP.

Since aspiration of microorganisms in oropharyngeal secretions is a major cause of pneumonia in the elderly and swallowing disorders are the major risk factor for aspiration, clinical assessment of oropharyngeal hygiene and swallowing problems may be beneficial. Evaluation for swallowing disorders, which are common after cerebral infarction, may be performed by observation of oral movement and swallowing of various foods. Potential approaches to reduce aspiration in such patients include dietary modification and compensatory swallowing techniques, though controlled studies that have shown a reduction in associated pneumonia are lacking. Furthermore, since poor oral/dental hygiene is associated with increased bacterial colonization of oral secretions and of dental plaque, attempts to improve dental hygiene may reduce the infectious consequences of aspiration. The relatively easy act of daily teeth brushing may help to prevent pneumonia, but carefully conducted studies are needed. In addition to potentially reducing dental plaque, one study showed that the simple procedure of daily brushing stimulates sensory nerves that improve the swallowing reflex in elderly patients (48).

Until carefully controlled studies of these interventions have been conducted, definitive recommendations are not possible. Such studies should assess multiple outcomes rather than CAP alone, because a single disease-oriented study or guideline may not recognize potentially undesirable consequences of the intervention for coexisting conditions. Randomized clinical trials need to be designed to account for the variable effect of multiple comorbidities. However, because CAP is one of the most common reasons for hospitalization and is associated with significant morbidity and mortality, it is vital to conduct such studies.

One intervention for comorbid illness for which no further study is needed is smoking cessation. In one study, nearly one-third of pneumonia episodes in senior adult smokers could be attributed to smoking (49). Smoking is also associated with a substantial risk of pneumococcal bacteremia; one report showed that smoking was the strongest risk factor for invasive pneumococcal disease in immunocompetent nonelderly adults. Counseling patients to quit smoking and providing them with materials to assist with smoking cessation are essential. In summary, numerous risk factors and underlying conditions affect the susceptibility to and prognosis of CAP in elderly individuals. Physicians can intervene to modify some of the associated risk factors for CAP in the elderly. Administration of preventive vaccines, counseling about smoking cessation, stabilization of underlying conditions, and promotion of appropriate nutrition may help to reduce the risk of CAP and thereby promote longer and healthier lives for elderly patients.

References

1. Talbot GH, Bradley J, Edwards JE, et al. Bad bugs need drugs: an update on the development pipeline from the antimicrobial availability task force of the infectious diseases society of America. Clin Infect Dis 2006; 42:657–668.
2. File TM Jr. Clinical implications and treatment of multiresistant Streptococcus pneumoniae pneumonia. Clin Microbiol Infect 2006; 12(suppl 3):31.
3. Moore MR, Gertz RE Jr. Woodbury RL, et al. Population snapshot of emergent Streptococcus pneumoniae serotype 19A in the US. J Infect Dis 2008; 197:1016–1027.
4. Mandell LA, Wunderink RG, Anzueto A, et al. Infectious Diseases Society of America/ American Thoracic Society consensus guidelines on the management of community-acquired pneumonia in adults. Clin Infect Dis 2007; 44(suppl 2):S27–S72.
5. San Pedro GS, Cammarata SK, Oliphant TH, et al. Linezolid versus ceftriaxone/cefpodoxime in patients hospitalized for the treatment of Streptococcus pneumoniae pneumonia. Scand J Infect Dis 2002; 34:720–728.
6. Wunderink RG, Rello J, Cammarata SK, et al. Linezolid vs vancomycin: analysis of two double-blind studies of patients with methicillin-resistant Staphylococcus aureus nosocomial pneumonia. Chest 2003; 124:1789–1797.

7. Bernardo K, Pakulat N, Fleer S, et al. Subinhibitory concentrations of linezolid reduce Staphylococcus aureus virulence factor expression. Antimicrob Agents Chemother 2004; 48:546–444.

8. Fowler VG Jr., Boucher HW, Corey GR, et al. Daptomycin versus standard therapy for bacteremia and endocarditis caused by *Staphylococcus aureus*. N Engl J Med 2006; 355: 653–665.

9. Pertel, et al. Effects of prior effective therapy on the efficacy of daptomycin and cefriaxone for the treatment of community-acquired pneumonia. Clin Infect Dis 2008; 46:1142–1151.

10. Ellis-Grosse EJ, Babinchak T, Dartois N, et al. The efficacy and safety of tigecycline in the treatment of skin and skin structure infections: results of 2 double-blind phase 3 comparison studies with vancomycin-aztreonam. Clin Infect Dis 2005; 41(suppl 5):S341–S353.

11. Dukart G, Dartois N, Cooper CA. Integrated results of 2 phase 3 studies comparing Tigecycline with levofloxacin in patients with community-acquired pneumonia. Abstract L-1450 of the 46th Interscience Conference of Antimicrobial Agents and Chemotherapy. San Diego, CA, September 2006.

12. Maroko R, Cooper A, Dukart G, et al. Results of phase 3 study comparing a tigecycline regimen with an imipenem-cilastatin regimen in treatment of patients with hospital-acquired pneumonia. Abstract L-730 of the 47th Interscience Conference of Antimicrobial Agents and Chemotherapy, Chicago, IL, September 2007.

13. File TM Jr. Telithromycin new product overview. J Allergy Clin Immunol 2005; 115:S1–S13.

14. Zhanel GG, Wiebe R, Dilay L, et al. Comparative review of the carbapenems. Drugs 2007; 67(7):1027–1052.

15. Rea-Neto A, Niederman M, Prokocimer P. Efficacy and safety of intravenous doripnem vs. piperacillin/tazobactam in nosocomial pneumonia. Abstract L-731 of the 47th Interscience Conference of Antimicrobial Agents and Chemotherapy. Chicago, IL, September 2007.

16. Chen AY, Zervos MJ, Vazquez JA. Dalbavancin. a novel antimicrobial. Int J Cin Pract 2007; 61:853–863.

17. Stryjewski ME, O'Riordan WD, Lau WK, et al. Telavancin versus standard therapy for treatment of complicated skin and soft tissue infections due to Gram-positive bacteria. Clin Infect Dis 2005; 40:1601–1607.

18. Bhavnani SM, Passarell JA, Owen JS, et al. Pharmacokinetic-pharmacodynamic relationships describing the efficacy or oritavancin in patients with *Staphylococcus aureus* bacteremia. Antimicrob Agents Chemother 2006; 50:994–1000.

19. Noel GJ. Clinical profile of ceftobiprole, a novel β-lactam antibiotic. Clin Microbiol Infect 2007; 13(suppl 2):25–29.

20. Hawser S, Lociuro S, Islam K. Dihydrofolate reductase inhibitors as antibacterial agents. Biochem Pharmacol 2006; 71:941–948.

21. Hammerschlag MR, Sharma R. Use of cethromycin, a new ketolide, for treatment of community-acquired respiratory infections. Expert Opin Investig Drugs 2008; 17:387–400.

22. Advanced Life Sciences. About cethromycin. Woodridge, IL: Advanced Life Sciences, 2008. Available at: http://www.advancedlifesciences.com/product.php?id=1. Accessed October 2009.

23. Dalhoff A, Janjic N, Echols R. Redefining penems. Biochem Pharmacol 2006; 71: 1085–1095.

24. Craig WA. Pharmacokinetic/pharmacodynamic parameters: rationale for antibacterial dosing of mice and men. Clin Infect Dis 1998; 26:1–10.

25. Dunbar LM, Wunderink RG, Habib MP, et al. High-dose, short-course levofloxacin for community-acquired pneumonia: a new treatment paradigm. Clin Infect Dis 2003; 37(6): 752–760.

26. Lodise TP, Lomaestro B, Drusanoo GL. Piperacillin-tazobactam for Pseudomonas aeruginosa infection: clinical implications of an extended-infusion dosing strategy. Clin Infect Dis 2007; 44:357–363.

27. Chastre J, Wunderink R, Prokocimer P, et al. Efficacy and safety of intravenous infusion of doripenem versus imipenem in ventilatory-associated pneumonia: a multicenter, randomized study. Crit Care Med 2008; 36:1089–1096.

28. Wood GC, Boucher BA. Aerosolized antimicrobial therapy in acutely ill patients. Pharmacotherapy 2000; 20(13):166–181.

29. Niederman M, Chastre J, Corkery K, et al. IV Antibiotic use with adjunctive NKTR-061 (inhaled amikacin) treatment in intubated mechanically ventilated patients with gram-negative pneumonia. Abstract A241 of the International Symposium on Intensive Care and Emergency Medicine. Brussels, Belgium, 2007.

30. Mohr AM, Sifri ZC, Horng HS, et al. Use of aerosolized aminoglycosides in the treatment of Gram-negative ventilator-associated pneumonia. Surg Infect 2007; 8:349–357.

31. Michalopoulos A, Fotakis D, Virtzili S, et al. Aerosolized colistin as adjunctive treatment of ventilator-associated pneumonia due to multidrug-resistant Gram-negative bacteria: a prospective study. Respir Med 2008; 102:407.

32. Ioannidou E, Siempos II, Falagas ME. Administration of antimicrobials via the respiratory tract for the treatment of patients with nosocomial pneumonia: a meta-analysis. J Antimicrob Chemother 2007; 60:1216–1226.

33. Cassola M, Matera MG, Pezzuto G. Inflammation—a new therapeutic target in pneumonia. Respiration 2005; 72:117–126.

34. Danzinger LH. Beyond bacterial killing: immunopharmacologic effects of macrolides. Infect Med 1999; 16(suppl E):17.

35. File TM Jr., Tan JS. International guidelines for the treatment of community-acquired pneumonia in adults. The role of macrolides. Drugs 2003; 63(2):181–205.

36. Giamarellos-Bourboulis EJ, Pechere JC, Routsi C, et al. Effect of clarithromycin in patients with sepsis and ventilator-associated pneumonia. Clin Infect Dis 2008; 46:1157.

37. Meduri GU, Yates CR. Systemic inflammation-associated glucocorticoid resistance and outcome of ARDS. Ann N Y Acad Sci 2004; 1024:24–53.

38. Confalonieri M, Urbino R, Potena A, et al. Hydrocortisone infusion for severe community-acquired pneumonia: a preliminary randomized study. Am J Respir Crit Care Med 2005; 171(3):242–248.

39. Meduri GU, Golden E, Freire AX, et al. Methylprednisolone infusion in early severe ARDS: results of a randomized controlled trial. Chest 2007; 131:954–963.

40. Wunderink RG, Waterer GW. Genetics of community-acquired pneumonia. Semin Respir Crit Care Med 2005; 26:553–562.

41. Jackson LA, Neuzil KM, Yu O, et al. Effectiveness of pneumococcal polysaccharide vaccine in older adults. N Engl J Med 2003; 348:1747–1755.

42. Koivula I, Stén M, Leinonen M, et al. Clinical efficacy of pneumococcal vaccine in the elderly: a randomized, single-blind population-based trial. Am J Med 1997; 103:281–290.

43. Simberkoff MS, Cross AP, Al-Ibrahim M, et al. Efficacy of pneumococcal vaccine in high-risk patients. Results of a Veterans Administration Cooperative Study. N Engl J Med 1986; 315:1318–1327.

44. Nichol KL, Nordin J, Mullooly J, et al. Influenza vaccination and reduction in hospitalizations for cardiac disease and stroke among the elderly. N Engl J Med 2003; 348: 1322–1332.

45. Riechert TA, Sugaya N, Fedson DS, et al. The Japanese experience with vaccinating schoolchildren against influenza. N Engl J Med 2001; 344:889–896.

46. File TM Jr., Tan JS. Pneumonia in older adults: reversing the trend. JAMA 2005; 294: 2760–2763.

47. McAlister FA, Majumdar SR, Blitz S, et al. The relation between hyperglycemia and outcome in 2,471 patients admitted to the hospital with community-acquired pneumonia. Diabetes Care 2005; 28:810–815.
48. Yoshino A, Ebihara T, Ebihara S, et al. Daily oral care and risk factors for pneumonia in older patients in nursing homes. JAMA 2001; 286:2235–2236.
49. Nuorti JP, Butlser JC, Farley MM, et al. Cigarette smoking and invasive pneumococcal disease. Active Bacterial Core Surveillance. N Engl J Med 2000; 342:681–689.

Index

Printed and bound by CPI Group (UK) Ltd, Croydon, CR0 4YY

18/10/2024

01776263-0001